Reforming food in post-Famine Ireland

MANCHESTER
1824
Manchester University Press

Reforming food in post-Famine Ireland

Medicine, science and improvement, 1845–1922

IAN MILLER

Manchester University Press
MANCHESTER AND NEW YORK

distributed in the United States exclusively
by Palgrave Macmillan

Published by Manchester University Press
Oxford Road, Manchester M13 9NR, UK
and Room 400, 175 Fifth Avenue, New York, NY 10010, USA
www.manchesteruniversitypress.co.uk

Distributed in the United States exclusively by
Palgrave Macmillan, 175 Fifth Avenue, New York,
NY 10010, USA

Distributed in Canada exclusively by
UBC Press, University of British Columbia, 2029 West Mall,
Vancouver, BC, Canada V6T 1Z2

British Library Cataloguing-in-Publication Data
A catalogue record for this book is available from the British Library

Library of Congress Cataloging-in-Publication Data applied for

ISBN 978 0 7190 8886 5 hardback

First published 2014

Typeset
by Action Publishing Technology Ltd, Gloucester
Printed in Great Britain
by CPI Group (UK) Ltd, Croydon, CR0 4YY

For my family

Contents

Figures and tables

Figures

Tables

Acknowledgements

The research in this monograph was supported by an Irish Research Council Fellowship. Upon moving to Dublin in 2009, I became intrigued by the question of how and why Irish dietary customs adjusted so dramatically after the Famine. While developing this initial idea, I discovered a rich array of printed and archival documents relating to food in Ireland since the Famine. The topic of consumption and production in post-Famine Ireland transpired to be one of deep complexity and enormity. This monograph recaptures some of the key areas of debate between the Famine and Irish independence in 1922.

I wish to thank Dr Catherine Cox for her support for my project. The Centre for the History of Medicine in Ireland where I pursued this research provided an active environment in which I learnt about, explored and began to appreciate modern Irish medical history. In particular, David Durnin, Sarah York, Mary Daly, Lindsey Earner-Byrne, Kirsten Mulrennan, Fiachra Byrne and Tom Feely proved to be excellent colleagues to work beside. I especially wish to thank Anne Mac Lellan for her enthusiasm for my research and the discussions which we regularly shared about Irish medical history. Further afield, Leanne McCormick, James Vernon, Michael Worboys, Hilary Marland, Carol Helstosky, James Kelly, Keith Smith, Philomena Gorey and Sean Lucey provided ongoing support for my research and academic career as did Ian Burney who I particularly wish to acknowledge.

I am indebted to Juliana Adelman for our in-depth discussions about late nineteenth-century Irish abattoirs; Christopher Hamlin for our enthusiastic conversations about the Irish stomach; Ciara Breathnach for directing me towards historical resources relating to Irish tea-drinking habits; David Gentilcore for sharing his research on the history of the potato; and Senia Pašeta for discussing her research on Maud Gonne's Ladies School Dinners Committee with me.

The archival staff at the British Library, National Library of Ireland, Public Record Office of Northern Ireland (PRONI), Royal College of Physicians of Ireland, Royal College of Surgeons in Ireland and the Wellcome Library were always helpful, accommodating and efficient. In particular, Harriet Wheelock and Robert Mills at the Royal College of Physicians of Ireland Heritage Centre and Mary O'Doherty at the Royal College of Surgeons in Ireland were particularly supportive and accommodating. I am particularly grateful to the Deputy

Keeper of Records, Public Record Office of Northern Ireland for allowing me to reproduce my cover image. Images have also been reproduced courtesy of the National Library of Ireland.

I wish to acknowledge Manchester University Press for being extremely supportive and efficient throughout the entire process of publishing this monograph. An earlier draft of Chapter 1 was previously published in *Medical History*. I am indebted to the editor of the journal, Sanjoy Bhattacharya, and Cambridge University Press for allowing me to reproduce aspects of this research that directly discuss the Famine. I presented various aspects of this monograph at workshops, conferences and events at University College Dublin, the Institute of Historical Research in London, Mater Dei Institute of Education, University of Limerick and City University London. I would like to thank the organisers and audiences for their suggestions and thoughts.

Finally, I especially wish to thank Kevin Miller, Pauline Miller, Sarah Miller, Katie Miller and Miriam Trevor.

Introduction

When inaugurating the Dublin-based Health and Industries exhibition Ui Breasail in 1911, Lady Aberdeen, wife of the Lord Lieutenant of Ireland and founder of the Women's National Health Association, declared: 'Better food, greater energy; better economy, greater prosperity; better health, fuller life; these sequences give sense and truth to a relation which sounds at first incongruous and ridiculous – national well-being.'[1] Aberdeen's statement is complex. She presented food as integral to national interests, illustrating how improvement of the self through healthy eating was historically interpreted as a prerequisite for achieving full social, economic and national potential. Food supplied bodily energy which, in turn, optimised the productive capacities of labourers, according to Aberdeen. In her view, the anticipated increase in national wealth that would naturally result could not fail to promote communal health. Combined, these processes held the potential to improve Ireland on multiple levels. Aberdeen privileged personal acts of consuming as a basis of personal health, economic fecundity and national well-being. In short, she upheld food as integral to the organisation of Ireland. But why did Aberdeen link food consumption to so many domains of Irish existence? Why did she imbue it with levels of significance that extended so far beyond the physical and biological? And how, in the first place, did the issue of diet capture her attention?

Historiographical studies understate the complex meanings ascribed to food in post-Famine Ireland. Unsurprisingly, accounts of the striking adjustments in consumption and production customs from the 1850s onward coalesce around the Famine (c.1845–52), after which Ireland is routinely portrayed as having steadily progressed to a safer dietetic modernity marked by declining dependency on the potato as a dietary staple. This seemingly instinctual communal response to the stark warning afforded by the Famine is often presumed to have later shielded the Irish populace from the ominous, but resonant, threat of a further major famine; an outcome only made possible by the consumption of a more diverse diet in what transpired to be a critical period of reform in national food practices. Shifting trading patterns have also routinely been depicted as having helped to reshape Irish food cultures. In the decades that followed the Famine, exports of beef, butter, dairy produce and eggs increased while imports of goods such as tea, bacon and cheap American ham rose.[2]

Historians often assess this shift quantitatively. Statistical analysis has proved valuable for categorising post-Famine dietary change in terms of calorific intake or fluctuating import and export figures. Yet, when used alone, this approach bears inherent limitations. For instance, in terms of consuming, historians have meticulously described what the Irish population probably ate in the past. Leslie A. Clarkson and E. Margaret Crawford offer the most detailed survey. Assessing available historical data through the lens of modern nutritional reasoning, in their *Feast and Famine: A History of Food and Nutrition in Ireland, 1500–1920*, the authors determine the nutritional status of the Irish population at various historical junctures. Notably, they demonstrate that the Irish diet became identifiably closer to its equivalents in other regions of the United Kingdom after the Famine. As they astutely assert, this constituted a dramatic cultural and social change given that in 1845 close to 45 per cent of Ireland's population (mostly the poor) subsisted principally upon potatoes. After the Famine, the Irish enjoyed far greater dietary variety as monotonous potato-heavy diets were replaced by, or at least complemented with, the consumption of bread, meat, butter, tea, Indian meal and oatmeal, although a physiological price was admittedly paid in terms of lower levels of nutritional intake.[3]

Although immensely valuable, Clarkson and Crawford's study is less informative on precisely *how* and *why* Irish diet changed after the Famine. Nor does it fully grapple with the intricacies of an undeniably profound social and cultural adjustment. We are left uninformed on which social agencies sought to guide, direct and influence the path of dietary change. How successful were they? What motivated them? By posing questions such as these, a fuller account of what I term 'food reform' can be configured. Dietary change bore important meanings for both the consuming Irish public and for those critically observing them; factors that the methodologies of nutritional analysis less persuasively explore. Food, after all, is a bio-cultural phenomenon. Eating and digesting are not solely undertaken to fulfil the energy and nutrient needs of the body: they are physical acts laden with certain meanings when undertaken in particular social, cultural, economic and political contexts.[4]

Significant changes were also made in Irish food production after the Famine. To a certain extent, potato cultivation can be understood as having encouraged a solitary, hand-to-mouth subsistence existence that gratified immediate human needs. Gradually diminishing dependency on the crop paved the way for new regimes of agricultural production which, it was hoped, would ensure fuller Irish participation in an international capitalist market economy. Agricultural development, so would-be improvers insisted, would be marked by commercialisation.[5] To facilitate this, human, animal and biological material needed to be harnessed and rendered productive, so they argued.[6] Intensified agricultural practices relied upon strong, healthy and well-fed bodies to undertake production while a technical knowledge of how to exploit animal and plant life was required. Efficient and successful functioning in a market economy depended upon farmers and producers gaining access to agro-biological knowledge, so scientific agriculturists insisted after the Famine.[7]

Analysis of these powerful and pervasive ideas is mostly absent from accounts of post-Famine agricultural reconstruction which tend to explore economic and political factors alone. As corn prices dropped from the late 1840s onward, many farmers in Ireland chose to rear livestock to accrue profit. British markets acted as a prime driving force for Irish agricultural change. As Michael Turner demonstrates, in the 1850s approximately 35 to 40 per cent of Irish-produced cattle were exported (alive) to Britain to be retailed as meat. This figure increased dramatically to 50 per cent in the mid-1860s and close to 70 per cent by the end of the century.[8] Although historians have statistically mapped this trend, they have mostly shied away from distilling the contemporary meanings once attached to post-Famine agricultural reconstruction.

Pre-existing narratives of post-Famine food reform often obscure its intricacies, not to mention the persistence of food as a central, often troublesome, element of a society under intense social, economic and political reconfiguration until well into the twentieth century, if not beyond. Ireland is understood to have steadily advanced towards a healthier, safer and recognisably modern relationship with food and away from a somewhat basic subsistence existence towards agricultural diversity and fuller integration into modern economic trading systems. Even if the post-Famine population often failed to attain the high levels of nutritional value once gleaned from the potato, then at least they were no longer exposed to the tumultuous human, social and national cost of mass starvation. Notions of progression are paramount in this established narrative. When Louis Cullen depicted dietary change as synonymous with improvement in 1981, he asserted that 'the evolution of diet corresponds closely to the general profile of transition in Irish society'.[9] By propagating notions that shifting food behaviour automatically generated advancement, statements such as these lend a cogency to Irish food history that is in many ways illusory in nature. They also impart a sense of socio-economic progression not always felt by contemporaries themselves. Gleanings from the work of social historians hint at the potential for a more nuanced portrait of post-Famine food reform to be drawn. Well into the twentieth century, under-nutrition was endemic not only across poverty-stricken slums in major cities such as Dublin but also throughout vast rural areas in the west of the country; a scenario which indicates that dietary reconfiguration was a process not altogether smooth in nature.[10] On the contrary, food reform emerges from the historical record as a fragile, complex and fragmented process that, when reconstructed, reveals inherent complexities.[11]

The striking shifts in food practices that followed the Famine demand and deserve rigorous historical analysis, not least because the absence of a rounded rendering of Ireland's modern dietary past conceals a crucial element of a critical transitional phase in Irish social, economic and political life. In response, this study sets out to unearth the workings of post-Famine food reform. More specifically, it situates Irish historical food discourses within a broader framework of post-Famine politics of the body and life more generally. If we return to Aberdeen's statement, it becomes apparent that food reform was often interpreted as a mechanism for enabling physical, social and economic improvement. According to this perspective, private and personal acts of consumption were imbued with broader national significance meaning that interventions in the self could be construed as beneficial, if not pivotal, to Irish national vitality. Broadly analogous processes, I suggest, occurred in food production. The application of new scientifically focused understandings of animals, crops and other foodstuffs in food production was equally understood as a likely harbinger of personal, economic and national development.

Regulating consumption and production

The governance of food and diet by state bodies and the medical profession in the modern period is often presented as an all-pervasive mechanism. Sociologists, in particular, depict nineteenth- and twentieth-century sciences of nutrition as a driving force behind pervasive techniques of 'nutritional policing' endorsed by state bodies under the auspices of producing healthy citizens.[12] They point to the increasing regulation of dietary behaviour that formed part of the rise of social and medical modernity. Michael Foucault's concept of biopolitics is helpful here. Although Foucault said relatively little about food, historians have since framed dietary regulation as an expression of biopolitics.[13] In particular, Bryan S. Turner, applying Foucauldian methodologies, suggests that industrial labourers were subject to higher levels of dietary regulation from the mid-nineteenth century onward as state bodies and other social agents formed responses to urban poverty and sought to maximise labour efficiency by promoting nutritional health and healthy eating.[14]

Broadly speaking, biopolitics refers to forms of political governance that initially materialised in the eighteenth century. According to Foucault, it was in that century that new expressions of liberal governance evolved that were less concerned with managing territory and controlling inhabitants and more interested in the biological regulation of individuals and populations.[15] Accordingly, statecraft techniques emerged that targeted both individual and collective (or 'social') bodies.[16] Individual bodies were to be improved by optimising their capabilities and increasing their economic utility. Individuals were encouraged to self-regulate and self-govern to effect both personal and collective development. Simultaneously, a burgeoning state and expert interest in assessing the size, quality and health of populations developed. This encouraged collective efforts to be made to maintain the physical and psychological well-being of political units, as exemplified by the emergence of statistical mechanisms designed to measure local and national health and morbidity levels.[17] Health was something that could now be carefully measured and assessed to identify potential personal, socio-economic and national arenas in need of improvement. The appearance of these political forms coincided with both the transformation of biology into a discrete scientific sub-discipline and the professionalisation of orthodox medicine. Biopolitics placed life itself at the centre of political activity. In turn, health became transformed into a legitimate object of political governance in the sense that governments, for the first time, defined one of their remits as being to bolster, monitor and regulate the physical and mental well-being of national populations.[18] Today, we take for granted the role played by the state in regulating food and encouraging its production, as well as enabling legislation and forms of social welfare that protect citizens from starvation.[19] In the past, the state adopted a more ambiguous stance to assuming responsibility for the feeding of citizens. Nonetheless, this scenario changed significantly throughout the period under analysis in this study. From the 1840s, as James Vernon persuasively details, hunger became widely agreed upon as an unacceptable bodily condition and as a problem that should be a matter of state interest.[20]

Nonetheless, and importantly, food intake was something that non-official individuals and groups also sought to shape, define and regulate, as evidenced by Aberdeen's presence in the area of Irish nutritional health. Biopolitics does not necessarily refer to formal state action. In fact, it is often complemented by – indeed, is often reliant upon – action in non-governmental sectors. Vernon also convincingly posits that the historical efforts of non-state bodies to manage hunger produced their own networks of power, political constituencies, understandings of state responsibilities and forms of statecraft. In short, food regulation was not simply a top-down process. This, Vernon insists, occurred due to an array of actors – including political activists, social scientists, journalists, nutritionists, dietary reformers, philanthropists and the victims of hunger themselves – having contributed to a continual flow of new perspectives on, and solutions to, food-related problems.[21] Historically (and currently), a range of interacting factors impacted on and shaped public attitudes to food including education, medicine, media information, health policies, changes in physical or social environments, acculturation to the norms and values of foreign cultures, technological innovation and shifting expert ideas pertaining to food.[22] Together, these produced diffuse systems of power that targeted, and ostensibly sought to improve, the self by promoting certain forms of dietary behaviour.

In addition, this monograph suggests that post-Famine agricultural life was also subject to new biological and political imperatives. In his seminal text *Ways of Knowing: A New History of Science, Technology and Medicine*, John Pickstone suggests that, historically, different types of scientific activity were intimately related to one another. By this, he means that broadly analogous forms of analysis impacted simultaneously at any given time on how life – human, animal, mineral and social – was understood, institutionalised and actualised in certain forms of social, cultural and economic behaviour.[23] Following this lead, this study demonstrates that the attempted regulation of life extended beyond the realm of the human in Ireland after the Famine. State and non-state bodies made efforts to harness and optimise animal and plant life, as well as human life, to achieve full economic potential by referring to broadly similar forms of inquiry into nutrition and physiology. In short, food production was scientifically targeted in the post-Famine period at the very same time that human life evolved into an object of medical, scientific and political scrutiny.

By the time of the Famine, a range of mechanisms were in place throughout Ireland that conveyed food-related information. Physicians advised their patients and the public on the most suitable foodstuffs to consume. Scientists provided an expert rationale that underpinned this advice and were increasingly called upon to co-operate with government bodies in advisory capacities. Agricultural scientists also provided expert knowledge on food production. Journalists conveyed information relating to imports and exports as well as the most up-to-date thoughts on diet. In fact, as Vernon posits, journalistic interventions in food concerns proved to be remarkably central to the transformation of starvation and hunger into conditions of humanitarian concern from the mid-nineteenth century onward.[24] Finally, philanthropy served as a powerful tool used to ameliorate the condition of the less affluent, a social grouping who most frequently formed the target of reform strategies. To fully appreciate the intricacies of post-Famine food reform therefore depends upon examining the interplay between a diverse set of social forces and adopting an analytical approach that integrates consumption and production. It also necessitates synthesising various fields of inquiry rather than focusing on, say, medicine, science or politics as food discourses typically cut across these disciplinary boundaries. This raises important questions: who sought to guide food reform and why? Who held socio-cultural authority over food in post-Famine Ireland, if anyone? Did these individuals or groups amicably interact or, conversely, was food a contested terrain? And how did the different actors interested in food publicly present their interests, and for what purposes?

Improvement

Importantly, post-Famine discussion of the reconstruction of food customs was consistently framed in terms of improvement, a secondary theme of this study. As a term, improvement encompassed virtually all areas of activity including the moral, intellectual and physical enhancement of both the self and society. Across the period in question, the idea of improvement was upheld due to an unshakeable belief in progress inherent in social thought across the British Isles between the eighteenth and early twentieth centuries. According to this perspective, society was in a constant state of development and advancement, becoming increasingly refined and civilised.[25] Those interested in stimulating social and economic progress emphasised the importance of individual effort in bettering both the self and the larger community, an approach adopted by Aberdeen in Ireland when she linked individual action to the enhancement of national socio-economic life.[26] The concept of improvement was multifaceted. Helen O'Connell argues that nineteenth-century improvement agendas were characteristically framed by a desire to stabilise Irish society, subdue political unrest and promote engagement with modern social and economic practices. Prior to the Famine, the disintegration of Ireland's mono-crop culture was widely understood as an important step towards the country's integration into an international nexus of trade and commerce. According to O'Connell, the encouragement of a culture based upon restraint (dietary or otherwise) and the quelling of emotions were seen as necessary steps towards fostering a spirit of industriousness and, in turn, stimulating national development.[27] Consumption and production were seen as two disparate, yet intertwined, arenas that, if developed, would productively contribute to the broader project of improving Ireland.

Accordingly, Part I of this monograph focuses on the formation of new medical and scientific understandings of food consumption and production in the mid-nineteenth century and the efforts made to apply them in Ireland to ameliorate adverse social and economic conditions. Importantly, it asserts that food was thought about differently from around the 1830s and increasingly appreciated in terms of nutritional consistency for the first time. This development impacted profoundly on discussion of dietary change. Chapter 1 explores expert opinion on the pre-Famine potato diet. It demonstrates that scientists with an interest in nutrition began to examine the potato diet in new physiological and nutritional terms during the 1840s, allowing them to input into contemporary discussion among political economists on the Irish social condition. The issue of famine relief afforded them an opportunity to assert their perspectives in an official capacity. Importantly, this encouraged a subtle, but significant, shift in discussion of the Irish diet as debates on the quantity of potatoes being consumed by the Irish gradually gave way to a more nuanced discussion of how the population could still obtain nutritional quality if reliance upon the potato as a dietary staple diminished. Chapter 2 demonstrates that a contemporaneous shift occurred in expert opinion on Irish food production practices. Animal and plant life, so agriculturists insisted in the 1840s and 1850s, could be understood with reference to organic chemistry; as composed of complex combinations of chemical elements. In turn, the practical application of this knowledge would enrich agricultural productivity and create national prosperity. These two opening chapters are particularly concerned with the production of new knowledge of food in the 1840s and 1850s, the efforts made to apply that knowledge in Ireland during the Famine and beyond, and the reasons why these initiatives ultimately floundered due to being viewed unfavourably by the Irish public.

Despite an initial optimism about national prospects immediately following the Famine, the late nineteenth century was marked by deep apprehension about Irish well-being. Rather than presuming that food-based anxieties receded as dependency on the potato lessened, even despite the persistence of minor famines in the west of Ireland, Part II of this monograph asserts that Irish consumption and production customs continued to be targeted as areas of necessary reform and improvement long after the Famine. In fact, the remainder of the nineteenth century saw sustained alarm about the socio-economic path that the country seemed to have traversed since the Famine. Although fears about national communal starvation mostly diminished, concern persisted about the nutritional health of the poor and the quality of foodstuffs being consumed in place of the potato. Chapter 3 explores post-

Famine apprehension about the long-term dangers of subsisting on nutritionally insufficient diets; a concern that first became particularly pronounced during the 1850s and 1860s in debates on institutional feeding. Critics castigated scanty institutional feeding as they perceived it to be weakening and debilitating the bodies of the institutionalised. Given the high numbers of younger residents being raised in Irish institutions, it is unsurprising that workhouses and prisons came to be viewed as institutions imbued with the potential to permanently damage the health of the future generation of Ireland.

Chapter 4 expands upon the theme of nutritional health by exploring post-Famine anxieties about the poor nutritional quality of food consumed by the less affluent as an alternative to the potato. It posits that the gradual replacement of the potato diet with a more diverse one created intense debate about the trajectory of post-Famine dietary change. Concerned individuals routinely queried whether this adjustment was in fact hindering socio-national development instead of promoting advancement. For many physicians and medical writers, poor diet had contributed to a chronic condition of downward-spiralling national physical decline caused, in part, by adverse eating habits, excessive tea drinking and the commercialisation of the Irish diet. Contemporaneous fears emerged about national economic decline in food production, producing debates about national economic vitality that tied in to discussion of physical decline. By the turn of the twentieth century, it seemed to many contemporaries that post-Famine Ireland was trapped in an unremitting condition of economic decline and deterioration. Chapter 5 considers the impact of emerging awareness of the presence of germs and bacteria in foodstuffs from around the 1870s and argues that this played an important role in post-Famine debates on the standard of food production. Economic stagnation could now be partly blamed on the relative impurity of Irish dairy produce in comparison to that of other countries and a perceived failure of Irish food producers to adhere to the new standards of purity imposed by contemporary bacteriologists and public health reformers.

Part II concludes by demonstrating that significant adjustments were made to the structure of domestic and agricultural education in 1900 in direct response to post-Famine apprehension about physical and economic decline. Chapter 6 demonstrates that the issue of food underpinned these structural changes. From 1900, female pupils were encouraged to improve their cookery skills to bring improvement to the Irish domestic sphere and, hopefully, end practices of subsisting upon innutritious products such as tea and white bread. Simultaneously, instructors showed male agriculture pupils how to produce food in ways attentive to both purity and productivity in response to pressing economic concerns. Overall, Part II of this monograph explores concepts of national decline in post-Famine Ireland, the centrality of food to the discourses produced by this apparent decline and the formation of pedagogic responses designed to resolve ongoing concerns about what the less affluent ate and produced.

Imperialism and the Irish body

Medical historians have often veered away from explicitly assessing past representations of the Irish body. Nor have they fully analysed how Ireland's political, social and quasi-colonial circumstances were once viewed as having a detrimental impact on Irish physical and mental well-being. Oonagh Walsh provides a notable exception in her analysis of how late nineteenth-century Irish asylum psychiatrists were prone to framing their pre-dominantly Catholic subjects as more irrational and prone to mental illness than their Protestant counterparts. In turn, Walsh suggests, castigating the Catholic Irish as mentally vulnerable automatically implied their unsuitability for political self-governance.[28] Catherine Cox, Hilary Marland and Sarah York explore the bodily and mental implications of post-Famine emigration by demonstrating high levels of asylum admissions among Irish emigrants to mid-Victorian Lancashire.[29] Catherine Cox also demonstrates that a perceived rise in incidences of insanity in late nineteenth-century Ireland was often understood and explained through racial stereotypes of the Irish and Celtic races being prone to mental illness.[30]

A historiographical absence of analysis of how Irish health was historically viewed as tied to imperialism results partly from a lack of consensus on whether Ireland actually was a colony or, indeed, a reluctance to admit that it was so.[31] Certainly, medical historians of Ireland have failed to inquire into the potential connections between the health of the body and imperialism with the enthusiasm shared by historical geographers such as David Nally or medical historians interested in colonialism in countries including India and South Africa.[32] In relation to food production, some historians have argued that Ireland was part of a colonial economy or, at least, benefited unfavourably from being part of the liberal market economy supported by the British state in the period under analysis.[33] A key intention of this monograph is not to form a decisive opinion on whether Ireland was part of a colonial economy but rather to explore the meaning of historical views on Irish import/export patterns and their connection to broader personal, social, economic and political domains. Considering Ireland in these terms reveals much about the physical experience of living in post-Famine Ireland and, importantly, broadens our understanding of a critical phase in modern Irish history.

Ireland was incorporated into the United Kingdom when the Act of Union of 1800 took effect. The nineteenth century witnessed the rise of Catholic nationalism and the Land Wars that took place between the 1870s and 1890s (which, at their simplest, were a struggle between the long-established landlord class and their tenant farmers). Assertive forms of nationalism evolved in the early twentieth century prior to the attaining of national independence (albeit without what is now known as Northern Ireland) in 1922. Physical improvement was presented as a crucial strategy of expansion into Ireland. Reformers ostensibly sought to improve the condition of the Irish poor by rearing them into healthy individuals capable of interacting with modern social and economic systems.[34] For instance, if, for many critical observers, pre-Famine reliance upon the potato embodied Irish backwardness, then by default a transition towards a varied diet automatically implied the lifting of peasants from adverse conditions of primitivism to biological and economic modernity. The modernisation of food production, too, was intended to instigate a mutually beneficial dialogue with international trading systems and allow Ireland to engage productively with a market economy. Colonial medicine could also be used to define the physical and psychological capacities of colonial subjects while often creating and perpetuating racial stereotypes; to measure the health of colonised populations through information gathering and statistical analysis; and to provide penetrative ideas about race, health promotion and disease management that ultimately informed how the Empire was governed. Colonising powers routinely depicted their subjects as weak and feeble and enthusiastically referred to medical and scientific ideas to validate that derogative perspective.[35]

Nonetheless, images of an oppressed colonised population are disrupted in Ireland as the country was not only European and Christianised but also significantly contributed to the Empire by providing soldiers, administrators and medical professionals.[36] As Sikata Banerjee observes, Ireland was less of an 'other'. British expansion into Ireland in fact created diverse ideological and cultural contexts and a highly complex circulation of social power.[37] Furthermore, issues of medical and scientific authority acquire considerable intricacy in modern Irish history. Binaries between western and non-western medical knowledge, and the imposition of the former onto the latter, were less relevant in Ireland in comparison to countries such as India. From around 1790, orthodox medical science emerged from the hospitals of Paris in a recognisably modern form; as a discipline characterised by an adherence to empirical knowledge and the professionalisation of groups who sought to differentiate themselves from their non-orthodox counterparts.[38] This process was also apparent in Ireland where, as James McGeachie skilfully demonstrates, medicine developed in a 'normal' fashion (equivalent to other areas of Western Europe) in what he terms an 'abnormal' place.[39] In fact, the early nineteenth-century prominence of the Dublin School of Medicine and its contributions to an international nexus of medical activity provided a framework in which diffuse systems of biopolitical, colonial and social power could simultaneously operate under the aegis of improvement. Irish medical and scientific communities were interested in applying expert knowledge to improve the Irish condition for different reasons, sometimes connected to Empire, sometimes connected to Irish needs. Regardless of their views on Union, Irish medical men were also connected to an international movement to professionalise orthodox medicine and increase its presence in the management and resolution of social concerns.[40] They also formed part of an emerging Irish middle-class culture that was often highly concerned with resolving the problem of the poor and in reforming the classes below.

Nonetheless, regardless of the diverse motivations for promoting food reform, lifting Ireland into dietary modernity was a deeply problematic agenda. In England, the displacement of 'traditional' or 'simple' dietary forms had resulted from the dramatic social changes that had accompanied eighteenth-century industrialisation.[41] As urban centres had expanded, industrial workers became detached from agricultural food bases while food markets commercialised; developments that precipitated the growth of new trading patterns and innovations in production. Imperialism, and an interlinked opening of international trade routes, also guaranteed the English population access to a wider array of foodstuffs.[42] Contemporaneously, the emergence of a relatively wealthy middle class who shared particular values and attitudes to food carried important implications for traditional food customs. As Norbert Elias details, certain consumption habits acquired social acceptability and came to be viewed as part and parcel of the processes of becoming civilised and modern while other habits and tastes (such as eating with fingers and spitting on the floor during meals) were reconstituted as remnants of a less sophisticated, primitive inheritance.[43] Inherent in these trends was a profound sense that dietary modernisation was a marker of becoming civilised. However, the modernisation of diet had not been without its problems even in Britain. Widening class inequalities often meant poor nutrition and decreasing physical stature lower down the social scale.[44] This created powerful social anxieties about under-fed urban populations and prompted numerous enquiries into food quality, supplies and dietetic health.[45] Regardless, would-be improvers continued to view dietary change as something necessary and unavoidable within modernisation. Despite its detrimental ramifications for the less affluent, developments in consumption and production continued to serve as an index of social modernity.

Ireland presented a remarkably different terrain for promoting a move towards a modern, civilised diet. At its simplest level, British food reform was concerned with resolving the dietary problems that had emerged as part of the social fallout of industrialisation.[46] Yet industrialisation mostly failed to occur throughout much of Ireland during the period in question, at least to the same extent as it had in Britain.[47] Although it appeared obvious that a transition into modernity had hardly created a dietetic paradise in Britain where the fruits of colonisation and industrial wealth meant food and good health for all, this failed to quell speculation on how to draw Ireland into the spectrum of modernity, a step seen in the mid-nineteenth century as dependent upon removing the potato diet from Ireland's social infrastructure. Promulgators of improvement rarely paused to consider the potential ramifications of connecting Ireland to international modernising patterns or to question the suitability of Ireland as a site of modernisation and the potential of resistance to techniques of governance to emerge. After all, Irish dietary and productive behaviour might well have been brought closer into line with its British counterpart following the Famine, but Britain itself was contemporaneously experiencing a turbulent relationship with food. As this monograph demonstrates, the implications of this adverse predicament were not lost on many Irish contemporaries who often opted out of venerating modernisation and industrialisation as the preferred path of national progression.

Resistance

This monograph also traces how dominant food discourses were often resisted as a means of further illustrating the multifaceted nature of post-Famine food reform and, by extension, the concept of 'nutritional policing'. Importantly, the health of the Irish body served as a key point of contention in post-Famine Ireland; as a concern recurrently articulated through the lens of food and dietary change. Notably, the Famine raised (and still does raise) intricate questions about whether the state allowed the Irish population to starve under a misguided belief that the blight afforded a providential opportunity to permanently adjust national dietary patterns, stem population increase and stimulate socio-economic development.[48] At the heart of these assertions lie important insinuations on the physical effects of imperial governance and Ireland's social structure on the Irish body. Although historical allegations of deliberate state-led and landlord-supported starvation were perhaps unfounded – certainly exaggerated – those calling attention to them were successfully, often deliberately, forming responses to the very real implications of British expansion upon physical experience.[49] Critical questions recurrently surfaced between the Famine and independence about the authenticity of state interest in improving Ireland's physical, economic and social fabric and whether its relative inefficacy in stimulating improvement was actually helping to maintain Ireland in a disadvantageous socio-economic condition.

Improvement was central to the rhetoric of the imperialist 'civilising mission' and Irish middle-class thought in the nineteenth and early twentieth centuries.[50] Nonetheless, this policy of providing welfare to imperial subjects was rarely fully adhered to in practice.[51] Nally sceptically suggests that 'improvement' was routinely invoked to falsely justify Britain's presence in Ireland and also lambasts the insincerity of British interests in supporting socio-economic progression.[52] Certainly, those who challenged food-related policies in Ireland consistently contested the integrity and validity of improving strategies initiated by state bodies. At worst, opponents of British rule in Ireland, as well as those who benefited unequally from the nature of the Irish class structure, routinely referred to the state's allegedly inadequate food policies in their rhetorics of political resistance. As this study demonstrates, their critiques often focused intently on bodily concerns.

This situation shares parallels with colonial Egypt where, as Omnia El Shakrey suggests, nationalist groups publicly rejected hierarchical civilising discourses by expending considerable energy insisting that colonial expansion was the root cause of backwardness, not its remedy. In these adversarial discourses, imperialism itself was delineated as a hindrance to national development and a barrier to progress and modernisation. Both imperialists and nationalists agreed on the need for development but disagreed on the terms upon which it could be effected.[53] In Ireland, those opposed to British governance – and, indeed, even some of those in favour of the Union but who wished to strengthen Ireland's imperial role – portrayed the inefficacy of imperial governance, tied up as it was with issues such as landlordism and Catholic–Protestant relations, as the root cause of relative under-development. This perspective, as demonstrated in this monograph, was palpable in critiques of famine relief, workhouse dietary provisions, limited financial assistance given to agricultural science and, later, an absence of school meals legislation in Ireland and wartime food policies. The forms of resistance that emerged were multi-layered. Food producers questioned the authority of medical scientists in attempting to regulate dairy and meat production; farmers resented scientific food production as they perceived it as associated with landlordism while issues such as excessive tea drinking became gradually entangled with broader discussion of the rise of the Irish grazier community and the production in Ireland of foodstuffs intended for exportation rather than domestic consumption. At their most extreme, critics insisted that the state was pursuing a policy of weakening Ireland at its core – its diet – as part of a broader strategy of subjugation. At the risk of over-simplifying a complex situation, the pervasive question of who should govern Ireland depended heavily for some upon determining whether the Irish body remained weak due to alleged defaults in the Irish character that required external governance or, conversely, whether imperialism itself had unfairly castigated the Irish body as frail while maintaining socio-economic conditions detrimental to physical and, by extension, national vitality.

The striking changes in consumption and production that occurred after the Famine in fact offered an important lens for assessing Ireland's role within the British Isles and Empire; offering insight into the importance of day-to-day matters during a period of accumulating tensions in Irish social, economic and political relations. In fact, public opinion on food gained considerable complexity in post-Famine Ireland because of the country's intricate political and social culture.[54] Resistance to, or disinterest in, modernising processes in food production and consumption was rife in post-Famine Ireland. Consumers and producers tended not to act as passive recipients of medical and scientific information on food. For instance, throughout the early nineteenth century political economists had persistently lambasted Irish potato-eating habits, yet this had achieved little, if anything, in terms of stemming potato consumption. As William Wilde, prominent eye and ear surgeon and father of Oscar, asserted in 1857:

> To effect any sudden alteration in the dietary of a people is a matter of greater difficulty than a change in either their religious or political institutions – the former under excitement may become as contagious as an epidemic, and the latter be enforced by the strong arm of power, while a revolution in diet, especially in Ireland, where the accustomed food had been easily raised and was comparatively palatable, and, moreover, had become the basis of habits so firmly fixed as to influence the entire social condition of a people, required even more than the stern necessity of want before it could be accomplished, or the inhabitants brought to relish any other descriptions of food.[55]

Wilde perceptively recognised potato consumption as an integral component of Irish national identity; as a deeply ingrained social practice. Even despite the nationally felt consequences of the Famine, potato consumption remained culturally tenacious despite its catastrophic potential. Since the early 1700s, the potato had defined who the Irish peasant was, shaping his cultural identity and his social interactions.[56] Despite prevailing hopes in the early 1850s that Irish dietary patterns would naturally adjust now blight had receded, Wilde remained astutely aware of the capacity of Irish labourers to reject all suggestions that they should abandon the potato and thereby, in essence, sacrifice part of their sense of selfhood.

In reality, the success of state-led (and voluntary) efforts to effect change depended upon public consensus. Yet, as this study demonstrates, in post-Famine Ireland, approaches to new forms of consuming and producing were negotiated through a range of factors including, among others, scepticism about the accuracy of nutritional science; associations forged between agricultural science and landlordism; wariness towards an encroaching medico-scientific authority; and an ever-complex web of Anglo-Irish relations. For instance, even despite her close connection to the monarchy, Lady Aberdeen faced consistent hostility from Unionists who disregarded her viceroyalty for being sympathetic to nationalism.[57] Many nationalists, meanwhile, resented Aberdeen's obvious connections with imperialism and viewed her castigation of Ireland as an unhealthy country as damaging to the image of Ireland abroad and, importantly, to their political cause.[58] Citizens repeatedly displayed resistance to medical and scientific input into their consumption and production behaviour on a range of practical, intellectual and political levels, and for multifaceted reasons. Furthermore, British rule was a routinely contested system of governance – increasingly so during the period in question – meaning that state-directed intervention in food risked being subject to scepticism or opposed due its alleged Anglo-centric, quasi-colonial nature. Colonial issues aside, the validity of nutritional knowledge (and medical authority) itself was repeatedly challenged as inaccurate; as too rigid, scientistic, moralistic, sexist and class prejudiced; and as too intent on diagnosing populations as sick rather than strong and healthy.[59]

Although omnipresent throughout this study, the theme of resistance is particularly prominent in Part III, a section that reveals some of the ways that early twentieth-century nationalist rhetoric referred to the health of the Irish body with direct reference to post-Famine changes in consumption and production patterns and referred to an apparent development of a colonial economy to expose the apparent inadequacy of imperial liberal governance. Chapter 7 explores how and why Maud Gonne interpreted an absence of school meals legislation in Ireland for much of the 1910s as a deliberate policy of 'school-day starvation'. In essence, her narrative purported an inverted form of biopolitics; one that weakened imperial subjects instead of promoting health and generating economic wealth. Similarly, during the First World War, Sinn Féin members insisted that the imperial state had, since the Famine, deliberately created an economic system where the most nutritious foods were being exported to Britain leaving Irish citizens to consume less nutritious imported products – a scenario with adverse implications for Irish health. Food, this monograph suggests, persistently served as a key arena in which resistance to both imperial and medical governance was formed and where the complexities of Anglo-Irish relations, as well as internal Irish social relations, were played out between the Famine and independence.

Overall, this study argues that post-Famine food reform was contingent on factors other than shifting economic patterns and a need felt to consume foodstuffs other than the potato to guard against further major famines. On the contrary, food was something that historical actors concerned with the Irish condition saw as crucial to well-being and development in all aspects of national life. Food was routinely upheld as pivotal to the Irish national condition. It is in this context that food became central to the medical, scientific, social, political and cultural narratives formed in this critical period of modern Irish history.

Notes

1 'Ui Breasail: Increasing Popularity, the Food Section, What to Eat and How to Cook it', *Irish Times* (27 May 1911), p. 8.

2 D. E. Jordan Jr., *Land and Popular Politics in Ireland: County Mayo from the Plantation to the Land War* (Cambridge: Cambridge University Press, 1994), pp. 160–1; A. Gibson, *The Strong Spirit: History, Politics and Aesthetics in the Writings of James Joyce, 1898–1915* (Oxford: Oxford University Press, 2013), p. 55. For an in-depth account of post-Famine dietary change, see L. A. Clarkson and E. M. Crawford, *Feast and Famine: A History of Food and Nutrition in Ireland, 1500–1920* (Oxford: Oxford University Press, 2001), pp. 109–10.

3 Clarkson and Crawford, *Feast and Famine*, pp. 88–110.

4 P. Fieldhouse, *Food and Nutrition: Customs and Culture* (London: Chapman and Hall, 1986 [1991]), pp. 1–2.

5 D. Nally, '"That coming storm": the Irish Poor Law, colonial biopolitics, and the Great Famine', *Annals of the Association of American Geographers*, 98:3 (2008), 714–41.

6 D. Nally, 'The biopolitics of food provisioning', *Transactions of the Institute of British Geographers*, 36:1 (January 2011), 37–53 on p. 38.

7 See Chapter 2.

8 M. Turner, *After the Famine: Irish Agriculture, 1859–1914* (Cambridge and New York: Cambridge University Press, 1996), p. 58.

9 L. M. Cullen, *The Emergence of Modern Ireland 1600–1900* (London: Batsford Academic and Education, 1981), p. 140.

10 J. Prunty, *Dublin Slums, 1800–1925: A Study in Urban Geography* (Dublin: Irish Academic Press, 1998), pp. 34–5; C. Breathnach, *The Congested Districts Board, 1891–1923: Poverty and Development in the West of Ireland* (Dublin: Four Courts Press, 2005), pp. 37–42.

11 Modern-day analysis still pits dietary change against the Famine. See, for instance, *Changes in the Food Chain since the Time of the Great Irish Famine* (National Nutrition Surveillance Centre, University College Galway, 1995).

12 See J. Coveney, *Food, Morals and Meaning: The Pleasures and Anxiety of Eating* (London: Routledge, 2nd edn, 2006).

13 A. Bobrow-Strain, 'White bread bio-politics: purity, health, and the triumph of industrial baking', *Cultural Geographies*, 15:1 (January 2008), 19–40; Nally, 'The biopolitics of food provisioning', p. 38.
14 B. S. Turner, 'The government of the body: medical regimens and the rationalization of diet', *British Journal of Sociology*, 33:2 (June 1982), 254–69 on p. 266.
15 M. Foucault, *The Birth of Biopolitics: Lectures at the Collège de France, 1978–79* (New York: Palgrave Macmillan, 2008).
16 T. Lemke, *Bio-Politics: An Advanced Introduction* (New York: New York University Press, 2011), p. 37.
17 D. Padovan, 'Bio-politics and the social control of the multitude', *Democracy and Nature*, 9:3 (November 2003), 473–94 on pp. 473–4.
18 S. Hodges, *Contraception, Colonialism and Commerce: Birth Control in South India, 1920–1940* (London: Ashgate, 2008), p. 4.
19 W. A. McIntosh, *Sociologies of Food and Nutrition* (New York and London: Plenum Press, 1996), p. 195.
20 J. Vernon, *Hunger: A History* (Cambridge, MA and London: Belknap Press, 2007), p. 8.
21 Ibid., p. 8.
22 Fieldhouse, *Food and Nutrition*, pp. 8–16.
23 J. Pickstone, *Ways of Knowing: A New History of Science, Technology and Medicine* (Manchester: Manchester University Press, 2000), pp. 106–34.
24 Vernon, *Hunger*, pp. 18–40.
25 S. Tarlow, *The Archaeology of Improvement in Britain, 1750–1850* (Cambridge: Cambridge University Press, 2007), p. 16.
26 A. B. Rodrick, *Self-Help and Civic Culture: Citizenship in Victorian Birmingham* (Aldershot: Ashgate, 2004), pp. 2–3.
27 H. O'Connell, *Ireland and the Fiction of Improvement* (Oxford: Oxford University Press, 2006).
28 O. Walsh, 'The designs of providence: race, religion and Irish insanity', in J. Melling and B. Forsythe (eds), *Insanity and Society: The Asylum in its Social Context* (London: Routledge, 1999).
29 C. Cox, H. Marland and S. York, 'Emaciated, exhausted and excited: the bodies and minds of the Irish in nineteenth-century Lancashire asylums', *Journal of Social History*, 46:2 (August 2012), 500–24.
30 C. Cox, *Negotiating Insanity in the Southeast of Ireland* (Manchester: Manchester University Press, 2012), pp. 53–64.
31 See, for instance, the debates contained within T. McDonough (ed.), *Was Ireland a Colony? Economics, Politics and Culture in Nineteenth-Century Ireland* (Dublin: Irish Academic Press, 2005).
32 e.g. W. Ernst, *Mad Tales from the Raj: The European Insane in British India, 1800–1858* (London and New York: Routledge, 1991).
33 See, for instance, D. O'Hearn, 'Ireland in the Atlantic economy', in McDonough (ed.), *Was Ireland a Colony?*
34 O'Connell, *Ireland and the Fiction of Improvement.*
35 W. Anderson, *Colonial Pathologies: American Tropical Medicine, Race and Hygiene in the Philippines* (Durham, NC: Duke University Press, 2006), p. 69.
36 J. Wright, *Ireland, India and Nationalism in Nineteenth-Century Literature* (Cambridge: Cambridge University Press, 2007), p. 16.
37 S. Banerjee, *Muscular Nationalism: Gender, Violence and Empire in India and Ireland, 1914–2004* (New York: New York University Press, 2012), p. 14.

38 See, for instance, E. H. Ackerknecht, *Medicine at the Paris Hospital, 1794–1848* (Baltimore, MD: Johns Hopkins Press, 1967).
39 J. McGeachie, '"Normal" development in an "abnormal" place: Sir William Wilde and the Irish school of medicine', in G. Jones and E. Malcolm (eds), *Medicine, Disease and the State in Ireland, 1650–1940* (Cork: Cork University Press, 1999).
40 G. Jones, 'The Border in Irish Medicine'. Paper given to the Centre for the History of Medicine in Ireland Seminar Series, University College Dublin, 22 November 2012.
41 D. J. Oddy, 'The paradox of diet and health: England and Scotland in the nineteenth and twentieth centuries', in A. Fenton (ed.), *Order and Disorder: The Health Implications of Eating and Drinking in the Nineteenth and Twentieth Centuries* (Edinburgh: Tuckwell Press, 2000).
42 D. J. Oddy, 'Food, drink and nutrition', in F. M. L. Thompson (ed.), *The Cambridge Social History of Britain, 1750–1950: Volume Two, People and their Environment* (Cambridge: Cambridge University Press, 1990).
43 N. Elias, *The Civilising Process*, trans. E. Jephcott (Oxford: Blackwell, 1978–82); B. S. Turner, *The Body and Society: Explorations in Social Theory* (London: SAGE Publications, 2nd edn, 1996), pp. 169–71.
44 H. A. Levenstein, *Revolution at the Table: The Transformation of American Diet* (New York and Oxford: Oxford University Press, 1988), p. 23.
45 I. Miller, *A Modern History of the Stomach: Gastric Illness, Medicine and British Society, 1800–1950* (London: Pickering and Chatto, 2011), pp. 11–38.
46 J. Burnett, *Plenty and Want: A Social History of Diet in England from 1815 to the Present Day* (London: Methuen, 1966 [1979]), pp. 30–47.
47 Mass industrialisation occurred only in pockets, especially in the north-east. See A. Bielenberg, *Ireland and the Industrial Revolution: The Impact of the Industrial Revolution on Irish Industry, 1801–1922* (London: Routledge, 2009).
48 For providence, see P. Gray, 'Potatoes and providence: British government responses to the Great Famine', *Bullán: An Irish Studies Journal*, 1:1 (Spring 1994), 75–90. For recent discussion of Britain's role in the Famine, see T. P. Coogan, *The Famine Plot: England's Role in Ireland's Great Tragedy* (New York and Basingstoke: Palgrave Macmillan, 2012).
49 For comparison, see E. M. Collingham, *Imperial Bodies: The Physical Experience of the Raj, c.1800–1947* (Cambridge: Polity Press, 2001).
50 For discussion of the civilising mission, see M. Mann, '"Torchbearers upon the path of progress": Britain's ideology of a "moral and material progress" in India, an introductory essay', in H. Fischer-Tiné and M. Mann (eds), *Colonialism as Civilizing Mission: Cultural Ideology in British India* (London: Anthem Press, 2004), p. 8.
51 J. Midgley and D. Piachaud, 'Introduction', in J. Midgley and D. Piachaud (eds), *Colonialism and Welfare: Social Policy and the British Imperial Legacy* (Cheltenham: Edward Elgar Publishing, 2011), p. 28.
52 Nally, 'That coming storm', p. 716.
53 O. E. Shakry, *The Great Social Laboratory: Subjects of Knowledge in Colonial and Postcolonial Egypt* (Stanford: Stanford University Press, 2007).
54 M. Hechter, *Internal Colonialism: The Celtic Fringe in British National Development, 1536–1966* (London: Routledge, 1975).
55 W. Wilde, 'Epidemic disease in Ireland', *Dublin Review*, 42 (March 1857), 76–95 on p. 91.
56 Clarkson and Crawford, *Feast and Famine*, p. 59.
57 E. Reilly, 'Women and voluntary war work', in A. Gregory and S. Pašeta (eds), *Ireland and the Great War: 'A War to Unite us All'?* (Manchester: Manchester University Press, 2002), p. 51.

58 V. McLeish, 'Sunshine and sorrows: Canada, Ireland and Lady Aberdeen', in D. Lambert and A. Lester (eds), *Imperial Lives across the British Empire: Imperial Careering in the Long Nineteenth Century* (Cambridge: Cambridge University Press, 2006), p. 277.

59 See also P. Crotty, *Good Nutrition? Fact and Fashion in Dietary Advice* (St Leonards: Allen and Unwin, 1995).

I

Science, improvement and food, c.1845–80

1

The chemistry of famine: nutritional discourse and dietary transformation

In 1845, approximately 45 per cent of the Irish population depended on the potato as a dietary staple, consumed with buttermilk, water, fish or whiskey.[1] In stark contrast to countries such as Italy where, as David Gentilcore demonstrates, state bodies actively encouraged potato consumption, British politicians and social commentators criticised Ireland's mono-crop existence, routinely blaming it for the country's intransigent lack of socio-economic development.[2] Political economists derided the potato as easy to produce. In doing so, they affirmed their stereotypical, self-produced views of the Irish peasantry as inherently idle. Easy cultivation meant less time labouring, so they insisted, which, in turn, caused over-population as peasants were left with excess free time spent procreating rather than labouring.[3] Political economists and improvers sought to halt this mono-crop existence to stabilise Irish society, steer the country's inhabitants into modernity and promote moral values of restraint.

Abstract economic theory aside, the potato was undeniably prone to recurrent failures – a challenging concern given the relative lack of availability of alternative foodstuffs. Poor nationwide harvests occurred in 1740–1, 1800–1, 1816–18, 1822 and 1831 while partial, regional potato scarcities were common in intermittent years.[4] In this context, dietary transformation came to be widely agreed upon as an indispensable mechanism for resolving deep-rooted problems in Ireland's socio-economic infrastructure.[5] This chapter explores the emerging interest in the potato diet among certain groups of scientists with an interest in nutrition in mid-century Ireland and how they used their ideas on food, diet and nutrition to input into broader debates on national dietary regeneration. Prior to and during the Famine, nutritional scientists produced new knowledge of the physiology of food and its nutritional impact in the human body; a step that ultimately granted them opportunities to engage with famine relief activities between 1845 and 1847. Importantly, a new nutritional consciousness emerged in this period meaning that discussion of the large quantities of potatoes being consumed in Ireland gradually gave way to debates on how the Irish populace could obtain the nutritional quality previously attained from the potato. This chapter also explores the surfacing of public resistance to nutritional science, a discipline that became popularly dismissed in

Famine-period Ireland as a woefully inadequate tool being used by a state disinterested in forming an adequate response to widespread starvation. Overall, this chapter explores the mid-century production of empirical knowledge on the potato, the complex ways in which it was applied for the purpose of improving and the layers of resistance that formed to medico-scientific ideas during the Famine.

Analysing the peasant body

Throughout the early nineteenth century, the Irish potato diet was increasingly considered in biological and physiological terms, a development that added important new contours to contemporary discussion of the fabric of Irish socio-economic life. Shifting medico-scientific approaches to food provided a key impulse. Traditionally, physicians had tended to assess the ways in which human bodies respond to food with reference to constitution. They were less concerned with identifying the specific properties of individual foodstuffs as they understood the manner by which food was assimilated as variable from person to person and as contingent on a range of factors such as lifestyle, health and environment. In contrast, from around the 1820s, physicians and medical scientists subjected human food intake to new, empirically driven analytical investigations. The physiology of digestion now captured the attention of numerous medical investigators who sought to configure nuanced, empirically grounded understandings of how the human body digests and processes food.[6] Physicians, pathological anatomists and physiologists speculated on how food was taken into the bodily system, assimilated into the blood and passed into the tissues. They explored the mastication of food, its admixture with saliva, its digestion by the stomach's muscular powers, how it was propelled into the bowels, its assimilation into human blood and its transformation into excrement.[7] Methods of chewing, stomach sizes, the ideal time spent by the body digesting, and so on, all came to be scrutinised by new techniques of internal exploration.[8] Importantly, this allowed physicians to establish new norms of healthy digestion and to deem deviation from these as unhealthy and unnatural.

Given the unique nature of Irish dietary customs, it is unsurprising that the Irish peasant gradually fell under the gaze of ever more sophisticated forms of digestive analysis. Ireland's curious mono-crop tradition – characterised by remarkably high levels of potato consumption – clashed profoundly with the ideals of a burgeoning dietetic science whose proponents venerated variation, restraint and moderation.[9] In response, physicians sought to determine new ways of measuring and describing Irish digestive health. Considerable attention was awarded to the potato diet in Derry-born physician James Johnson's widely read *A Tour of Ireland* (1844). Although best remembered for attending the Duke of Clarence and editing the popular *Medico-Chirurgical Review*, Johnson also penned a series of influential works on digestion. It was perhaps Johnson's interest in exploring the workings of the stomach, combined with his Irish background, that fostered his enthusiasm for linking the potato to Irish physiology.[10] In *A Tour of Ireland*, Johnson expressed bewilderment at a widespread habit of only half-boiling potatoes, leaving the centre so solid that it was colloquially referred to as the 'bone of the potatoe'. This custom no doubt made sense to the Irish peasant as consuming harder material allayed hunger for longer. However, it fitted uneasily with Johnson's opinion on healthy digestion. Accordingly, in his text, he proclaimed that 'there is scarcely a more indigestible substance taken into the human stomach than a half-boiled potatoe; and, to, a moderately dyspeptic Englishman – such diet would be little less than poison'.[11]

Johnson insisted that over-reliance on the potato maintained the Irish peasantry in a realm akin to primitive culture. By perpetuating a rudimentary lifestyle of hand-to-mouth subsistence, the peasant, so Johnson insisted, was unconsciously sustaining an agricultural system obstructive to Ireland's anticipated progression into socio-economic modernity. Johnson's unabashed views on Irish cultural primitivism reached a notable climax when he attributed popular beliefs in fairies, goblins, daemons and kelpies to gastric phenomena. For Johnson, the stomach and digestive organs were a rich epicentre of nerves from which, through internal nervous connections, abdominal problems could present themselves in other parts of the body, in this instance in the mind.[12] This model allowed Johnson to ascribe the sightings of fantastical creatures to the potato diet and to argue that indigestion – stimulated by excessive consumption of poteen (an extremely strong distilled alcoholic beverage) and potatoes – caused vivid nightmares later recalled as actual sightings.[13] Johnson's contentions were imbued with a profound sense that the British stomach was a far healthier organ than its Irish equivalent. In turn, he referred to the apparently deviant composition of Irish digestive physiology to sequentially explain socio-economic and cultural backwardness. Unsuitable dietary arrangements, it seemed, held implications that extended far beyond the confines of individual bodies. Johnson's depictions served little purpose in terms of disseminating health advice. However, they did add expert weight to broader political and economic debates on Irish society. Medico-scientific opinion, in this instance, became fashioned as compatible with politico-economic agendas.

Medical literature such as Johnson's undoubtedly influenced the views of lay figures such as Thomas Campbell Foster who, in the early 1840s, announced that the Irish peasantry had an unnatural craving for large quantities of food. Potatoes, so Foster believed, contained very little nourishment, meaning that large amounts needed to be eaten to fulfil the human system's nutritional requirements. Yet by perpetually subsisting on excessive food quantities, the Irish peasant's stomach had become engorged, constantly craving quantity, so Foster proclaimed. Foster even asserted that pathological investigation had revealed the size of the potato-fed Irish peasant's stomach to be double that of the average stomach, although his source for this weighty claim remains elusive.[14] In Foster's writing, as with Johnson's, the concept of communal abnormal digestion offered a trope that affirmed impressions of an inferior culture by expressing profound difference between centre and periphery. Foster drew upon notions of a normative digestive system that rendered that of the Irish peasant as essentially pathological – an allegoric device predicated to imply social primitivism and cultural backwardness. Notably, when not penning travel literature, Foster contributed regularly to *The Times*, a newspaper prone to promulgating unsympathetic attitudes to Irish poverty by specifying its root cause as national idleness. Foster's observations of the peasant body can therefore be seen as one element of his broader agenda of promoting Irish socio-economic reform and development. Both of these examples reveal that physiological ideas were amenable to contemporary political and economic thought that dismissively targeted the unregulated Irish body as a physical site in need of urgent improvement.

As a tool, however, digestive physiology was less useful for suggesting which foodstuffs might replace the potato should the elusive goal of dietary transformation ever be effected. Nonetheless, new forms of nutritional chemistry had emerged in the 1830s that took food itself as an analytical starting point. In the 1830s, internationally renowned German chemist Justus von Liebig had successfully drawn attention to the high social and economic utility of chemistry.[15] Liebig had also acquired considerable influence across the United Kingdom in the late 1830s.[16] By empirically analysing the chemistry of an array of foodstuffs, Liebig found himself able to decipher a comprehensive list of which chemicals entered the body during digestion. This placed him in an authoritative position to offer public advice on consumption. He understood physiological phenomena as predominantly chemical in nature and demonstrated that organic nitrogenous constituents were derived from plant proteins, that protein could be obtained by consuming meats and vegetables, and that protein strengthened flesh and cellular tissue. Overall, Liebig's key contribution to an already rich medical and scientific literature on diet was the development of the precept that chemical transformations occur during digestion and that foodstuffs were best chosen with an awareness of chemical behaviour in mind.[17] The public profile of Liebig's research significantly increased in the 'hungry '40s' when he was able to convincingly present his work as bearing high social value in terms of alleviating hunger and under-nutrition.[18]

Evidently, by the eve of the Famine a strong intellectual framework was in place that allowed digestion and nutrition to be empirically examined. This coincided with a more general drive: the dissociation of science from its origins as a gentlemanly hobby and amateur pursuit into something approaching a profession. Chemistry, in particular, was routinely upheld in the 1840s as a socially beneficial force and scientific cookery promoted as a helpful civilising agent.[19] Importantly, as Juliana Adelman argues, during the 1840s the British state and Dublin Castle eagerly valued, embraced and promoted scientific endeavour in the belief that it might help to effect Irish socio-economic improvement.[20] It is in these interwoven contexts that proponents of food chemistry found themselves well placed to exert an intellectual and practical sway in state-managed famine relief practices. Like the study of digestion, nutritional science offered a convincing rationale with the potential to be harnessed by state bodies to make sense of Irish dietary habits and to devise a blueprint for dietary reform.

Salvaging the potato

In 1845, Irish potato yields were 33 per cent less than in previous years; in 1846 75 per cent less. By 'Black '47', the number of acres under potato cultivation had fallen from over two million to only 284,000.[21] From the onset, chemical theories influenced understandings of blight. In October 1845, Prime Minister Robert Peel established a Scientific Commission to determine the causes of crop failure and to develop solutions. Historians have rebuked this official group for their mistaken conclusions on the cause of blight (established as fungal only in the 1890s).[22] Ciarán Ó Murchadha, for example, insists that the Commission was hampered by a lack of expertise in plant biology and passes judgement on its members for ignoring suggestions that the blight might have fungal origins.[23] Yet Ó Murchadha's perspective is retrospective, reliant upon hindsight and, for those reasons, ultimately fails to inquire into why it was that the Commission consistently pursued an approach anchored in the theory of chemistry. Fungal theories were certainly proposed and remedies to exterminate fungi with acids, alkaline liquors and chlorine were well circulated.[24] Yet chemistry was, in many respects, a more theoretically and practically developed discipline than mycology in the 1840s, and a more socially active one. Furthermore, the composition of the Commission reflected the high confidence placed in chemistry in official circles. It was comprised of a group who overtly subscribed to, and promulgated faith in, organic chemistry. Lyon Playfair was a Scottish Professor of Chemistry at the Royal Manchester Institution, John Lindley was an accomplished English botanist and Robert Kane was the President of Queen's College, Cork.[25] Playfair was eminent in political circles and was a personal acquaintance of Peel.[26] An often un-noted, but highly significant, point about the Commission is that Playfair was a former pupil of Liebig.[27] Kane had also studied organic chemistry in Giessen under Liebig and, at the onset of the Famine, was actively engaged in promoting Liebigian agricultural science in Ireland.[28] Given Liebig's weighty influence, it is unsurprising that the Commission's members focused intently upon exploring the chemistry of famine and remained disinclined to engage with suggestions that ran counter to their expert presuppositions.[29]

Peel established the Scientific Commission shortly after the publication of George Phillips's *The Potato Disease: Its Origin, Nature and Prevention.* Phillips had gained prominence as a highly active member of the London Chemical Society and was respected in political circles for his scientific prowess. In 1842, he had set up a chemical laboratory to help enforce the Pure Tobacco Act.[30] This was not the first time that the potato had come under scientific scrutiny. Indeed, Enlightenment scientists had eagerly pursued a project of better understanding the crop.[31] Yet the Famine added new urgency to such investigations. In his work, Phillips reconsidered the potato in a Liebigian framework. The crop emerged from Phillips's work analysed and dissected into its constituent parts: water, starch, sugar, potateine, gum, albumen, ligneous fibre, silica, alumina, lime, potash, magnesia and so on. He also portrayed these highly specific agents as serving individual purposes in the human system once ingested. Problematically for political economists, Phillips's analysis indicated that the crop was in fact a highly nutritious food article that contained all the essential constituents of healthy digestion and nutrition: starch, gum, sugar and albumen, which provided the body with a healthy supply of carbon, oxygen, hydrogen and nitrogen.

Phillips also sought to define how blight-ridden potatoes had evolved from healthy to diseased. Blight, in his view, had decreased the potato's sugar, potateine, gum, albumen and ligneous fibre levels. Accordingly, Phillips outlined a subtle transformation from healthiness to rottenness involving the decomposition of albumen; the colouring of potatoes with oxygen; the browning of diseased crops with alkalis; the consistency of potatoes shifting from acid to alkali; and ammonia being produced by putrid fermentation. He pinpointed rain as the primary cause of these chemical alterations and explained that excess moisture had encouraged surplus tubers to form. These had subsequently ceased to be supplied with nutriment once rain had prostrated the crop's powers. In Phillips's view, newly formed pendulums and tubers had therefore been left unsupported by the plant. This had caused the living principle to cease to exist and chemical processes of decomposition to commence. Phillips concluded that rain and moisture had stimulated the potato beyond its ability, overpowering it and producing putrefaction.[32]

The influence of Phillips's findings was palpable in the Commission's optimistic suggestions of 1845 that nutritional elements could be salvaged from diseased potatoes. Kane confidently asserted that starch could in fact be retrieved from diseased potatoes, although he appended a warning that extracted starch could not act as a substitute for the potato itself as potatoes contained an array of other constituents that were essential to human health.[33] Accordingly, Kane proposed that the poor could be educated and taught how to manufacture starch at home. The success of this strategy depended upon the techniques of chemistry being precisely imitated in domestic settings.[34] However, the Commission's instructions for extracting starch were intricate to say the least. They recommended that peasants make a rasp or grater by punctuating a tin sheet with holes. The pulp produced from grating a diseased potato could then be drenched with water, and the remaining pulp and starch separated. The pulp was then to be dried on a griddle over a fire and put aside while the wet lumps of starch were being dried on a shelf over a number of days. Through leaflets, posters, and talks given in churches, the Irish peasantry were informed that wholesome bread could be made by mixing starch and pulp with peas-meal, bean-meal, oatmeal or flour.[35]

Ultimately, the dispersion of such intricate advice created negative public perceptions of nutritional science. Furthermore, the apparent collusion of scientists with the state in dispensing seemingly ineffectual advice did little to bolster the public repute of those working in the discipline. Some sporadic evidence exists of localised enthusiasm for the Commission's remedies. In October 1845, Henry John Porter, land agent to the Duke of Manchester of Tanderagee, Co. Kildare, held meetings at the school houses on his estate to instigate the domestic conversion of potatoes.[36] However, in the view of more critical observers, the Commission's advice held little worth. The Commission persisted in advocating domestic starch production despite receiving an influx of letters lamenting its impracticalities. Some of these implicated peasant culture as a restrictive factor. Reverend Edward Hoare of Ballymore, Co. Kildare, wrote to the Commission expressing his doubts that the peasantry could ever be persuaded to produce starch.[37] A paper read to the Natural History Society of Dublin in December envisaged problems with starch production as residing in 'the apathy and indifference of the peasantry' who disliked new innovations in potato storage. Peasants, so the speaker suggested, did 'not look much beyond the present hour' and, in any case, believed that public funds would soon be made available to cover their loss.[38]

Others saw problems in implementing starch production schemes as resting more in financial limitations than with peasant conservatism or apathy. Further letters sent to the Commission and the Famine Relief Commissioners insisted that Dublin Castle and the state were oblivious to the financial circumstances of the peasantry. One of these stressed that cottiers could not afford the lime recommended by the Commission for drying potatoes.[39] Similarly, Reverend William Fisher, rector of Killmore, Co. Cork, estimated that 2,500 peasants in his parish could not afford to buy the oatmeal recommended as a mixer for starch, adding that financial aid would be more appropriate.[40] Further letters expressed indignation at the state's reluctance to prohibit corn exports, a seemingly more realistic solution than encouraging peasants to resort to complex processes of extracting chemical elements from their diseased potatoes.[41] On a sub-textual level, these conflicting accounts of peasant conservatism and calls for financial support reflected far broader debates about self-help and state intervention. Underpinning this discussion of financial aid were strong implications that Ireland deserved fuller state support and that a system of scientifically guided starch production based on self-initiative was impractical, insufficient and inferior to financial aid.

Public confidence in science was hardly bolstered by public intra-professional disputes. Edward Carroll, agricultural superintendent on the estates of William Wrexon Beecher, Mallow, Co. Cork and member of the Royal Agricultural Society of Ireland, wrote to the *Freeman's Journal* in October dismissing advice on converting potatoes as a collection of 'silly nostrums' created by men who 'knew little of practice applicable to the circumstances of this country'. He denounced Kane's idea of drying potatoes in the open air on the basis that the Irish weather, especially in autumn, was such that barely two days passed without rain. Carroll also regretted the Commission's suggestions that potatoes could be dried in uninhabited rooms by angrily exclaiming that most small Irish labourers did not have the luxury of space in their huts.[42] Although Carroll's statements pointed to tensions within science, they were also resonant of wider concerns felt that a government located in distant London (and Dublin Castle) was proving inattentive to Irish needs. Carroll's articulation of this issue in a nationalist-minded newspaper guaranteed a potentially receptive audience who might have adapted the ambiguity of science's function in relief practice into a trope for articulating more general apprehension about centralised approaches to pressing Irish needs.

These public critiques left nutritional science vulnerable to being seen as synonymous with political inefficacy. Reverend Richard Walsh of Headford, Co. Galway, returned the recommendations that had been dispatched to him as a measure not only of his lack of confidence in the Commission but also of his horror at state indifference to the want and distress of the Irish nation.[43] Unsurprisingly, the Commission's activities quickly generated anger in nationalist-orientated newspapers. In November 1845, *The Nation* called for the rejection of all official recommendations as, if anything, they seemed to have accelerated the decomposition of potatoes.[44] Journalistic hostility intensified in the following month after the Commission circulated a questionnaire requesting information on the spread of the blight. It seemed to critics that although some months had now passed, all Kane and his colleagues had so far achieved was to meet and theorise rather than undertake more practical tasks such as collating information on the extent of loss of the potato, when scarcity was likely, the state of the food markets and the availability of alternative foodstuffs. This predicament sharpened public hostility to the Commission, as evidenced by the *Freeman's Journal*'s declaration that 'this negligence – this apathy – this carelessness of the obligations of humanity is so shameful'.[45] The *Cork Examiner* vociferously announced that the government was 'mocking the Irish' with this 'unaccountable delay' and pronounced that 'our rulers would lavishly squander public money on itinerant "Commissioners" who came here to abuse us, but are deaf to our cries for bread'.[46] Similarly, at a public meeting held in Co. Mayo in January 1846 (later recorded in the *Freeman's Journal*) one speaker announced that 'the learned pundits, if anything, had recommended a course of action which was the complete opposite of that which would have been wisest', and that 'such is the dependence to be placed on the theories of those self-sufficient gentry who take upon themselves so dogmatically to point out the causes of and the remedies for the visitations of Providence'.[47] In all of these examples, nutritional science became entangled in a wider web of simmering anti-Union sentiment and scorned as an integral, but illustrative, component of British political neglect during a national crisis.

Anger peaked as the high cost of the Commission became apparent during summer 1846. Despite a costly financial outlay, it seemed to sceptics that all the vast expense surrounding the Commission had resulted in was scientific confirmation of the somewhat obvious fact that the potato crop had failed. Although acknowledging Lindley's profound understanding of vegetable physiology, *The Nation* asserted: 'we defy anyone to point out a single physiological reason advanced on the subject by him, or even the smallest exhibition of scientific knowledge, from the appearance of the celebrated manifestoes of the Potato Commissioners to the present day'. The newspaper also declared that Lindley 'has scarcely advanced a single opinion on the disease which he has not renounced at a subsequent period'.[48] In November, the *Tuam Herald* castigated the so-called 'Potato Commission' for being 'the greatest farcical humbug ever got up even in Ireland' and promptly renamed it 'The Commission for the Destruction of Potatoes' on the basis that 'it is a notorious fact that in every instance where the direction of the Commissioners was followed, the potatoes were utterly destroyed!'[49] Clearly, some months into the operations of the Commission, attitudes to the Commission had evolved from scepticism to anger.

Nonetheless, the approaches adopted by the Commission demonstrate the new visibility of nutritional theory in the 1840s and the popularisation of contemporary views on the importance of choosing foods with nutritional value. The Famine afforded Liebig's disciples opportunities to publicly display their intellectual and social prowess and to promulgate their unswerving faith in chemistry's social usefulness. Advice to convert diseased potatoes was a misguided expression of the excitement and confidence then being placed by some in contemporary nutritional science. Science had now confirmed the nutritional quality of the potato diet, to some surprise, and it could now be hypothesised that the Irish peasantry could subsist if they salvaged the nutritional goodness still present in their otherwise diseased crops. Nutritional science's entanglement with political critique ultimately served to undermine public perceptions of the discipline in Ireland. Its solutions were publicly rebuked as further confirmation of governmental neglect, offering those opposed to the Union a rich resource for political critique. For critics, the most that officially sanctioned research into the chemical constitution of the potato seemed to have proved was something that the Irish had instinctively known all along: that a peasant population could subsist healthily on the potato. As William Wilde recalled in 1851:

> The Potato Commission did not effect much good, although it was said thirteen thousand pounds were expended upon the inquiry – an extravagance which very much annoyed the doctors, who only got five shillings a day without meat or drink . . . for doctoring a hundred or two starving wretches in typhus fever. The chemists then took up the question, and found that there was too much phosphorus in one description of food, and too much sulphur in another, and too much or too little lime in a third; and, in fine, that, with few exceptions, man could not live on bread alone. Then the fact became evident to the chemists, which had long ago been practically demonstrated by the people, that the potato, bad as it was, contained more life-sustaining elements, added to more palatable qualities, and less deleterious constituents, when taken for any length of time into the system, than any other vegetable that could be procured.[50]

According to Wilde, scientific conjecture had proved itself to be of limited utilitarian worth as a state tool, having merely reiterated forms of knowledge – in a language steeped in the technicalities of expert analysis – already intuitively known by the Irish peasantry through day-to-day experience, but which political economists had routinely dismissed. Although the capacity of the potato to sustain human life may have been a momentous revelation to chemical scientists, from the perspective of the Irish peasant and other critics, the financial costs incurred discovering what was inside a potato and how to extract its elements might have been better spent providing food for an increasingly destitute population.

Replacing the potato

Despite the Commission's lack of practical success, its members undoubtedly heightened public awareness in Ireland of the relatively nascent science of nutrition, albeit in an unintentionally damaging way. Nutritional imperatives continued to surface in the more sustained discussion of famine relief that took place from 1846 onwards. The onset of widespread famine-related diseases in the winter of 1845–6 suggested that links existed between innutritious diets and epidemic disease. During the winter, physicians also came to appreciate that diseased potatoes were altogether unsuitable for consumption. In late 1845, prominent Catholic physician Dominic Corrigan wrote to the Commission warning that the consumption of extracted starch had in fact increased the susceptibility of the population to epidemic diseases as the practice lowered nutritional and bodily health.[51] Corrigan's advice was mostly ignored. However during that winter, Irish physicians found themselves caring for individuals presenting worrying symptoms of rigors, hot skin, abdominal pain, diarrhoea and swollen muscles after consuming diseased potatoes.[52] They initially considered the possibility of the existence of an entirely new form of gastro-enterite.[53] However, in April 1846, the *Dublin Hospital Gazette* linked these symptoms to those recently observed in outbreaks of land scurvy during Indian famines.[54]

In the meantime, Corrigan aggressively reiterated his views, first published in reformist medical journal *The Lancet* some fifteen years earlier, on the correlation between innutritious diets and epidemic disease, a relationship not universally agreed upon. Alternative explanations for 'Famine Fever' highlighted apparent interconnections between poverty and fever, and the potential role of atmospheric or electrical phenomena in generating disease.[55] Corrigan reprinted his findings in pamphlet format in 1846, warning ominously that fever was likely to strike again. To solidify that point, in his *On Famine and Fever*, he detailed the experiences of over one hundred years of Irish famines and posited that famine had been present each time a fever epidemic had struck, regardless of season or climate. Cynically, he suggested that those who linked fever with filth had done so to justify withholding the most appropriate type of aid to the starving: food.[56]

Corrigan's critics dismissed his ideas as conjecture and asserted that fever had also recurred in times of plenty.[57] Nonetheless, Corrigan became prominent during the Famine after being appointed as a key member of the Central Board of Health which, in response to changes in patterns of Famine Fever, was established in March 1846, disbanded in August and reappointed in

February 1847. The Board served as an advisory body empowered to instruct Poor Law Boards of Guardians to establish, equip and staff fever hospitals.[58] Corrigan found himself well positioned to project his views on the connections between fever and innutritious diets. The Board also consisted of esteemed Dublin medical practitioner Philip Crampton, Kane, and two civil servants: Randolph Routh and Edward Twistleton.[59]

Drawing directly from Liebig's principles, the Board developed advice based upon the by-now familiar precept that nutritional elements previously obtained from the potato could be obtained from a rigidly defined combination of meats, vegetables and grains. Importantly, the Board heralded the anticipated adoption of a new national diet as a positive precursor of permanent social and economic improvement. For its members, only a scientifically determined diet should replace the potato, a perspective implicit in their view that ignorance of this tenet had led voluntary relief providers to make erroneous decisions. Philanthropic Quakers, the Board observed, were dispensing rice as they understood that rice was consumed as a sole dietary article in oriental countries. In response, the Board publicly insisted that rice was not in fact consumed alone anywhere in the world but was always instinctually prepared with vegetables, oil, butter, meat or fish to allow consumers to obtain from other sources the important nutritional elements which it did not contain. The Board also disregarded suppositions that the bulk of rice could supply the missing quantities of food required by the seemingly overly large Irish stomach. Rice, the Board maintained, certainly swelled into a visible mass of food. However, that mass contained a disproportionately smaller amount of nutritional value.[60]

In many ways, this critique of the operations of unofficial relief schemes affirmed a sense of the superior nature of dietetic knowledge derived from laboratory analysis and empirical observation. Unlike Johnson and Foster, the Board was less intent on judging the *quantity* of potatoes consumed in Ireland and more concerned with promoting alternative dietary regimes that would allow the Irish to obtain the nutritional *quality* once drawn from the potato. In this context, the Board looked favourably on Indian meal (maize) and oatmeal as fitting substitutes for the potato. Its members understood these as highly nutritious foodstuffs and viewed the more advanced forms of agricultural production required to produce them as a potential enabler of modernisation in Irish food production. This vision was noticeably evident in the Board's optimistic claim that the introduction of meal had already transformed how food was thought about in Ireland. On this matter, they stated:

> It has often been desired, that the people of Ireland could be induced to turn from the potato to grain as their food, as tending to produce improvement in their habits and as rendering them less liable to suffer from periodic famines. All attempts to effect this have hitherto failed. However, the knowledge that they have now acquired of the very superior nutritious qualities of oatmeal, and its price continuing to bear such a relation to the cost of potatoes, as to render its consumption often more economical than that of the potato, will, it would seem to us, eventually and certainly lead to the desired end.[61]

This statement clearly demonstrates a faith in the providential good that the Board foresaw as likely to result from the blight once it had receded: a change in crop culture would simultaneously protect against future famines and promote positive adjustments in social and economic behaviour.

In autumn 1845, Robert Peel purchased £100,000 worth of Indian meal from America. Sales commenced in March.[62] Initially, its introduction was greeted enthusiastically. The *Freeman's Journal* published recipes for tasty puddings and bread that could be made from Indian meal, describing it as not only highly nutritious for humans but also as an admirable food for fattening pigs and oxen. Dogs reportedly relished it.[63] However, the famine-stricken poor tended not to be in a position to read the *Freeman's Journal*. Furthermore, practical difficulties punctuated the public distribution of meal; a development that ultimately encouraged the Board to criticise indoor relief policies. From 1846, Poor Law Unions were granted permission to substitute potatoes for alternative foodstuffs.[64] By 1848 only three out of 140 workhouses served neither type of meal while fifty-four served a mixture of oatmeal and Indian meal; the remainder serving one or the other.[65] However, workhouse staff encountered various problems when preparing dishes containing meal. When meal was introduced at the South Dublin Union Workhouse in April 1846, the baker reportedly did not know how to mix it with flour to produce bread; a telling scenario that demonstrated the pitfalls of policies of simply providing food without clear instructions on how to prepare it in a country whose inhabitants were often accustomed to preparing only potatoes.[66]

The provision of meal in workhouses created public concern. In May 1846, the South Dublin Union Relief Committee publicly asserted that the pound of bread made from Indian meal and three liquid pints of porridge allocated per day by Boards of Guardians was enough to feed only two people rather than the officially suggested six. On this, one member stated, 'we do not think that sixteen ounces of food, the allowance given by the South and by the North Union Committees, has been recognised by physiologists as sufficient for the healthy sustenance of an adult man', adding that the economic savings were insufficient to justify keeping pauper populations in a precarious balance between healthy and diseased existence.[67] These provisions were also unpopular among workhouse paupers. When the Lord Mayor of Dublin toured the city's workhouses in May 1847 to personally taste the dishes on offer, paupers complained to him that they would prefer bread to porridge as the latter played havoc with their stomachs.[68]

Pressing financial demands placed further pressure on workhouse administrators.[69] As institutions became swamped and as epidemic disease rapidly spread, the Board's members became ever more perturbed by the limitations of relief policies, in one instance announcing that institutionalisation was an even greater evil then allowing the poor to fend for themselves in the community.[70] This was probably an exaggeration predicated to fortify the case for more interventionist forms of state relief but it did raise pertinent questions about the sites where peasant health was best preserved. Meal supplies in the community were often so lacking that the impoverished continued to eat diseased potatoes. A limited understanding of how to prepare and cook meal seemed just as rife in the community as it was in the workhouse kitchen. Indian meal had initially been imported un-milled and had not always been sufficiently ground by millers.[71] The Board insisted that insufficient cooking had resulted in a failure to assimilate a full supply of nutriment, predisposing entire communities to dysentery and diarrhoea.[72] As the dispersion of recipes had proved ineffective, the Board supported closer dietary regulation to halt the tide of epidemic disease; an idea which, in their view, depended upon scientifically informed guidance. Accordingly, its members began calling for forms of official relief policy involving the provision of *cooked* food. Only by doing so could consumption patterns be nutritionally regulated and safeguards against disease established, so they insisted.

The Board clearly strove, perhaps unsuccessfully, to bridge the chasm between nutritional theory and nutritional practice. As well as promulgating an awareness of the potential connections between disease and innutritious diet, its members stressed the importance of food quality. In that way, they helped to establish a sense that expert nutritional interventions were imbued with the potential to spark reform in spaces ranging from the bodily to the economic and national. During the Famine, Corrigan and Crampton actively enaged with wider politico-economic discussion of promoting permanent societal change in Ireland via a carefully directed dietary adjustment. Drawing inspiration from established narratives of Irish improvement, they demarcated a move away from a mono-crop diet as a process best regulated with reference to nutritional science although, in the short term, their efforts to realise this aim were obstructed by the intensity of famine conditions and popular distaste for some of the new foodstuffs being brought into Ireland. Nonetheless, their visions reflected the increasing presence of biologically driven impulses in debates on how best to bring improvement to the Irish social, economic and national condition through the medium of food reform.

Soup controversies

The Board's aspirations were thwarted when state bodies finally consented to embark on a scheme of dispensing cooked food. Overwhelming applications for indoor relief in 1846 led the government to sanction the nationwide establishment of soup kitchens, despite that policy diverging significantly from pervasive *laissez-faire* ideologies of minimal intervention. The soup kitchen scheme was initiated under the Temporary Relief Act.[73] In 1847, the government consulted Alexis Soyer, famed French chef of the prestigious Reform Club, and soon dispatched him to Dublin where he set to work co-ordinating the construction of a network of kitchens. The Board approved, in part because its members were becoming increasingly exasperated by observing famine-stricken peasants devouring raw meal.[74] Yet the scheme was immediately stricken with controversy, in part because the very notion of the soup kitchen was popularly associated with the stigma and social degradation of pauperism. This had been evident in Germany some decades earlier when Count Romford had established soup kitchens only to be met with public chagrin.[75]

From the outset, the grandiose ceremonial opening of the scheme caused public consternation. The *Freeman's Journal* expressed nationalist fury at the opening of Dublin's first soup kitchen as the Union Jack was 'flaunted from the top of the soup kitchen ... proclaiming to the Heavens the degradation of our provincialism, but unfolding a tale, as it flaps in the listless air, of a union with England brought about by force, stained by corruption, cemented in blood, and now consummated in famine'. The *Journal* presented the soup kitchen as emblematic of the extension of an unwelcome foreign power into Ireland, embodying a distinct lack of sensitivity to the needs of a vulnerable, subjugated populace.[76] For the *Freeman's Journal*, the public feeding of the poor at the scheme's opening ceremony served as an inappropriate, but telling, articulation of English attitudes to the Irish poor. 'Five shillings each to see paupers feed!', exclaimed the newspaper, 'five shillings each to watch the burning blush of shame chasing pallidness from poverty's wan cheek! – five shillings each! When the animals at the Zoological Gardens may be inspected at feeding time for sixpence!'[77] Rejecting the ostensibly charitable ideals of soup kitchen schemes, infuriated nationalists condemned the structures as unwelcome emblems of British expansion. For them, the very act of eating and digesting food in these establishments carried meanings of subjugation to an imperial power, of colonial unjustness and inhumane treatment. These accounts portrayed soup kitchens not as benevolent structures but instead as sites founded to ease the conscience of those in power; buildings masquerading as symbols of British kindness but in reality serving concoctions devoid of nutritional or palatable value. The physical act of consuming food in them carried symbolic meanings of subjugation and a shunning of state responsibility to adequately care for starving citizens.

Prominent medical figures also took issue with Soyer's use of nutritional science. Allegations of the dishonesty and public spectacle of Soyer's soups coloured medical responses. While constructing his Dublin kitchen, Soyer penned a booklet entitled *The Poor Man's Regenerator* in which he recorded his economical recipes intended to raise the health of the Irish poor.[78] Soyer proudly proclaimed to have personally discovered that existing soup providers (including the Quakers) were ignorant of the nutritional quality of their ingredients. Proper seasoning, Soyer maintained, was needed to restore and strengthen the digestive organs of the famine-stricken.[79] Soyer would have been better positioned to publish such strong claims had he actually been equipped with a firm understanding of contemporary scientific cookery. In the view of outraged critics from the orthodox medical community, the digestive organs of famine-stricken peasants certainly needed more than the addition of herbs to their soups. Critical medical experts in both Ireland and Britain spotted Soyer's precarious comprehension of the basic principles of modern food science and angrily denounced his suggestions as fraudulent and his soups as deficient.

Prominent Edinburgh physician James Simpson wrote immediately to Henry Labouchere, Chief Secretary of Ireland, to condemn Soyer's assertions. Drawing from Liebig's doctrines, Simpson asserted that most of Soyer's soups did not contain meat, despite nutritional scientists having established meat to be more nutritious than vegetables. Reciting Liebigian theory, he advised against the provision of soup unless it was prepared with reference to valid scientific principles.[80]

In similar fashion, *The Lancet* derided Soyer's recipes as 'soup quackery' and as 'soups of pretence ... taken by the rich as a salve for their consciences' as part of 'a spasmodic feeling of benevolence'. The journal noted that other clubs, committees and relief associations had dispensed food without any public boasting or ostentation, in sharp contrast to the government's public spectacle. *The Lancet* then undertook a thorough chemical analysis of the contents of each soup, dismissing some of them – turnip parings, celery tops and salt – as items not even worthy of being described as food. Soyer's soups were determined to contain less than three ounces of solid aliment per quart despite nutritional chemistry having stipulated that healthy individuals needed between twelve and fourteen ounces per day. On this, *The Lancet* sardonically warned that 'organic chemistry will not, we fear, bend to the receipts of the most miraculous cookery book'. Continuing its scathing attack, *The Lancet* complained that both Soyer and the government had wrongly assumed that a bulk of water could compensate for a deficiency of solid aliment, stating:

> No culinary digestion, or stewing, or boiling, can convert four ounces into twelve, unless, indeed, the laws of animal physiology can be unwritten, and some magical power be made to reside in the cap and apron of the cook for substituting fluids in place of solids, and *aqua pura* for solid aliment, in the animal economy.

The journal concluded by asserting that although the public mind had been satisfied by developments in relief provision, this was unlikely to extend to the public stomach. 'Marquises, and lords and ladies, may taste the meagre liquid, and pronounce it agreeable to their gustative inclinations', announced the journal, 'but something more than an agreeable titillation of the palate is required to keep up the manufactory of blood, bone and muscle which constitutes the strong healthy man.'[81]

What most angered *The Lancet* was a clear misappropriation of accumulated scientific knowledge. After all, important questions were at stake in these debates relating to medical respectability and professionalism, as well as questions of authority in knowledge of food. *The Lancet*'s accusation of quackery was certainly not accidental. In a period when orthodox medicine was embroiled in the process of professionalising and extending its social influence, the public application of inaccurate scientific knowledge was potentially damaging, especially when seemingly sanctioned by a London-based government and Dublin Castle. Furthermore, the interest aroused by the Famine meant that relief practices were now being widely discussed on an international level. The medical profession had remained notably silent when the Scientific

Commission had dispensed publicly challenged advice on starch production at the commencement of the Famine. Then, state policy was at least ostensibly attempting to make good use of analytical knowledge, even if in a seemingly misguided fashion. Yet two years later, the government appeared to be relying upon nutritional knowledge espoused by a figure that they regarded as a medical charlatan. Concerned medical figures staunchly denied that nutritional science had informed the workings of soup kitchen schemes and denigrated the forms of knowledge that underpinned soup provision as false. After all, this was the sort of 'quack' activity that medical reformers were eager to distance themselves from. Medical critics in Britain instead articulated the prowess and social utility of 'proper' nutritional science.

Importantly, these debates reached far beyond the pages of the medical press. Even Queen Victoria's doctor Sir Henry Marsh suggested in a widely distributed pamphlet that soup was an unhealthy, dangerous relief mechanism. Instead, he insisted, only semi-liquid diets could maintain the health of children and sedentary adults. The labourer's food, Marsh also advised, needed to be at least partly solid as healthy digestion depended upon mastication and insalivation whereas liquid soups naturally digested too quickly, producing hunger and debility. To confirm this point, Marsh argued that eating the 'bone of the potatoe' had in fact long fulfilled this bodily requirement as it involved the slow digestion of a solid substance. 'The consideration of the diet best calculated to uphold his [the labourer's] strength and maintain his health', wrote Marsh, 'is at all times one of the highest national importance – at the present time, and in the existing disastrous state of the country, it is one which claims the utmost amount of attention, scientific and practical, which can be devoted to it.' However, for Marsh, soup provision dangerously violated established scientific laws.[82] The final publication produced on the soup kitchens was commissioned by the Royal Dublin Society, compiled and penned by Irish chemist John Aldridge.[83] Aldridge analysed the nutritive values of the soups offered in Soyer's soup kitchen and compared these with the dietary laws outlined in contemporary nutritional chemistry. He praised just one of Soyer's soups as it contained fish and concluded that to sustain healthy animal life, the Irish poor needed to combine flesh, seeds and vegetables in a bulky preparation of food proportionate to the capacity of the digestive organs.

Notably, like many of his contemporaries, Aldridge perceived the onset of blight as a suitable occasion to spur Irish industriousness. These visions about Irish improvement had not been entirely discarded by 1847 even despite the urgent need to offer short-term solutions to famine. Revealingly, Aldridge argued that orthodox forms of scientific knowledge, rather than those espoused by Soyer, had much to offer the Irish situation in both the short term and long term. He noted that carnivorous animals living on highly concentrated food were energetic and lively while herbivorous animals, tending to eat more gradually, were almost always sluggish and idle. Industrial exertion, Aldridge asserted, could never occur if the Irish poor were fed similarly to cows and sheep. Yet he considered the Irish poor to have been even worse fed than cattle for decades as hay, he believed, was a far more concentrated food than the potato.[84] In sharp contrast to the dominant iconography of the Famine that routinely emphasised the skeletal, starved rural peasant, Aldridge depicted a potentially empowered peasant invigorated by a precise comprehension of nutritional science, only if he was shielded from false forms of nutritional knowledge. Aldridge, like many contemporaries, remained eager to position nutritional science as a discipline replete with potential long-term benefits to Ireland provided that expert forms of scientific knowledge based upon analysis and deduction were appropriately utilised.

Conclusion

The Famine offered crucial opportunities for scientists with a specialism in nutrition to enter into a productive dialogue with political economists and social reformers by connecting their work to broader agendas of Irish social change and economic development. They helped to identify and target the Irish body as a suitable site of reform. The Famine afforded them further opportunities to debate how to regulate dietary patterns and guarantee future dietary and national well-being. Despite this interaction between nutritional science and the state, the application of nutritional knowledge was intricate and ultimately resisted. In fact, those promoting scientific dietary adjustment faced considerable public scepticism. The overwhelming intensity of famine conditions also disrupted the efficient implementation of scientifically guided relief schemes. This was particularly evident in the responses formed to state-sanctioned schemes, particularly Alexis Soyer's soup kitchen network. Soyer's comprehension of diet differed significantly from analytically driven forms of scientific knowledge.

Nonetheless, the Famine was an important moment when expert nutritional knowledge began to exert influence on discussion of Irish dietary behaviour. A shift in tone in discussion of the Irish body occurred as dismissive representations of the *quantity* of food consumed in Ireland gave way to debates on the *quality* of food that ought to be consumed once blight receded. The Famine coincided with a period when new empirical forms of knowledge were in formation and when serious efforts were being made to apply these to alleviate adverse social circumstances. As further chapters will reveal, the issue of nutritional quality was to pervade post-Famine critiques of Irish diet from hereon as idyllic hopes of post-Famine dietary regeneration were replaced by sustained concern about poor nutritional health.

Notes

1 Clarkson and Crawford, *Feast and Famine*, pp. 59–87. See also C. Ó Gráda, *Ireland Before and After the Famine: Explorations in Economic History* (Manchester and New York: Manchester University Press, 1993), pp. 1–97.

2 D. Gentilcore, *Italy and the Potato: A History, 1550–2000* (London and New York: Continuum, 2012), pp. 64–91.

3 P. Gray, *Famine, Land and Politics: British Government and Irish Society 1843–1850* (Dublin and Portland, OR: Irish Academic Press, 1999), pp. 4–9.
4 Ó Gráda, *Ireland Before and After the Famine*, pp. 2–8.
5 C. Kinealy, *This Great Calamity: The Irish Famine, 1845–52* (Dublin: Gill and Macmillan, 1994 [2006]), pp. 1–3.
6 Miller, *Modern History of the Stomach*, pp. 11–38.
7 See, for instance, W. Beaumont, *Experiments and Observations on the Gastric Juice and the Physiology of Digestion* (Plattsburgh: F. P. Allen, 1833).
8 Representative texts include J. Abernethy, *Surgical Observations on the Constitutional Origin and Treatment of Local Diseases* (London: Longman, Hurst, Reese and Orme, 1809); J. A. Paris, *A Treatise on Diet* (London: Thomas and George Underwood, 1826); J. Johnson, *An Essay on Morbid Sensibility of the Stomach and Bowels* (London: 1827); A. Combe, *The Physiology of Digestion* (Edinburgh: MacLachlan and Stewart, 1836).
9 *Miller, Modern History of the Stomach*, pp. 11–38
10 Johnson, *Essay on Morbid Sensibility.*
11 J. Johnson, *A Tour in Ireland* (London: S. Highley, 1844), p. 313.
12 See Miller, *Modern History of the Stomach*, pp. 11–38.
13 Johnson, *Tour in Ireland*, pp. 311–2.
14 T. C. Foster, *Letters on the Condition of the People of Ireland* (London: Chapman and Hall, 1846), pp. 558–9.
15 W. H. Brock, *Justus von Liebig: The Chemical Gatekeeper* (Cambridge: Cambridge University Press, 1997), p. 176.
16 Ibid., pp. 94–115.
17 J. von Liebig, *Research on the Chemistry of Food*, trans. W. Gregory (Lowell: Daniel Bixby and Company, 1848).
18 M. R. Finlay, 'Early marketing and the theory of nutrition: the science and culture of Liebig's extract of meat', in H. Kamminga and A. Cunningham (eds), *The Science and Culture of Nutrition, 1840–1940* (Amsterdam: Rodopi, 1995).
19 R. H. Kargon, *Science in Victorian Manchester: Enterprise and Expertise* (Manchester: Manchester University Press, 1977), pp. 48–9.
20 J. Adelman, *Communities of Science in Nineteenth-Century Ireland* (London: Pickering and Chatto, 2009), pp. 1–5. See also E. G. Lengel, *The Irish through British Eyes: Perceptions of Ireland in the Famine Era* (London and Westport, CT: Praeger, 2002).
21 Clarkson and Crawford, *Feast and Famine*, p. 88.
22 C. Matta, 'Spontaneous generation and disease causation: Anton de Bary's experiments with *Phytophthora infestans* and late blight of potato', *Journal of the History of Biology*, 43 (Fall 2010), 459–91.
23 C. Ó Murchadha, *The Great Famine: Ireland's Agony, 1845–52* (London: Continuum, 2011), p. 34.
24 T. P. O'Neill, 'The scientific investigation of the failure of the potato crop in Ireland 1845–6', *Irish Historical Studies*, 5 (September 1946), 123–38.
25 J. S. Donnelly Jr., 'Famine and government response 1845–6', in W. E. Vaughan (ed.), *A New History of Ireland V: Ireland under the Union I, 1801–70* (Oxford: Clarendon Press, 1989), p. 274.
26 Kargon, *Science in Victorian Manchester*, p. 91.
27 Brock, *Justus von Liebig*, p. 183.
28 R. Kane, *The Industrial Resources of Ireland* (Dublin: Hodges and Smith, 1844).
29 O'Neill, 'The scientific investigation'.
30 N. G. Coley, 'Medical chemists and the origins of clinical chemistry in Britain (circa

1750–1850)', *Clinical Chemistry*, 50:5 (May 2004), 961–72.
31 Gentilcore, *Italy and the Potato*, pp. 42–52.
32 G. Phillips, *The Potato Disease: Its Origin, Nature and Prevention* (London: S. Highley, 1845).
33 *Nation* (1 November 1845), p. 36.
34 See, for instance, National Archives of Ireland, Dublin (hereafter NAI), Famine Relief Commission Papers (hereafter RLFC) 3/1/3417, Report by Joseph Rogers on production of flour and meal from potatoes.
35 *Nation* (8 November 1845), p. 54.
36 NAI, Chief Secretary Office Registered Papers (hereafter CSORP), RLFC2/Z14466, Letter from Henry John Porter.
37 NAI, CSORP, RLFC2/Z15556, Letter from Reverend Edward Hoare requesting copies of the report on preserving the potato crop.
38 O'B. Bellingham, 'Observations upon the potato disease as it prevailed in Ireland this year', *Dublin Medical Press*, 13 (1845), 359–64 on p. 364.
39 NAI, CSORP, RLFC2/Z14434, Letter from John Glasson.
40 NAI, CSORP, RLFC2/Z16624, Letter from Reverend William Fisher, Rector of Killmore.
41 NAI, CSORP, RLFC2/Z14888, Anonymous letter; CSORP, RLFC2/Z15316, Letter from William Cockburn, Cork.
42 'The Potato Malady', *Freeman's Journal* (31 October 1845), p. 3.
43 NAI, CSORP, RLFC2/Z15866, Letter from Reverend Richard Walsh, Headford.
44 *Nation* (1 November 1845), p. 36.
45 'The Government Commission: The Potato Disease', *Freeman's Journal* (19 December 1845), p. 2.
46 *Cork Examiner* (29 December 1845), p. 2.
47 'The Potato Disease', *Freeman's Journal* (15 January 1846), p. 2.
48 'The Potato Crop', *Nation* (8 August 1846), p. 16.
49 'Dr Kane on the Potato Commission', *Tuam Herald* (7 November 1846), p. 2.
50 W. Wilde, 'The food of the Irish', *Dublin University Magazine*, 43 (March 1854), 127–46 on p. 138.
51 NAI, CSORP, RLFC2/Z14518, Letter from Dominic Corrigan.
52 'Symptoms produced by eating diseased potatoes', *Dublin Hospital Gazette*, 23 (1846), 166.
53 J. D. O'Brien, 'Cases of a peculiar form of gastro-enteritis resulting from the use of diseased potatoes', *Dublin Hospital Gazette*, 24 (1846), 184–5.
54 M. J. McCormack, 'A case of land scurvy produced by eating diseased potatoes', *Dublin Hospital Gazette*, 29 (1846), 263–8.
55 L. M. Geary, '"The late disastrous epidemic"': medical relief and the Great Famine', in C. Morash and R. Hayes (eds), *Fearful Realities: New Perspectives on the Famine* (Dublin and Portland, OR: Irish Academic Press, 1996), pp. 49–50.
56 D. J. Corrigan, *On Famine and Fever* (Dublin: J. Fannin, 1846).
57 L. M. Geary, 'Famine, fever and the bloody flux', in C. Póirtéir (ed.), *The Great Irish Famine* (Cork: Mercier Press in association with Radio Telefís Éireann, 1995), p. 75.
58 Ó Murchadha, *The Great Famine*, p. 94.
59 Geary, 'Late disastrous epidemic', p. 51.
60 *Report of the Commissioners of Health, on the Epidemics of 1846 to 1850*, H. C. 1852–3 [1562] xli, pp. 19–20.
61 Ibid., p. 25.
62 Donnelly Jr., 'Famine and government response', p. 278.
63 'How to Convert Indian Corn into Food', *Freeman's Journal* (21 February 1846), p. 4;

'Indian Corn', *Freeman's Journal* (28 February 1846), p. 1.
64 *Twelfth Annual Report of Poor Law Commissioners*, H.C. 1846 [704] xix.1, p. 25.
65 Data collated from *Returns from County Gaols and Workhouses in Ireland of Daily Diet allowed to Able-Bodied Men*, H. C. 1847–8 [486] liii.
66 'South Dublin Union', *Freeman's Journal* (18 April 1846), p. 4.
67 'Pauper Rations', *Freeman's Journal* (13 May 1847), p. 2.
68 'South Union Relief Committee', *Freeman's Journal* (27 May 1847), p. 4.
69 V. Crossman, *The Poor Law in Ireland, 1838–1948* (West Tempest: Dundalgan Press, 2006), p. 20.
70 Geary, 'Late disastrous epidemic'.
71 Donnelly Jr., 'Famine and government response', pp. 279–80.
72 *Report of the Commissioners of Health*, p. 21.
73 Kinealy, *This Great Calamity*, pp. 120–1.
74 'The Rations for the Poor: Spread of Fever', *Freeman's Journal* (19 May 1847), p. 2.
75 See F. Redlich, 'Science and charity: Count Rumford and his followers', *International Review of Social History*, 16:2 (August 1971), 184–216.
76 'The Soup Fete: Degradation Consummated', *Freeman's Journal* (10 April 1847), p. 2.
77 'Finale of a Cook's Triumph', *Freeman's Journal* (14 April 1847), p. 2.
78 R. Cowen, *Relish* (London: Phoenix, 2006), p. 127.
79 A. Soyer, *Soyer's Charitable Cookery* (Dublin: Hodges and Smith, 1848), pp. 11–12.
80 J. Simpson, *On the More Effective Application of the System of Relief by Means of Soup Kitchens* (London: Whittaker and Co., 1847).
81 Editorial, *Lancet*, 49 (27 February 1847), 232.
82 H. Marsh, *On the Preparation of Food for the Labourer* (Dublin: James McGlashan, 1847).
83 Cowen, *Relish*, p. 130.
84 J. Aldridge, *On the Comparative Nutritive and Pecuniary Value of Various Kinds of Cooked Food* (Dublin, 1847).

2

Reforming food production: agricultural science and education

The immediate post-Famine period was marked by profound optimism about the potential of Irish agricultural development. In the space of just a few years, Ireland's socio-economic landscape had radically adjusted. By 1851, Ireland was a more desolate country, preparing itself for a gradual recovery from the socio-psychological scars left by the mass emigration, disease and death created by the Famine. Yet the country's inhabitants appeared, or were at least presumed, to be ready and willing to improve their socio-economic conditions. For some would-be improvers, agricultural practice offered a fertile ground upon which the seeds of modernisation could be planted to facilitate fuller Irish integration into an international capitalist market economy. Michael Turner meticulously details how, following the Famine, Irish agriculture became less dependent upon tillage and potato cultivation. Instead, many farmers chose to accumulate profit from livestock production.[1] Nonetheless, historians have paid relatively scant attention to the scientific ideas in circulation that agricultural improvers then hoped would inform and underpin agricultural rejuvenation.

During the Famine, potatoes, vegetable crops and meats had been scientifically re-envisaged. Nutritional scientists had reduced these foodstuffs to their chemical structures and fervently sought to extend their findings beyond the confines of their laboratories. To bolster their claims of the social value of their scientific findings, individuals such as Robert Kane had underscored the individual, socio-economic and national value of referring to, and making practical use of, empirical knowledge of food and nutrition. In many ways, this development was mirrored in scientific interventions in Irish agriculture, a terrain where reformers also privileged organic chemistry as a potential improving mechanism.[2] This chapter suggests that post-Famine agriculturists promoted new understandings of how to productively harness biological agro-material found on Irish farms during and after the Famine. In that way, the biological imperatives that had proved central to discussion of Irish dietary readjustment in the 1840s can be seen to have impacted in spheres other than the bodily. Scientists also empirically reassessed and redefined animal and plant life using broadly analogous techniques of chemical analysis, one outcome being the formation of new ideas about how to maximise Irish food production and foster economic development.

This chapter explores post-Famine scientific readings of the biology and physiology of crops, plants and animals and their subsequent promotion as an aid to Irish food production. Like those who sponsored new understandings of human nutrition, proponents of scientific food production consistently framed their ideas in terms of national advancement. They achieved this by firmly distinguishing between what was old and new, traditional and modern, and regressive and progressive. In the 1850s, agricultural science was institutionalised via a state-supported network of agricultural schools and model farms aimed at all social classes. Ultimately, however, small farmers exhibited resistance and apathy towards these educational schemes for an assortment of social, political and practical reasons, a factor that restricted the socio-economic effectiveness of agricultural schools. By exploring these themes, this chapter reveals further connections made between food and national improvement while demonstrating that food production, as with consumption, evolved into a site of deep contestation between different Irish social groups and, sometimes, between colonising and colonised powers.

Governing agricultural life

To produce food scientifically required thinking scientifically. And to do so productively depended upon Irish agricultural labourers absorbing radically new ideas about how to harness land and animals while internalising a psychological mindset geared towards productivity, not subsistence. Robert Kane's thoughts on agriculture outlined in his seminal *Industrial Resources of Ireland* (1844) offer an illustrative example of how reformers upheld agro-scientific knowledge as a key to refashioning the relationship between man and land. *Industrial Resources* blended Kane's nationalist perspectives with his broader economic ideologies and improving agendas.[3] As Juliana Adelman persuasively argues, his book received a remarkably favourable reception in part due to its buoyant promises of national advancement.[4] In it, Kane posited that Ireland had all of the natural resources needed to industrialise and modernise but lacked the skill and capital needed to fully exploit those resources. It was through education, Kane insisted, that Ireland's latent potential could be realised; a stance informed by having personally observed the economic value of education in France and Germany during periods of study in those countries.[5] *Industrial Resources* synthesised Kane's perspectives on the potential social utility of organic chemistry and his longing to bolster Ireland's economic and social performance. It proposed a unique form of economic nationalism; one perhaps more concerned with raising Irish potential for self-governance than with increasing output for the benefit of imperial interests.

Kane, as outlined in Chapter 1, was a prominent member of both the Scientific Commission and the Central Board of Health – expert groups that had promoted scientifically informed food consumption during the Famine. Kane echoed his framing of scientific consumption as a precursor of national advancement in his perspectives on food production. Mapping a linear path from primitivism to civilisation, as James Johnson and others had done in relation to Irish eating customs, Kane insisted that the uptake of sophisticated food production techniques would ultimately distinguish modern Irish farmers from their potato-driven counterparts. Accordingly, he openly criticised the simplistic lifestyle of cottier farmers for its primitivism but optimistically asserted that this socio-cultural backwardness was rectifiable if producers internalised agro-scientific knowledge. This, Kane maintained, would be economically and nationally advantageous. As the country progressed from 'agriculture' to 'manufacture', Irish soil would be mastered as modern agriculturists learnt how to maximise its productive capacities. 'His operations,' wrote Kane on the subject of the modern farmer, 'resembles a manufacturing chemist, except that his product is a palatable food instead of soap or oil of vitriol.' Kane also foresaw the potential commercialisation of Irish meat production as a signifier of advancement. In his view, Ireland's anticipated ascent into agricultural modernity depended upon a nationwide shift from 'watching cattle' to 'manufacturing food'.[6]

The scientific impulse for *Industrial Resources* stemmed from Justus von Liebig, under whom Kane had previously worked.[7] In addition to illuminating the chemical composition of foodstuffs and their workings in the human system, Liebig had pursued pioneering research into the chemical dimensions of food production. For both Liebig and Kane, the intellectual basis of the modern agriculturist's work needed to coalesce around the premise that the healthy growth of animals, plants and crops depended upon an appropriate supply of particular chemical elements. Liebig had categorised sixteen of these, identifying carbon, hydrogen, nitrogen and oxygen as the most important while acknowledging that smaller quantities of other chemicals were equally vital for healthy growth. These findings formed the basis of Kane's opinion that decisions on which crops to rotate on Irish soils should be made with reference to scientific estimations of their chemical composition. He noted, for instance, that corn thrived in soils replete with silica; turnips, beet and potato in soils with high potash content; and peas and clover in lime-abundant soils. For Kane, it was not just human bodies that needed to be fed with nutrients; the land itself also did. Furthermore, although plants and crops were known to naturally obtain chemical elements from the soil, Kane, following Liebig's lead, proposed that chemical elements could be artificially supplied to sustain productivity should natural supplies deplete.[8] From the 1840s, Liebig's disciples in Ireland eagerly promulgated these ideas and sought to adapt them to suit Irish geographical and geological circumstances. Importantly, they saw their activities as tied to the overarching project of ending Ireland's mono-crop culture and stimulating agricultural diversity.

Agriculturists also drew attention to the scientific enhancement of meat production. Following the repeal of the Corn Laws in 1846, corn prices fell dramatically while cattle and sheep prices rose. Combined, these factors persuaded many Irish to turn to grazing and livestock rearing.[9] In light of this, scientific communities endorsed new approaches to converting animal life into human food. An address delivered to the Royal Dublin Society by Edmund W. Davy, Professor of Agriculture and Agricultural Chemistry at the Carmichael School of Medicine, Dublin, in 1859 exemplified contemporary ideas on how to enhance Irish meat production. In this, Davy asserted that:

The animal, in fact, may be likened to a machine in many respects:-

> 1st. There is the constant wear and tear going on throughout every part of the system; for by every movement of the body a part of its substance is worn away or destroyed.
>
> 2nd. Like the machine, it requires its different parts to be renewed, and new matter take the place of that which has become (as it were) worn out, and unfit for further use.
>
> 3rd. We know that *heat* is the primary cause of the motive power of most of our machinery. The body of the animal, in like manner, requires to be kept at a certain temperature, and when, by any means, this falls below a certain point, life becomes extinct, and the motions of its complex and wondrous machinery ceases.
>
> The food which the animal takes may be regarded as the agent which keeps the several parts in motion.[10]

Davy evoked a mechanical image of the animal body as a site of energy preservation and conservation; as a structure composed of eroding, decaying parts requiring vigilant maintenance; and as a potential object of efficient rationalised production. He reconfigured the animal as a machine whose powers needed precise manipulation if producers were to successfully mould it into an article of production. Borrowing heavily from the language of mechanical engineering, Davy deconstructed the animal body into multiple, adjustable elements and parts to define it as a physical site that could be subject to expert analysis and modification. Notably, Davy's representation of the animal – an interactive system consisting of heat, power and energy flowing through the body, accompanied by internal wear, tear and repair, and a complex web of inputs and outputs – offered a radically different interpretation of animal life than most Irish small farmers would have encountered. It also demanded major adjustments in Irish animal–human interactions by articulating new, perhaps unfamiliar possibilities for the human exploitation of animals.[11]

Davy believed that animals needed to be fed with an appropriate input of foodstuffs. In his view, producers needed to provide animals with combinations of food containing rigorously defined quantities of chemical elements for the 'animal machine' to fulfil its maximum productive potential. In his address, Davy stipulated that producers should approach feeding animals with a thorough appreciation of the physiological functions of carbon, hydrogen and oxygen and an awareness of the physiological functions of sugars, oils, albumens, alkalis and water. Cattle fed with rich, nourishing food produced valuable manure and superior meat, he pronounced. According to Davy, food also repaired and nourished animal systems and impacted on internal temperature. Keeping animals at a temperature conducive to healthy growth demanded significant changes in the architecture of the farm. Davy urged farmers to remove cattle from damp weather and place them in indoor accommodation as he believed that exposure to cold, wet weather placed strain on respiratory systems, encouraging cattle to develop instinctual, but uneconomical, food cravings. Making firm distinctions between expert and lay knowledge, Davy disregarded the pre-existing stock of knowledge on cattle fattening and feeding instinctually accumulated by farmers through years of agricultural labour. Although he acknowledged that farmers had acquired this through years of practical toil and trial and error techniques, Davy insisted that non-empirical knowledge had failed to create general laws that could be universally applied.[12] By juxtaposing practical experience with analytical expertise, Davy also sought to carve out an important role for a new type of agricultural expert who might not necessarily have spent so much as a single day working on a farm but who could nonetheless claim and exert intellectual authority on production.

Davy's lecture signified his confidence in organic chemistry. He allocated science a pivotal role in the broader strategy of stimulating the Irish economy by defining what Irish agriculture could be and what it was not. Davy's illustrative example, as with Kane's, illustrates some of the ways in which scientists publicly presented agricultural science as a utilitarian mechanism of food reform. Both Davy and Kane demanded a complex reconfiguration of the relationship between Irish farmers and the natural world. The end result, so they hoped, would provide all classes of farmers with the intellectual and practical resources required to stimulate development.

Communicating agro-scientific knowledge

Agricultural reformers mostly agreed upon education as an appropriate impetus to progression or, as Richard Jarrell suggests, a conduit between scientific theory and practice.[13] Kane certainly saw agricultural development as dependent upon wider public access to educational resources. To reinforce that point, he asserted in *Industrial Resources* that it was not enough to simply offer money to small farmers to allow them to buy fertilising products as, so Kane lamented, these farmers would probably only use fertilisers inaccurately if they lacked an empirical knowledge of how to apply them.[14] Importantly, Kane identified Irish smallholders as the neediest recipients of agro-scientific knowledge.[15] Problematically, expert agricultural knowledge tended to be communicated only among elite scientific groups rather than being directed at small-scale farming communities. In the 1840s, pamphlets and public lectures served as important mediums of agro-scientific knowledge. For instance, in 1844 John Frederick Hodges published a pamphlet entitled *What Science can do for the Irish Farmer*. Hodges was Professor of Chemistry at the Royal Belfast Institution and had also completed his doctoral thesis with Liebig at the University of Giessen.[16] He was a prime example of an agriculturist who openly admitted to having no practical farming experience but who nonetheless chose to act as a spokesperson for Liebig's agricultural principles in Ireland. His pamphlet offered an evocative manifesto that campaigned for a radical overhaul of traditional production practices. Optimistically, Hodges presented agricultural chemistry as a rational mechanism for doubling, if not trebling, the produce of up to twenty million acres of Irish land. In his view, if knowledge was dispensed of the chemical elements needed by crops for healthy growth, and if Irish soils were analysed to determine their natural composition, then Irish farmers would be empowered with a precise understanding of the most suitable foodstuffs that could be produced in accordance with Ireland's specific physical and geological circumstances.[17]

Hodges served as a leading member of the Chemico-Agricultural Society of Ulster, a group established in 1846 to counteract a perceived lack of awareness of agricultural chemistry among small farmers. Although the Society's members contemplated expanding their activities across Ireland, their influence ultimately remained confined to northern regions where they engaged primarily with Ulster gentlemen and farming societies.[18] During the Famine, the Society regularly debated which foodstuffs might replace the potato, the failure of which it openly upheld as a blessing in disguise for Irish society.[19] It published numerous pamphlets which identified sites of potential agricultural improvement and detailed the myriad transformative purposes of scientific knowledge. In a pamphlet on crop rotation published in 1846, John T. Burnett reiterated how making practical use of organic chemistry could stop land from becoming exhausted.[20] Similarly, Hodges published a pamphlet on the subject of manure in which he urged small farmers to equip themselves with a precise knowledge of its chemical elements.[21] Cattle shows offered a further medium for dispensing agro-scientific knowledge. The Royal Agricultural Society of Ireland ran annual events where large prizes were awarded to entrants displaying the strongest, healthiest examples of livestock. These prizes were intended to offer a stimulus to other farmers who, the Society hoped, would be spurred on to produce superior animals, having witnessed the degree of perfection attainable with modern breeding and keeping techniques. These events also featured displays of produce such as grains, flax and artificial manures, as well as diagrams depicting modern drainage methods.[22]

Clearly, avenues of communication existed in the 1840s that allowed agricultural improvers to publicly engage. However, literacy levels were low among the less affluent, despite that group being routinely targeted in agricultural literature.[23] Pamphlets therefore proved relatively ineffective as instructional mechanisms for them. Furthermore, cattle shows and public lectures traditionally catered very much for middle-class interests. In fact, lectures had long acted as signifiers of civility and middle-class respectability and, in any case, were falling out of fashion by the 1840s, a period when lecturers became increasingly convinced that public speaking was achieving little in the way of popularising scientific knowledge.[24] During the Famine, journalists aggressively criticised cattle shows for having introduced improved husbandry among larger classes of farmers, but no one else.[25] The costly expense of these events, not to mention their implicit ethos of social exclusion, led to their gradual dismissal as vectors of modern agricultural knowledge intended for all. Indeed, cattle shows had initially developed as an interest of the higher classes alone. Stock breeding, and the ownership of large – often excessively fat – animals, served as potent reminders of social prestige but implicitly excluded those who could not afford the costs of attending them. At worst, experimentation in meat production carried strong associations with the governing classes and their quest to produce the 'ideal bovine'.[26] Agricultural shows came under particular fire during the Famine. In characteristically blunt fashion, in 1847 the *Tuam Herald* published an editorial entitled 'Are Human Beings as Well Fed as Bullocks?' that contained livid assertions that bullocks, cows, swine and sheep were better fed than the mass of impoverished Irish citizens afflicted by the Famine, all for the sake of being displayed at spectacular farming shows. Expressing profound disgust, the newspaper listed off the amount being fed to each animal in minute detail and calculated the numbers of humans who could have been comfortably fed with an equivalent amount of food.[27]

Efforts to promulgate agricultural development among small farming communities at ground level were also proving frustrating. This was apparent in the exasperated tone of the Royal Agricultural Improvement Society of Ireland's instructors during the Famine. In 1851 George Brennan, practical instructor in Dingle, Co. Kerry, recalled how he had felt compelled to advise a supplier in Tralee to stop supplying the local populace with bean seeds upon witnessing small farmers planting them too late in the season, despite having been given advice to the contrary. Brennan also listed his numerous fruitless efforts to encourage the local populace to sow unfamiliar crops such as parsnips and lamented the exhausting levels of energy that he had spent trying to establish the benefits of planting winter crops in the minds of local communities.[28] Outbursts such as these indicate that many small Irish farmers remained sceptical or apathetic towards new innovations. They also rendered visible the intricate psychological barriers that agricultural improvers needed to traverse to optimise food production. These anecdotal reports confirm Cormac Ó Gráda's suggestions that technological conservatism and excessive risk aversion delayed the diffusion of new agricultural innovations after the Famine.[29]

In response, prominent figures such as Kane expended considerable energy publicly stressing the need for a nationwide, state-supported system of agricultural education.[30] His ideas gained credence. In 1848, John Sproule of the Royal Horticultural Improvement Society of Ireland, and ex-editor of the *Irish Farmer's Journal*, wrote to MP and Duke of Leinster Charles William Fitzgerald, one of the largest landowners in Ireland and an active member of the Royal Dublin Society. In his letter, Sproule lamented that informal agricultural education had failed because farmers had been slow to follow dispensed instructions on agricultural practice. He depicted farmers as unswervingly attached to long-established practices and as individuals who obstinately refused to entertain new concepts. Sproule even observed that many small farmers had haphazardly engaged with new agricultural techniques without instruction and then ascribed their lack of success to the inefficacy of those techniques, a vicious circle that further intensified distrust to 'new-fangled plans'.[31] Sproule's stance was probably exaggerated given its appearance in a wider plea to implement new educational policies. However, it demonstrates the ways in which prominent scientific figures positioned education as a device that might counteract the rigid conservatism and ingrained backwardness that they stereotypically associated with Irish small farmers.

In this context, model farms came to be recognised as a potentially effective means of dispensing awareness of modern food production. During the Famine, Irish Quakers had stressed the usefulness of education in enacting permanent agricultural adjustment.[32] In 1848, the Society of Friends opened an experimental farm at Ballina, Co. Mayo. Then, Ballina was among the most impoverished of regions in Ireland. The new farm was intended to provide an educational resource that would equip destitute able-bodied men with the scientific expertise and skills needed to become permanently self-sufficient. Instructors introduced their students to the benefits of multi-crop farming.[33] The pinnacle of these experiments was a model farm constructed at Brookfield, Co. Fermanagh; an initiative comprised of an extensive network of large farm buildings and modern examples of land drainage.[34] The site aimed to serve as a visible example of high farming which, its managers hoped, would encourage surrounding communities to improve their own farms. In the view of the Quakers, a thriving, industrious neighbour was likely to influence his fellow farmers by example, thereby energising free competition among the less industrious.[35]

Glasnevin, a model farm located near Dublin, offered a further prototype. Founded in 1838, it contained fifty-two acres of land, all cultivated by modern systems of crop rotation. Young Dublin men training to teach at National Schools regularly visited Glasnevin to become acquainted with modern agricultural practice. Farming on all scales was taught at the institution meaning that even those with relatively small land allotments could, in theory, benefit. Importantly, Glasnevin was consciously upheld as a self-sufficient site entirely reliant upon its own resources with minimal need to purchase manure or food externally.[36] It therefore provided an emblematic site of mid-Victorian values of self-reliance. Its managers aspired to creating and moulding educated, refined and civilised types of farmers – individuals well versed in the technicalities of modern farming systems and dedicated to functioning productively in a modern capitalist economy.

Drawing from the success of the Quaker model farms and Glasnevin, the state established a national network of agricultural education in the late 1840s. Adelman details how the Queen's Colleges offered higher-level agricultural diplomas from 1849 onwards.[37] Yet the establishment of a nationwide network aimed at all social classes, relatively unexplored by Adelman, also held broad socio-cultural significance. This network served as a vector of scientific knowledge aimed primarily at small farmers. Jarrell goes so far as to suggest that the scheme constituted 'the most comprehensive state-supported system of agricultural instruction the world had seen to that time'.[38] Notably, when devising the network, the Commissioners of National Education adhered to the same mid-Victorian notions of self-help that had formed the ideological basis of pre-existing establishments. As well as dispensing agro-scientific information, these schools aimed to foster self-reliance and industriousness; values routinely, and often derogatorily, depicted as absent from traditional Irish culture. Political economists typically viewed self-help as preferable to state assistance although state bodies, in this instance, willingly allocated initial financial resources on the understanding that long-term self reliance would be stimulated.[39] In 1847, the Commissioners rented land throughout Ireland.[40] The following year, they allocated £4,600 to the erection of fourteen model agricultural schools. Thomas Kirkpatrick was appointed as the Commissioners' agricultural inspector, and held that position until well into the 1860s.[41]

Syllabuses fused scientific and practical agriculture and incorporated up-to-date topics such as the chemical composition of vegetables and plants, modern forms of husbandry and scientifically informed tactics of livestock rearing.[42] The content of the *Agricultural Classbook*, used extensively in this period, also reveals that educators aligned agricultural knowledge with broader improving agendas. The *Classbook* deeply problematised traditional production practices. It portrayed small farmers as having erred in the past by adhering to traditional practices and, accordingly, encouraged the replacement of older tillage systems with four-course systems of crop rotation.[43] Likewise, the *Classbook* warned that meat production levels had failed to keep pace with an ever-increasing demand. Accordingly, it encouraged the adaption of Irish farming systems to allow meat and dairy produce to be scientifically produced rather than grain crops alone.[44] As part of its persuasive rhetoric, the *Classbook* portrayed the quality of Irish livestock, particularly in smallholdings, as dismal. It tackled this concern by asserting that the most intelligent farmers in the country were convinced that the number of farm animals could be raised nationally by up to 25 per cent but only if farmers adopted improved modes of breeding and management.[45]

To help to enact this new capitalist-orientated agricultural utopia, the *Classbook* drew on the technical reconfigurations of animal life espoused by figures such as Davy. An emphasis on meat production was fitting given that the British market was beginning to act as a driving force for shifting Irish agricultural trends. In the 1850s, Irish producers exported approximately 40 per cent of cattle to Britain. This figure rose to 50 per cent in the mid-1860s and 70 per cent by the century's end.[46] Agricultural reformers were deeply sensitive to this development. In one instance, the *Classbook* asserted that the prime aim of modern improvements in cattle, sheep and pig rearing was 'to establish the supremacy of the stomach and dethrone the empire of the head; and at the same time diminish, as much as possible, the development of the nervous system, which would induce too much irritability, and destroy that indolence and quietness so essential for the fattening process'. To facilitate this, the *Classbook* revealed ways in which heads and bones could be made finer, offal diminished, and nervous systems controlled by influencing the actions of the stomach through scientifically defined feeding methods. These steps, so pupils learnt, would allow animal bodies to be transformed into perfect, efficient machines for manufacturing meat.[47]

Evidently, educators urged agricultural pupils to adopt a psychological mindset that depersonalised the animal: to perceive of it as a more abstract physical site governed by the physiological cravings of its stomach. They exposed students to approaches that reduced animal bodies to an internal interplay of starch, water, oil, flesh-forming materials and fibres; all of which could be modulated by appropriate combinations of grass, hay, roots, grains and oil-cakes.[48] Furthermore, they sought to restructure traditional animal–human interactions to allow farm animals to be likened to machines; objects of production whose internal physiology could be manipulated in a manner amenable to efficient production. In fact, the *Classbook* overtly presented the ideal modern farmer as an individual who pursued his work in a similar fashion to mechanics and factory operatives. It drew firm distinctions between those who had achieved this – elite farmers – and those yet to do so: the small farmers. The former, equipped with scientific expertise, served as an ideal from whom the 'primitive', smaller farmer could learn.[49]

These educational practices also contained important moral dimensions. As Helen O'Connell argues, the project of Irish improvement can be understood in part as an effort to curb the alleged excesses and hedonism then associated with the rural peasantry.[50] Reflecting this imperative, the *Classbook* sponsored forms of labouring behaviour based upon rational calculation, industriousness and an ingrained commitment to improving the national socio-economic order. Pupils learnt, in secular language, to grasp the laws of political economy, respect private property and to work hard for frugal competence; characteristics then routinely attributed to British industriousness.[51] The *Classbook* reminded pupils that farmers used few implements when the agriculture of a country was wedged in a backward condition, and that even these were of 'the rudest construction'. Yet as nations civilised, food production costs increased, encouraging farmers to use modern implements and techniques. In turn, large farms evolved to accommodate more sophisticated machinery and to reduce production costs.[52] In this narrative, the accumulation of profit and socio-economic progression were presented as firmly interlinked in a language which, like many improving texts, forged clear distinctions between the 'primitive' and the 'modern'. This persuasive rhetoric captured a capitalist mentality – rather than a subsistence one – and transmitted penetrative visions of a stable reformed social order. Notably, the *Classbook* dismissed opposition by labourers to modern machinery, and the formation of illegal combinations who sought to destroy machinery, as remnants of social primitivism.[53]

In practice, advice offered on scientific animal rearing only bore relevance to farmers who could afford livestock. Nonetheless, the *Classbook* did offer improving information intended to filter down to the smallest of farmers and propounded ways in which less affluent farmers could also partake in the national accumulation of agricultural wealth. It encouraged cottiers and farmers in possession of holdings of less than fifty acres to conceive of pigs as 'the poor man's saving bank' as these animals could be fed cheaply with offal. According to this doctrine, pig-rearing engendered habits of foresight and thrift. Rather than purchasing tobacco or alcohol, so pupils learnt, those who saved to the upkeep of their pigs would ultimately improve their own condition and impress the results of their moral lessons onto their offspring.[54] Evidently, education contained important moral and psychological dimensions predicated to modify the personalities and outlooks of small farmers. Agricultural reform therefore offered an all-encompassing programme that targeted various domains of Irish life ranging from the individual and personal to the social, economic and national.

Institutionalising and resisting agricultural education

The period 1854 to 1876 witnessed agricultural prosperity and innovation. Although fewer people remained to work the land after the Famine, the potential to accumulate individual wealth or to specialise sharply increased.[55] In this period, agricultural chemistry, as its proponents forged a new social identity for the sub-discipline, optimistically promised improvement for all. But how successfully did ideals of agricultural modernity map onto the traditional, rural terrain of Irish life which they sought to supplant? In 1870, just twenty years after the establishment of the agricultural school network, the *Freeman's Journal* proclaimed that 'next to the Land Act we know of no more powerful lever for raising the social condition of the peasantry of the country than the system of agricultural education'. As evidence, the newspaper cited 5,117 pupils who had so far received training in agricultural schools, and a further 50,000 pupils who had read agricultural textbooks in National Schools.[56] This stance seems out of place in a period when agricultural education schemes were being subject to widespread criticism, scepticism and even hostility. In 1865, Catholic Unionist MP William Monsell asserted in the House of Commons that the sooner they were got rid of the better as 'it was notorious that the minor agricultural schools were complete failures throughout Ireland'.[57] By the 1870s, the vast majority of agricultural schools had been closed and sold.[58] How, then, can the seemingly dramatic failure of a scheme that promised socio-economic regeneration and affluence be accounted for?

Jarrell suggests that most recipients of agricultural education emigrated; an outcome that limited its influence in reforming Irish agriculture.[59] Yet emigration was just one of a confluence of forces that impeded the uptake of scientific agriculture. Financial considerations partly explain this trend. Despite the large expenditure channelled into them, model farms tended to remain unprofitable; a bone of contention recurrently complained of in the House of Commons. By the 1860s, a consensus existed that model farms had failed to encourage self-sufficient farming. On the contrary, they had continued to rely upon a continual flow of state funding; a problematic scenario in an era dominated by *laissez-faire* politics and liberal notions of minimal state intervention. That decade saw a sharp curtailing of expenditure on agricultural training, partly in response to the heavy outlay needed to construct buildings and buy livestock and farming implements.[60] In 1863, the House of Commons voted for a large expenditure reduction of £700 per annum from the overall budget for all the model farms on the basis that model farms were 'an after-growth and a great abuse' of the national education system. In the discussion that surrounded this vote, critics dismissed the type of farming conducted at these institutions as overly expensive and, worse still, as 'no example whatever to anybody outside of them'.[61] Critics in the House of Commons called for further expenditure reductions in the following year.[62]

Uncertainty about the practical value of agricultural science permeated these debates. State bodies had certainly been willing to give agricultural science a fair test in the 1840s through their support of a new nationwide educational network. However, the pervasive scientific ethos of institutions such as Glasnevin irked critics who resolutely maintained that agricultural science was disconnected from agricultural practice and that, in consequence, the government was wasting valuable money on experimentation rather than genuine forms of social improvement. Of course, this sentiment echoed attacks made on scientific communities during the Famine when critics had publicly condemned starch extraction. The Irish public, as Adelman notes, lost faith in the improving capacities of agricultural education as early as the mid-1850s.[63] By the 1870s, the seemingly speculative nature of agricultural science provided a key rationale for deconstructing the system in place. Welsh MP William Williams exemplified this perspective when, in the House of Commons in 1856, he dismissed expenditure on 'fancy agricultural teaching' as a waste of resources, especially when granted to support the conducting of seemingly impractical agricultural experiments at Glasnevin.[64]

This open attack on Glasnevin was in many ways surprising given the recent successes of the institution. Following a visit by Prince Albert in 1853, Glasnevin's managers renamed the model farm the Albert National Agricultural Training Institution. Furthermore, the institution had acquired a formidable international reputation. In 1858, one of its pupils won first prize in an agricultural essay competition organised by the Massachusetts Society for Promoting Agriculture.[65] Dr Pugh, Principal of Pennsylvania State Agriculture College, visited in the following year and left so impressed that he instigated a plan of mutual co-operation.[66] Canadian authorities also used Glasnevin as a template when developing a similar system of agricultural education.[67] In the 1850s and 1860s, its managers developed up-to-date systems of draining, subsoiling, road construction and weed eradication alongside a sophisticated network of gardens and conservatories. Glasnevin purported to offer a prototype model of 'high farming' that provided an example and training ground for rural populations. It contained a complex network of under-land pipes that conveyed liquid from manure tanks to the hydrants in the several fields. Its managers purchased the most modern appliances to farm the land

and provided pupils with ample opportunities to test them. They also obtained a powerful steam engine for thrashing grain, bruising oats, beans and peas, and dressing flax. Glasnevin's cattle was purported to be of the highest quality.[68]

Nonetheless, critics such as Williams continued to dismiss Glasnevin as overly experimental in nature and to question the extent to which agro-scientific knowledge had successfully translated into efficient agricultural practice at the institution. Glasnevin was undoubtedly a site that embodied the aspirations of contemporary organic chemistry, that strove to make manifest its principles of social and psychological improvement and that emblematised a desired scientific revolution in food production. However, the farm's ongoing interest in experimentation riled critics. Although Glasnevin certainly had scientific research output related to food, the farm operated in a cultural milieu that increasingly found difficulty in reconciling the chasm between chemical theory and social practice.[69] For instance, in 1851, just a few years after the establishment of Ireland's agricultural education system, American Unitarian minister and agricultural expert Henry Colman, in his influential *European Agriculture and Rural Economy*, had claimed that the extreme confidence placed in organic chemistry in Ireland had been premature as the application of sulphuric acid to bones was by then the only well-established practice that had stemmed from chemical science. According to Colman, knowledge of how to apply lime to soil and the composition of manures still remained highly contestable. This is not to imply that Colman completely rejected the potential importance of chemistry to agricultural pursuits. However, he recommended that unquestionable confidence should not be placed in it until scientists developed more substantial, concrete principles.[70]

Students had mixed attitudes to a syllabus that fused analytical and practical approaches to food production. In 1850, Thomas Byrne left Glasnevin disappointed by the lack of practical ploughing instruction offered at the institution.[71] The fathers of Thomas Barney and Robert Burns resigned them from the school as they were dissatisfied with Glasnevin's lofty tactics of farm management.[72] These scenarios cannot be entirely ascribed to conservatism. As Jonathan Bell and Mervyn Watson persuasively demonstrate, practical Irish farming advanced in this period as farmers applied a mixture of what they term 'improved' and 'common' farming methods. Moreover, seemingly cruder farming implements could often be highly refined, sometimes even more efficient than newer techniques in local contexts where they had been long tried and tested.[73] Likewise, the Commissioners of National Education had little time for the aspirations of chemical scientists. As early as 1852, they argued that scientific elements of teaching should be awarded less importance than their practical aspects.[74] Paradoxically, experiments undertaken at Glasnevin had started to discredit some of the key theoretical constructs espoused by elite scientists, thus calling into question the analytical framework that had underpinned the establishment of agricultural education. In 1859, Thomas Baldwin, prestigious employee at the institution, publicly challenged Liebig's conclusions on the chemistry of manures. Speaking to the Royal Dublin Society, he announced that experiments undertaken by himself at Glasnevin on the nutritive value of potato manures had never quite realised the expectations of Liebig's disciples. Baldwin concluded that 'the value of chemical analysis has been very much over-rated by chemists little acquainted with agriculture and by those who merely read without studying treatises on agricultural chemistry'.[75] Constantly shifting perspectives on the theory of agriculture did little to quell public scepticism.

Kirkpatrick's retirement as agricultural inspector and manager of Glasnevin led to his replacement by Baldwin, a figure who sought to instil a more practical, and less costly, ethos to the model farm system. One of his first reforms, initiated in 1865, curtailed financial expenditure on food experimentation, a step possibly taken in response to public criticism. In his annual reports, Baldwin reminded readers that the state had not established the farm for experimentation but instead as an example of practical farm management. His actions also stemmed from fears that the use of public money for agricultural experiments had tarnished the institution's public reputation.[76] Baldwin continued by critiquing the imbalance of chemical education and practical instruction at agricultural schools by claiming that:

> I have found that young men who had spent a year or two at our agricultural schools, and who could answer with great readiness questions about the chemistry of air and water, as well as about nitrogen and phosphorus, knew little or nothing of the actual practice of farming, not even of the management of the farm on which they spent a year or more. In many cases I have met young men who could tell me the quantities of food consumed by horses or cattle on those farms, and who had actually got no hold of the facts of practical farming. It appears to me to be too much the fashion to put these young men through a course of study in the elements of science and to neglect altogether the application of this science to practice. I have met young men of eighteen and twenty who could tell the composition of milk and different feeding substances, but who were utterly ignorant of the points which distinguish a bad from a good milk, or a good feeder from an unprofitable one. This is not as it ought to be.[77]

Similarly, in 1870, Baldwin vehemently announced:

> Let us not make ourselves ridiculous by preaching the science of modern agriculture to men who have never seen the objects with which this science deals. It would look like mocking poor and ignorant farmers in remote districts of Ireland to fill their agricultural instruction with chemistry or botany. It is more useful to show them how to raise turnips than to give them a philosophic exposition of Liebig's theories.[78]

Baldwin's remarks highlighted the tensions in existence between agro-scientific theory and practice. Faced with mounting pressure to justify public expenditure, Baldwin sponsored more pragmatic educational techniques. His motivations remain somewhat unclear. His public statements and reforms may have stemmed from a genuine belief that analytical chemistry had failed to productively inform agricultural practice. Yet his rejection of over-indulgence in scientific theory was also conducted in an era where Irish scientific establishments more generally were under threat of closure by London-based authorities and when key establishments such as the House of Industry were becoming more closely directed from the British mainland.[79] Baldwin may have defensively adapted his views on the function of food experimentation at Glasnevin to comply with the financial and ideological needs of the mainland. As such, he may have forwarded his opinions as part of an attempt to ensure Glasnevin's survival.

The uptake of agricultural education was also restrained by an array of religious, political and social factors. Some critics saw agricultural schools as veiled manifestations of broader power relations between Protestant and Catholic cultures and between imperial rulers and colonised subjects. The religious dimensions of the agricultural schools certainly contributed to public antagonism. In the House of Commons in 1863, Vincent Scully, land reformer and MP for Co. Cork, delivered a diatribe in which he asserted that the mass of the Irish population objected to model farms as they perceived them as 'nests of proselytism'.[80] Scully's assertions were characteristic, given that he intently focused his political career on promoting reforms that benefited the Catholic community. In this instance, his concerns about religious conversion implied that, at least for some, agricultural schools threatened an unwelcome expansion of Protestant ideals and ways of life into rural Catholic regions. Certainly, agricultural instruction contained moral dimensions to food production that privileged ideals broadly analogous to those venerated in Protestant culture. Apprehension over proselytism had been common during the Famine in response to fears that the organisers of certain relief schemes sought to convert Catholics in exchange for food.[81] Furthermore, the Irish education system more generally was hampered by opposition to its ethos of providing non-denominational education; a scenario that raised accusations from the Catholic community that state education was a 'Godless education experiment'.[82]

Similarly, Catholic critics often saw agricultural schools and model farms as sites where religious conversion might take place, despite ostensibly purporting to be non-denominational and secular.[83] Roman Catholic propaganda routinely attacked the system by insisting that the entire staff of Glasnevin – from the directors to the housekeepers – were non-Catholic.[84] Although historical data on the institution's staff that might corroborate this perspective does not exist, Glasnevin's surviving registers reveal that out of 816 pupils who enrolled between 1850 and 1869, 549 of these were of Roman Catholic origin. This constituted just over 62 per cent of the total number of pupils. Of the other students, 19.6 per cent were Protestant, 2.57 Presbyterian, and 3.06 per cent of other religious denomination or of unknown religious persuasion.[85]

Critical Catholic figures saw the ethos of mixed denomination model farms as morally problematic on the basis that the young age of pupils, their occupation and living circumstances all encouraged 'sensuality'. At their most emotive, critics portrayed Glasnevin pupils as leading 'lives of almost absolute Godlessness' and 'the lives of libertines'. Although managers made arrangements for religious instruction at Glasnevin, critics continued to denounce the establishment as a 'system of unmitigated paganism'. Managers took few steps to ensure that students ever attended Divine Worship, so Catholic propaganda asserted. On one occasion a Catholic layman accused the Protestant Kirkpatrick of being disinclined to interpret a Catholic neglect of worship as a serious offence. Further concerns were raised about modern agricultural training, even when undertaken in predominantly Catholic areas, being essentially a cultural force of Presbyterian and Protestant origin, having originated in Ulster.[86] The fear that Protestant ideals underpinned Catholic agricultural education was omnipresent in these accounts.

Non-religious imperatives also impacted profoundly on public perceptions of agricultural school initiatives. In fact, an enduring panoply of wider social and cultural forces impacted negatively on agricultural education. Models that likened animals to machines and privileged chemical visions of soil structures fitted uneasily with the Irish social and cultural landscape for an array of reasons including class tensions and broader attitudes to imperial power. In Ireland, the rejection of, or disinterest in, agricultural science was deeply entangled with the country's unique, but fraught, system of agricultural power relations. Meat production, for instance, was associated in the public eye with landlordism and the self-serving interests of wealthier grazier communities, not to mention imperial interests given that much of the meat produced in Ireland was ultimately shipped to Britain. Following the Famine, a new breed of capitalistic landlords had emerged, many of whom had acquired bankrupt estates under the 1849 Encumbered Estates Act. They proved far more determined than the previous generation of gentrified landlords to make their estates pay. Many of them hired ranchers or graziers.[87] At worst, graziers found themselves being publicly accused of having taken land away from the peasantry. In addition, grazing tended not to produce employment as it was not a labour-intensive form of work.[88]

Agricultural school managers also faced accusations that they produced men fit for employment only as stewards to Irish landlords instead of individuals likely to transform Irish farming cultures from below.[89] In this context, agricultural chemistry could be dismissed as both a by-product of an alien culture and an intrusive element of a class system acting repressively on the Irish peasantry. This was certainly the view of Scully, who asserted in the House of Commons in 1863 that Irish model farms were 'English hobbies' and that 'the model school at Dublin [Glasnevin] was neither more nor less than a nest for a Scotch family'.[90] Scully's contentions demonstrated that model farms and analytically driven forms of food production symbolised, for some, an unwelcome extension of mainland and Protestant ideals. They implied that even if agricultural science did eventually fulfil its improving potential, the fruits of that advancement would be unlikely to be evenly dispensed across Irish society as would-be improvers had promised.

An indication of the types of employment secured by pupils can be gleaned from the *Report of the Commissioners of National Education* for the year 1861.

Table 2.1 Employment destinations of Glasnevin students, 1858–61

Destination	*Number*
Farming at home, either for themselves or their relatives	68
Land stewards and assistant land agents	41
Clerks in the office of merchants, land agents, in Customs	14
National School teachers	10
Left in delicate health, and from other causes	10
Nurserymen, gardeners and assistant gardeners	9
Planters in the islands of Jamaica and Antigua	9
Entered the Queen's and Catholic Colleges	6
Emigrated to the Cape of Good Hope and Australia	5
Agricultural teachers	3
Total	**175**

Table 2.1 demonstrates that of the 175 students who graduated between 1858 and 1861, 38 per cent (the majority) found work on farms at home by 1862 while 23 per cent had secured employment as land stewards or land agents. Only 5 per cent went on to employment as National School teachers and only 3 per cent found work as agricultural teachers. Eight per cent emigrated to the West Indies, the Cape of Good Hope or Australia. Accusations that the system primarily benefited landlords were not entirely ungrounded in reality. However, those who supported this view underestimated the number of pupils who did return to their farms equipped with some degree of agro-scientific knowledge. Regardless, these statistics lend weight to contemporary claims, as well as suggestions made by Adelman, that students in model farms were often middle-class individuals who tended not to choose to secure employment as practical farmers.[91]

Negative perceptions of agricultural science and its institutionalisation increased alongside the accumulating tensions between landlords and tenants that ultimately led to the Land Wars of the 1870s, 1880s and 1890s, an agitation that sought to better the position of tenant farmers through land redistribution.[92] In the 1850s, movements such as the Tenant League demanded that improvements made to land or buildings by tenant farmers should be legally recognised as the property of the tenant, not the landlord.[93] With its Tenant Compensation Bill, the League argued that compensation should be sought for costs incurred in erecting new buildings, reclaiming wasteland and draining land.[94] Until tenant improvements could be seen as truly beneficial to tenants, small farmers had little incentive to improve land and increase food productivity because they knew that the benefits of those actions would most likely be reaped by their landlords.

Given the high levels of distrust between tenant farmers and landlords, it is unsurprising that schemes purportedly associated with landlordism proved unpopular. Some agricultural communities thought that model farms served a similar purpose to farming societies – networks also commonly believed to have been established by landlords for their own benefit.[95] These clubs had proved unpopular as peasants feared that if they improved their land, then they risked being turned out of their holdings to make room for larger proprietors or being forced to pay extra rent in consequence of their own initial outlay.[96] In 1871, even the Commissioners of Education conceded that the land question had created indifference, if not disfavour, to model farms and schools, widely regarded as instruments constructed by the gentry.[97] Although improvers promoted agricultural instruction as intended for all social classes, and despite the scientific community having made efforts to distance itself from perceptions of its work as of interest only to an enlightened middle- and upper-class elite, many small tenant farmers still associated modern agricultural science with a repressive class system. It seemed to them that raising food productivity would ultimately work against their interests.

Conclusion

In 1878, the *Freeman's Journal* commented on the subject of scientific education that 'the Commissioners of National Education, if they ever seriously dreamed of supplying it, have utterly and confessedly failed. If they deliberately conspired for the failure of their Model Farms, the collapse could not have been more complete.'[98] In the same year, the *Irish Farmer's Gazette* announced that the Commissioners were 'as competent to deal with Irish agricultural education as they would have been to negotiate the Treaty of Berlin'.[99] Evidently, the application of organic chemistry to post-Famine food production was a remarkably intricate process that failed due to a confluence of mitigating factors. New agricultural sciences sponsored novel ways of knowing food and the means by which it could be efficiently produced. This allowed advocates of organic chemistry to partake in far broader debates about the structural reform of Irish society, economic and national life. Yet, as had been the case with nutritional science in Famine-period relief policies, the institutionalisation of organic chemistry in an impressive state-supported agricultural education network ultimately did little to bolster the reputation of agricultural science and plans to maximise food production.

Agricultural education was intended to enhance public understandings of how to productively harness the resources available on Irish farms. Although scientific agriculturists had routinely castigated Irish farmers for their apparent conservatism, backwardness and primitivism, it was ultimately not conservatism that impinged upon the success of agricultural schools but a broad set of social, political and religious issues. Irish agriculture did follow a new path following the Famine yet it was not, as hoped, to be guided by the prescriptions of agro-scientific knowledge. Nonetheless, these debates on agricultural chemistry and education further reveal the new ways in which food was re-thought and reconsidered in mid-nineteenth-century Ireland, as well as how many scientists in Ireland consciously connected their ideas on food to the broader project of encouraging socio-economic development. This initial post-Famine optimism, as Part II of this monograph demonstrates, was soon to be superseded by profound pessimism about the direction that Irish society had traversed since the Famine.

Notes

1 Turner, *After the Famine*, p. 58.
2 Adelman, *Communities of Science*, p. 79.
3 C. Cullen, 'The Museum of Irish Industry (1845–1867): research environment, popular museum and community of learning in mid-Victorian Ireland' (Unpublished PhD thesis, University College Dublin, 2008), p. 72.
4 J. Adelman, '*The Industrial Resources of Ireland* by Robert Kane', in J. H. Murphy (ed.), *The Irish Book in English, 1800–1891 Volume IV* (Oxford: Oxford University Press, 2011), p. 551.
5 Cullen, 'The Museum of Irish Industry', pp. 65–6.
6 R. Kane, *The Industrial Resources of Ireland* (Dublin: Hodges and Smith, 1844), p. 248.
7 Brock, *Justus von Liebig*, p. 80.
8 J. von Liebig, *Animal Chemistry, or Organic Chemistry in its Application to Physiology and Pathology* (London: Taylor and Walton, 1842). For public reception, see Brock, *Justus von Liebig*, pp. 145–82.
9 R. D. Crotty, *Irish Agricultural Production: Its Volume and Structure* (Cork: Cork University Press, 1966), p. 66.
10 E. W. Davy, 'On the scientific principles involved in the feeding and fattening of stock', *Natural History Review*, 6 (1859), 261–8 on p. 262.
11 For shifting animal–human interactions, see K. Thomas, *Man and the Natural World: Changing Attitudes in England 1500–1800* (London: Allen Lane, 1983).
12 Davy, 'On the scientific principles', p. 261.
13 R. Jarrell, 'Some aspects of the evolution of agricultural and technical education in nineteenth-century Ireland', in P. J. Bowler and N. Whyte (eds), *Science and Society in Ireland: The Social Context of Science and Technology in Ireland, 1800–1950* (Belfast: Institute of Irish Studies, 1997), p. 101.
14 Kane, *Industrial Resources*, p. 279.
15 T. W. Freeman, 'Land and people c.1841', in Vaughan (ed.), *A New History of Ireland V*, pp. 252–3.
16 Adelman, *Communities of Science*, p. 79.
17 J. F. Hodges, *What Science can do for the Irish Farmer* (Dublin: W. Curry, 1844).
18 *Annual Report of the Chemico-Agricultural Society of Ulster* (Belfast: Francis D. Finlay, 1847).
19 *First General Meeting and Council Dinner of the Chemico-Agricultural Society of Ulster* (Belfast: Francis D. Finlay, 1846), p. 5.
20 J. T. Burnett, *The Chemico-Agricultural Society of Ulster on Rotations of Cropping* (Belfast: Francis D. Finlay, 1846).
21 J. F. Hodges, *Report of the Composition and Agricultural Value of Kelp* (Belfast: Francis D. Finlay, 1846).
22 H. Colman, *European Agriculture and Rural Economy* (Boston: Phillips, Sampson and Company, 4th edn, 1851), pp. 175–7.
23 M. E. Daly, 'Literacy and language change in the late nineteenth and early twentieth centuries', in M. E. Daly and D. Dickson (eds), *The Origins of Popular Literacy in Ireland: Language Change and Educational Development* (Dublin: Department of Modern History,

TCD, Department of Modern Irish History, UCD, 1990), p. 153.

24 E. Leaney, '"Evanescent impressions": public lectures and the popularisation of science in Ireland, 1770–1860', *Éire-Ireland*, 43 (Winter 2008), 157–82.

25 See, for instance, 'Royal Agricultural Improvement Society of Ireland', *Irish Farmer's Gazette*, 10 (March 1851), 157–8.

26 H. Ritvo, *The Animal Estate: The English and Other Creatures in the Victorian Age* (Harvard: Harvard University Press, 1987 [London: Penguin, 1990]), pp. 45–81.

27 'Are Human Beings as Well Fed as Bullocks?', *Tuam Herald* (17 April 1847), p. 3.

28 'Royal Agricultural Improvement Society of Ireland', pp. 157–8.

29 Ó Gráda, *Ireland Before and After the Famine*, p. 164.

30 Kane, *Industrial Resources*, pp. 403–4; R. Kane, *On the Importance of Agricultural and Industrial Education* (Dublin, 1845).

31 J. Sproule, *Model Farms as Leading to an Improved System of Cultivation: The Appropriate Remedy for the Present Distressed Condition of Ireland* (Dublin: James McGlashan, 1848), p. 10.

32 *Transactions of the Central Relief Committee of the Society of Friends during the Famine in Ireland in 1846 and 1847* (Dublin: Hodges and Smith, 1852), pp. 3–4.

33 Ibid., pp. 415–16.

34 Ibid., p. 96.

35 Ibid., p. 106.

36 Colman, *European Agriculture*, pp. 182–3.

37 See Adelman, *Communities of Science*, pp. 71–100.

38 Jarrell, 'Some aspects', p. 105.

39 A. Kidd, *State, Society and the Poor in Nineteenth-Century England* (London: Macmillan Press, 1999), p. 2. See also P. H. J. H. Gosden, *Self Help: Voluntary Institutions in the Nineteenth Century* (London: Batsford, 1975); E. Hopkins, *Working Class Self Help in the Nineteenth Century: Responses to Industrialisation* (New York: St. Martin's Press, 1995).

40 *Fourteenth Report of the Commissioners of National Education in Ireland*, Reports of Commissioners, Commons, 1847–48 [981], vol. xxix.219, pp. 12–13.

41 *Fifteenth Report of the Commissioners of National Education in Ireland*, H. C. 1849 [1066] xxiii.91, pp. 8–9.

42 Colman, *European Agriculture*, pp. 179–80.

43 Commissioners of National Education in Ireland, *Agricultural Classbook, or How Best to Cultivate a Small Farm or Garden: Together with Hints on Domestic Economy* (Dublin: Thom, 1853), p. 117.

44 Ibid., pp. 205–6.

45 Ibid., p. 206.

46 Turner, *After the Famine*, p. 58.

47 Commissioners of National Education, *Agricultural Classbook*, pp. 206–7.

48 Ibid., p. 211.

49 Ibid., p. 208.

50 O'Connell, *Ireland and the Fiction of Improvement*, p. 6.

51 J. M. Goldstrom, *The Social Content of Education 1808–1870: A Study of the Working Class School Reader in England and Ireland* (Shannon: Irish University Press, 1972), pp. 67–74.

52 Commissioners of National Education, *Agricultural Classbook*, p. 74.

53 Ibid., p. 75.

54 Ibid., pp. 273–4.

55 Ó Gráda, *Ireland Before and After the Famine*, pp. 151–2.

56 'Exhibition of Farm Produce at the Albert Institution', *Freeman's Journal* (2 December 1870), p. 4.

57 'Supply: civil service estimates', *House of Commons Debates*, 2 June 1865, 179, cc. 1248–60.
58 Jarrell, 'Some aspects', pp. 101–17.
59 Ibid., p. 113.
60 *Twenty-Seventh Report of the Commissioners of National Education in Ireland*, H. C. 1861 [2873] xx.91, pp. 148–9.
61 'Supply: civil service estimates', *House of Commons Debates*, 5 June 1863, 171, cc. 450–72.
62 *Thirtieth Report of the Commissioners of National Education in Ireland*, H. C. 1864 [3351] xix Pt.II.1, p. 33.
63 Adelman, *Communities of Science*, pp. 98–9.
64 'Supply: miscellaneous estimates', *House of Commons Debates*, 4 April 1856, 141, cc. 523–43.
65 *Twenty-Fifth Report of the Commissioners of National Education in Ireland*, H. C. 1860 [2593] xxv.1, p. 326.
66 *Twenty-Sixth Report of the Commissioners of National Education in Ireland*, H. C. 1860 [2706] xxvi.1, p. 298.
67 'Report of L'Abbé J. O. Godin on his mission to Europe', *Statement of the Public Accounts of the Province of Quebec for the Fiscal Year Ended 30th June 1869* (Quebec: Augustin Cote, 1869), pp. 21–62.
68 'The Albert Model Farm, Glasnevin', *Farmer's Magazine*, 36 (July 1869), 20–2 on p. 21.
69 C. A. Cameron, *The Stock-Feeders Manual: The Chemistry of Food in relation to the Breeding and Feeding of Livestock* (London and New York: Cassell, Petter and Galpin, 1868), pp. 203–4.
70 Colman, *European Agriculture*, pp. 226–7.
71 Data collated from University College Dublin Archives, IE UCDA AAC1/14, Records of the Albert Agricultural College, Albert Agricultural College Admission Registers.
72 Ibid.
73 J. Bell and M. Watson, *A History of Irish Farming, 1750–1950* (Dublin: Four Courts Press, 2009), pp. 293–302.
74 *Eighteenth Report of the Commissioners of National Education in Ireland*, H. C. 1852–3 [1582] xlii.1, p. 157.
75 T. Baldwin, 'On the application of artificial manures part one', *Journal of the Royal Dublin Society*, 2 (October 1859), 309–21.
76 *Thirty-First Report of the Commissioners of National Education in Ireland*, H. C. 1865 [1582] xlii.1, p. 311.
77 Ibid., p. 312.
78 *Thirty-Seventh Report of the Commissioners of National Education in Ireland*, H. C. 1871 [C.360] xxiii.7, pp. 386–7.
79 See R. A. Jarrell, 'The department of science and art and control of Irish science, 1853–1905', *Irish Historical Studies*, 23:92 (November 1983), 330–47; N. Whyte, *Science, Colonialism and Ireland* (Cork: Cork University Press, 1999).
80 'Supply: civil service estimates', *House of Commons Debates*, 5 June 1863, 171, cc. 450–72.
81 For prosetylism, see I. Whelan, 'The stigma of souperism', in Póirtéir (ed.), *Great Irish Famine*.
82 For religious tensions in education, see T. J. McElligott, *Secondary Education in Ireland, 1870–1921* (Dublin: Irish Academic Press, 1981).
83 'Report of L'Abbé J. O. Godin', p. 55.
84 A Catholic Layman, *Mixed Education: The Catholic Case Stated, or Principles, Working and Results of the System of National Education* (Dublin: John Mullany, 1859), pp. 339–43.
85 Data collated from Albert Agricultural College Admission Registers.
86 Catholic Layman, *Mixed Education*, pp. 339–43.

87 D. S. Jones, *Graziers, Land Reform and Political Conflict in Ireland* (Washington DC: Catholic University of America Press, 1995), pp. 99–100.
88 Ibid., p. 254.
89 'Supply: miscellaneous estimates', *House of Commons Debates*, 29 June 1857, 146, cc. 564–601.
90 'Supply: civil service estimates', *House of Commons Debates*, 5 June 1863, 171, cc. 450–72.
91 Adelman, *Communities of Science*, p. 74.
92 See S. Clark, *Social Origins of the Irish Land War* (Princeton, NJ: Princeton University Press, 1979).
93 For work specifically dealing with the Tenant League, see J. H. Whyte, *The Tenant League and Irish Politics in the 1850s* (Dundalk: Dublin Historical Society, 1963).
94 'The Tenant League: Address to the People of Ireland', *Freeman's Journal* (17 June 1853), p. 3.
95 *Thirty-Sixth Report of Commissioners*, p. 1331.
96 'Tenant-Right in Parliament', *Freeman's Journal* (7 April 1862), p. 3.
97 *Thirty-Seventh Report of the Commissioners*, p. 383.
98 'Agricultural Education', *Freeman's Journal* (21 September 1878), p. 7.
99 Reprinted in 'Agricultural Education in Ireland', *Freeman's Journal* (28 September 1878), p. 6.

II

Food and national decline in post-Famine Ireland, c.1845–1910

3

Food and improvement in the mid-nineteenth-century institution

The late nineteenth century was marked by profound concern about national social and economic well-being. Despite initial optimism in the 1850s about the prospects of dietary reconstruction and agricultural prosperity, pessimism about the Irish condition quickly re-emerged. Part II of this monograph explores the centrality of food in post-Famine debates on socio-economic stagnation and decline. Physical health seemed to suffer as the poor gradually replaced the potato with less nutritious foodstuffs. At the same time, Irish food production mostly failed to fully modernise, a problem that steadily limited the appeal of Irish imports abroad. Combined, these circumstances ensured that food retained a pivotal role in public discussion of national well-being after the Famine. Food-related issues inflected social, economic, political, medical and scientific discourses, providing further evidence of the ways in which contemporaries upheld food as integral to virtually all aspects of national life.

To introduce this theme, this chapter focuses on mid-century feeding in institutions and maintains that critics of institutional dietary policies invoked this seemingly internal institutional matter as a concern with national implications. Following the Famine, expert ideas on the relationship between diet, nutrition and illness became increasingly nuanced. Physicians paid closer attention to the issues of nutritional quality and deficiency and sought to firmly establish the potential long-term physical and mental consequences of consuming an insufficient diet. In doing so, they significantly advanced the Liebig-influenced debates on nutrition and the Irish diet that had been central to medico-scientific interventions in famine relief in the late 1840s. Institutions were replete with opportunities for physicians and medical witnesses to witness, monitor and better understand the negative physical and mental effects of poor nutrition. Their well-publicised observations and investigations helped to draw public attention to the idea that a nutritionally inadequate diet encouraged the onset of bodily conditions such as scrofula (or tuberculosis of the neck) and ophthalmia (or conjunctivitis). This forging of new links between illness and food consumption, or under-consumption, was an important development. As subsequent chapters demonstrate, it proved to be a characteristic feature of post-Famine discourse on the Irish body. Ultimately, questions about institutional feeding and nutritional health captured the attention of a range of individuals including physicians, institutional reformers, institutional staff, Catholic social reformers and journalists.

Accordingly, this chapter maintains that institutions – particularly workhouses, prisons, reformatories and industrial schools – were key sites in which anxieties about insufficient nutrition were robustly articulated, particularly between 1845 and 1880, a transformative period marked by public reflection on institutional living conditions. On the one hand, institutional managers intended feeding regimes to reflect and perpetuate the ethos of particular institutions. Broadly speaking, prisons aimed to punish, workhouses to deter and reformatories and industrial schools to reform. Institutional managers carefully regulated feeding arrangements to reinforce these imperatives. Restricting pauper and prisoner access to food was one of the simplest and most efficient ways to achieve these goals. On the other hand, institutions were ostensibly intended to improve. Whether managers should be principally chastising or reforming was a problematic question – one eloquently played out in debates on food provision. Although sparse feeding served the purpose of punishing and reforming, critics also pointed out that paupers and prisoners needed to remain physically healthy if they were ever to be returned to society as useful, productive citizens. This latter theme was most expressively played out in discussion of the institutionalised young, a group for whom, according to those concerned about institutional life, institutionalisation seemed inappropriate. They recognised children as the future adult population of Ireland and, for this reason, sought to preserve their health.

Advocates of institutional reform increasingly drew upon expert knowledge of nutrition as a useful resource. Many physicians who investigated workhouse and prison conditions sought to police the often fragile boundaries between under-feeding and adequate feeding and to monitor dietary regimes that, in their view, were designed to punish at the expense of sustaining health. They did so by drawing links between diet and illness, pursuing investigations into poor institutional health and experimenting with periods of nutritious feeding to decisively prove their ideas on diet and illness. Exploration of the ideological tensions that emerged between the need to preserve health while simultaneously perpetuating the ethos of particular institutions forms the basis of this chapter.

This nutritional discourse emerged in a transitional period of social thought on poverty and crime management. The number of institutions, and their residents, grew rapidly across nineteenth-century Europe. Political economists and institutional reformers came to view institutionalisation as an efficient means of maintaining social order. In workhouses, prisons, reformatories and industrial schools, anti-social behaviour could be monitored and rectified by managers and staff, the intention being to produce reformed, socially engaged individuals.[1] According to Oliver MacDonagh, the period 1830 to 1845 was marked by increased centralisation and social regulation in Ireland. He presents this era as fertile with new political ideologies, political techniques and inventive methods of observation.[2] Policing, prisons and public health all mutated into arenas where state bodies, MacDonagh suggests, 'intervened to a degree, and in a fashion, scarcely conceivable in contemporary Britain'. State bodies and private entrepreneurs built ever-larger complexes as the numbers of the institutionalised rose.[3] Various motivations underpinned this trend. Mark Finnane observes that by the 1830s the Irish gentry were widely seen as too incompetent or unwilling to adequately govern Ireland. In response, state bodies sought alternative options. Contemporaneously, fear mounted over apparently rising levels of Irish social disorder, which political economists often connected to over-population and an ailing economy. These issues further encouraged the state to rely upon institutionalisation to address and resolve critical social problems.[4]

Importantly, political economists tended to understand poverty and crime as expressions of ingrained moral and personality defects rather than as inevitable consequences of adverse social or economic conditions. Peter Gray persuasively argues that the period between the Famine and the Land Wars saw the development of a distinctly Irish brand of political economy that focused on reforming individual behaviours such as idleness and crime.[5] Society blamed individuals instead of considering crime and pauperism as products of inappropriate social, economic and political structures. Post-Famine institutions were intended to effect individual reform as character was seen as modifiable when subject to the moralising influences of institutional life.[6] Accordingly, institutional governors referred explicitly to the intellectual blueprint of 'moral reform', a pervasive ideological outlook intent on attacking the roots of poverty and crime by reforming the self.[7] By restricting dietary intake in the workhouse, paupers could be moulded into independent individuals who, upon release, had moral restraint and a new-found sense of self-governance; attributes needed to function independently in a capitalist economy.[8] Crime – similarly understood as a product of defective personality – came to be tackled through the inculcation of morally acceptable behavioural patterns in prisons. Nonetheless, the public often perceived institutions negatively. Reformers and journalists routinely castigated institutions as physically degrading environments that risked permanently damaging the physical and mental health of their residents due to their inadequate feeding and insanitary conditions. This stance allowed critics to challenge the idea that institutions served socially enhancing purposes. Discussion of these imperatives was particularly evident in four distinct sites: prisons, workhouses, reformatories and industrial schools. Importantly, public disapproval of institutional feeding formed an important part of broader debates about the true purposes of these institutions. Were they socially ameliorative sites as their advocates claimed or were they in fact places that weakened bodies and, in turn, contributed to, rather than resolved, problems in Ireland's socio-economic infrastructure?

Feeding the pauperised

The physical implications of subsisting on an innutritious diet were particularly apparent in the post-Famine workhouse. Although dubious workhouse feeding regimes had provoked public anger and disgust for some decades, a subtle shift in emphasis occurred in Ireland during the Famine.[9] Whereas the divisive issue of starvation had been particularly prominent in the late 1830s and early 1840s, it was during the Famine that physicians, medical authors and the Irish public also became attentive to the poor nutritional quality of workhouse food and its potential long-term impact on health.

State approaches to poverty realigned in the nineteenth century. The 1830s witnessed a radical redesigning of the pre-existing Poor Law. Poor relief was now channelled principally through workhouses – sites restructured in that decade to serve as deterrent environments. In many respects, the presence of the workhouse helped to transform poverty into a condition akin to crime, as something demanding punishment. The New Poor Law, implemented across England and Wales from 1834 and Ireland from 1838, sought to fulfil the ideological goal of deterrence by basing workhouse life around the premise that institutional living conditions needed to be considerably worse than those endured by the able-bodied poor living outside of the workhouse. This stigmatisation of poverty was expected to encourage the poor to engage more fully in modern economic existence and, in turn, render Ireland productive and wealthy. Dismal workhouse living conditions deliberately offered paupers an ominous reminder of the need to labour rather than depend on public funds.[10] Accordingly, from the 1830s the Poor Law Commissioners and Boards of Guardians recommended food provisions that were uniformly bland, unappealing and unappetising – more so, in theory, than the food consumed in the community.

Initially, the mono-crop nature of pre-Famine dietary customs had presented the Poor Law Commissioners with a fundamental ideological quandary. In 1836, Commissioner George Cornewall Lewis concluded that 'it is impossible that an Irish labourer could find any change for the worse which should continue to him the barest necessities of life'. According to Lewis, the Irish workhouse diet could scarcely be made less appealing than the monotonous potato diet. Nonetheless, the very effectiveness of the New Poor Law rested upon reducing physical comforts typically found at home. Lewis felt compelled to warn that the meagreness of Irish diet was seriously impeding efforts to implement the New Poor Law throughout the country. He ominously cautioned that 'in Ireland, the workhouse system can never act well, or even act at all, because it is impossible to make any reduction in the scale of the labourer's diet; and, consequently, the very hinge on which the entire system turns is wanting'.[11] The Commissioners agreed to limit adult Irish workhouse meals to just two per day, in contrast to the three allocated in England and Wales. In addition, they mostly excluded meat from Irish workhouse dietaries as it did not figure prominently in the diet of Irish labourers.[12]

Table 3.1 Workhouse dietary provisions in Ireland, c.1852.

Meal	*Males*	*Females*
Breakfast	8 oz. Oatmeal stirabout ½ pint new milk	6 oz. Oatmeal stirabout ½ pint new milk
Dinner	3 ½ lbs (raw weight) of potatoes 1 pint of skimmed milk	3 ½ lbs (raw weight) of potatoes 1 pint of skimmed milk

Table 3.1 outlines the recommended dietary allowances for workhouse paupers in Ireland from the 1830s onward and demonstrates that they consisted primarily of potatoes, oatmeal and milk. This was perhaps not too dissimilar from the normal diet of the pre-Famine poor. Nonetheless, the imposed two meals per day incited uncertainties – often grounded in reality – that paupers, once institutionalised, risked becoming susceptible to poor health, disease and even death while under state care. Virginia Crossman suggests that although hostility to workhouses was generally less intense in Ireland than in Britain, objections, when they did arise, were directed to specific aspects of workhouse management.[13] This argument is borne out in relation to food, a determining factor in public antagonism. Since its inception, critics had condemned the New Poor Law as unsuitable for Ireland for the reason that fewer employment opportunities existed there than in industrial Britain.[14] The Famine intensified public hostility in Ireland once the state began using workhouses to channel relief from 1847. The extent to which pauper inmates were deserving of severe food restrictions persisted as a thorny issue after the Famine; one that proved especially emotive as workhouses evolved from the 1850s into institutions that catered increasingly for individuals other than able-bodied labourers. Whether Famine victims, or the young, sick and elderly who filled post-Famine workhouses were responsible for their conditions of abject poverty was highly debatable.

Unsurprisingly, Famine-period criticism of workhouse dietaries coalesced around the sensitive topic of starvation. Identifying workhouses as sites of state-sanctioned starvation was commonplace in the early 1850s, particularly in relation to the west of Ireland.[15] In April 1852, food provision at Kilrush Union, Co. Clare, caused controversy when Reverend Sydney Goldolphin Osborne publicly rebuked the New Poor Law. Osborne was the rector of Durweston in Dorset and a prominent philanthropist whose interest in Irish social conditions had been sparked by a visit to the west of Ireland during the Famine in 1849. Importantly, he not only identified Irish workhouses as sites where managers permitted the starving of paupers but also sought to demonstrate that death could result from prolonged periods of restricted feeding should the bodily frames of paupers become gradually weakened and susceptible to disease.[16]

Osborne estimated that over 1,800 deaths had occurred in Kilrush workhouse over the previous year, noting a sharp rise after the Board of Guardians substituted milk with cocoa. He attributed disease outbreaks to this adjustment, claiming, on the subject of elderly residents, that 'they died in droves whilst being given cocoa'. Osborne also lambasted the introduction of 'artificial milk', as did the *Freeman's Journal* which alleged that 'the name is suspicious, but the thing is atrocious'. The *Journal* then lamented that 'nothing fills us with so much despair of our unfortunate peasantry as this deadly regimen which, under the name of "dietaries", and "breakfast", "dinner", and "supper" prepares him for the grave in a few months. No wonder that he should tremble at the idea of the workhouse'.[17] In accounts such as these, critics presented parsimonious workhouse policies as having overruled basic humane considerations by failing to guard against hunger, debilitation, disease and starvation.

Critics routinely alleged that Poor Law Commissioners and Boards of Guardians had referred to nutritional science to justify their meagre feeding policies. Following a medical inquiry into a number of institutional deaths in Co. Clare in 1851, the *Freeman's Journal* asserted that 'the workhouses are workshops for the rapid manufacture of pauper corpses, but Clare surpassed all others in the despatch with which it turned out the manufactured product'. The author maintained that paupers had formerly been provided with twenty-two ounces of meal per day, but that:

> The Commissioners, after some important experiments in animal chemistry, reduced the allowance to twenty ounces, ordering, in their dietetic wisdom, eight ounces for breakfast, and twelve for dinner. The person affected, one would suppose, should be the best judge of the relative value of any such experiments on his constitution. The paupers requested to have the meals equalised, and the Guardians urged the request on the commissioners, but the Liebigs of the head office were more filled with their quantitative theory of eight and twelve ounces, than the stomachs of the paupers with food, or their minds with satisfaction – and the poor request was rejected.[18]

This discussion of nutritional theory bore resonance given the existence of public scepticism to its use in official famine relief strategies. It seemed to some that a theoretical framework was in place that Poor Law Commissioners and Boards of Guardians had used to determine the bare minimum of sustenance possible for humans to subsist upon to justify minimal expenditure and rationalise starvation.

Importantly, many medical men operating in the Poor Law system did in fact persistently strive to highlight links – observed daily but not yet empirically proved – between scanty workhouse feeding and long-term physiological weakening. They sought to empirically confirm and add expert weight to lay observations such as those made by Osborne and the *Freeman's Journal*. Many of them actively partook in ongoing efforts to establish Irish workhouse dietaries as a gross assault on the bodies of the vulnerable. To achieve this, they sought to demonstrate that although workhouse dietaries theoretically kept bodies alive on a day-to-day basis, the Commissioners had resoundingly failed to consider the long-term chronic debilitation engendered by poor feeding. From the 1850s, would-be Poor Law reformers sharpened their case for the need to improve workhouse food by delineating more sophisticated links between innutritious diets and illness.

Many of these individuals expressed concern about the fate of the pauperised young. Representations of starving, poorly fed children were highly affecting.[19] By suggesting that the rising generation was being physically and morally weakened in a state-sanctioned relief system, critics positioned themselves to challenge and destabilise the ostensible improving rhetoric of the New Poor Law. For instance, in the 1840s, Dominic Corrigan investigated what he suspected to be a close correlation between inadequate workhouse dietaries and childhood scrofula. After noticing high incidence rates in Dublin's two workhouses, he recommended that Boards of Guardians increase food allocations for mothers and children. However, the Commissioners refused to humour Corrigan's suggestions, stubbornly, but characteristically, insisting that the percentage of scrofula-stricken children in workhouses corresponded with incidence rates among that group in the community. They apportioned blame to uncontrollable disease trends instead of adverse institutional arrangements.[20] Their arguments, which pointed to the natural course of disease patterns, failed to address the resonant point that once resident in a state-managed institution, some degree of preventative health care (via diet) was desirable, if not essential. Shortly afterwards, Arthur Jacob, prominent physician and co-founder of the *Dublin Medical Press*, made a strong case for the debilitating consequences of workhouse feeding by outlining specific connections between the onset of workhouse ophthalmia and poor nutrition.[21]

Childhood vulnerability permeated post-Famine criticism of the workhouse because the young could not easily be defined as idle or work-shy or, by extension, deserving targets of harsh regimes of bodily governance. Furthermore, and importantly, children could scarcely be perceived as to blame for their pauperised condition. Many young residents were famine orphans. Circumstance, not moral deficiency, had led to their institutionalisation.[22] Finally, children seemed pivotal to Ireland's post-Famine development, and needed to be strong and healthy if they were to contribute to future national life. Why then, critics posited, should children be given deterrent diets that, at worst, caused disfiguring illnesses and severe constitutional weakening? These issues called the efficacy of the socially improving rhetoric of workhouses further into question, articulating the tensions in play between the simultaneous functions of institutions as being to discipline and to preserve health.

Efforts to raise awareness of the unfavourable living conditions of the pauperised young were common in the 1850s but climaxed in 1859 in a nationally discussed scandal about Cork's workhouses. The debates that ensued reveal how critics framed the structure of workhouse life as producing only physical decline and deterioration instead of fostering personal and social improvement.[23] After observing remarkably high scrofula incidences among pauperised workhouse children, prominent entrepreneur and Lord Mayor of Cork John Arnott sparked a heated public dispute about conditions in the city's workhouses – sites where, in his view, insufficient feeding was causing high scrofula levels. Arnott insisted that scrofula resulted from a lack of proper nutriment. Scanty feeding wasted the blood, reduced vigour and health and rendered the young susceptible to disease, so Arnott insisted. These personal observations confirmed Arnott's opinion that vulnerable groups needed to be made exempt from the trial of the workhouse test. In relation to children, he emotively asserted that 'it would be a mercy to close the gates of the Union house against them, and let them attain the mercy of death, rather than be reared deformed, maimed and diseased objects, through the system of feeding them'.[24] The Poor Law Commissioners publicly refuted insinuations that their workhouse dietary regimes had been in any way responsible for institutional scrofula outbreaks, characteristically retorting that workhouse mortality rates broadly corresponded with the equivalent among that age group in the general community.[25]

Medical inspection of the food offered in Cork's workhouses cast substantial suspicion on these claims. Although these ultimately failed to decisively connect workhouse feeding to scrofula, they did expose suspiciously unsavoury discoveries about culinary practices. Local physician Albert Callanan described the workhouse soup that he saw in Cork's workhouses as virtually water, containing few solid ingredients such as rice, oatmeal and vegetables. He also noted that child residents left their porridge allocations uneaten while their bread supplies smelled sour and had a heavy, gluey texture as workhouse cooks had prepared them with coarse flour. Children also complained to him about regularly discovering insects floating in their soup.[26] Callanan's observations added weight to Arnott's estimation that Cork's workhouses had an average annual mortality rate among the young of 18 per cent due to subsistance on poor quality diets, a figure verified by prominent figures such as Robert Kane but which the Poor Law Commissioners quickly dismissed as an exaggerated rendering of a figure in reality closer to 6 per cent.[27]

Nonetheless, it proved empirically challenging to decisively link diet and scrofula. Although many physicians suspected that poor feeding somehow encouraged its onset, they struggled to decipher concrete connections. Instead, Arnott relied heavily upon circumstantial evidence offered by Cork-based physicians and institutional managers who shared and corroborated his views.[28] For instance, Reverend T. Lytons, chaplain of Spike Island Government Prison, recalled in his evidence that when he had provided beef, soup and vegetables to prisoners during a recent period of scrofula outbreaks, prisoner health improved and mortality rates lowered. Lytons used this evidence as part of an impassioned plea for improvement in the feeding of the pauperised young and for institutional managers to consistently offer solid food. 'The only moving thing with which the poor children in the Cork Union were acquainted', exclaimed Lytons, 'were the carogues which the children told Dr Callanan they got in their soup.'[29]

Although Arnott used the authority of medical evidence to effect, the Commissioners also made use of contrary expert evidence in the hope of being absolved of blame. Unsurprisingly, their expert witnesses, Dr Townsend and Dr

Harvey, came into Arnott's firing line after they explained that Cork Union food provisions fully satisfied the nutritional requirements recently outlined by Liebig. In response, Arnott vociferously announced:

> We give their chemical analysis for what it is worth, merely observing, that clover-hay, pea-straw and bran, possess each more carbon and nitrogen than wheaten flour; but we should never think of sending our children, or even our servants, to graze in a clover field, or of manufacturing bread from clover or pea straw. We are credibly informed that Doctor Franklin made a sawdust pudding; but very few would feel disposed to follow the Doctor into these departments of chemistry, or cookery. Some person who wrote to the *Constitution* showed, on Liebig's principles, that peas, beans and barley-meal, contain more solid matter than beef, mutton, veal or lamb. On the same principle I suspect that a paving stone contains more solid matter than wheaten bread.[30]

Arnott reprimanded the Union's dietaries for being based upon foundations of economy and cheapness and for having distorted and made inappropriate use of the findings of analytical chemistry 'to show that the cheapest food is the most nutritious'. Here, scientific knowledge was once again displayed as a tool being used to rationalise what Arnott saw as an unnecessary and unwarranted assault on Irish bodies. Instead of being purely objective, Arnott portrayed nutritional science as a more sinister mechanism of bodily governance that, when used by the wrong hands, proved physiologically hazardous.[31] Continuing his tirade, Arnott announced that:

> I have seen the water prettily analysed, to prove the existence of lime; I have listened to learned disquisitions on the constituent and nutritious properties of food in general, and workhouse food in particular, but have never seen the porridge, soup (a misnomer), skimmed milk, brown, bran, or Indian meal bread, carrion meat at 3 d., or arrow-root at 2 ½ per lb., put to the same interesting tests. The tests on these points are the tables of mortality and the fearful prevalence of a loathsome disease.[32]

Arnott concluded by associating workhouse dietary regimes with penality or, in his own words, 'capital punishment of death by starvation'.[33] Similarly, the *Freeman's Journal* referred to the scandal to affirm its long-standing argument that the New Poor Law was in reality a pervasive means of oppressing and degrading the destitute. Irish poverty, it asserted, was being wrongly treated as a crime deserving of punishment.[34] Adding to the debate, *The Nation* argued in relation to the scandal that managers were depriving able-bodied men and women, as well as children, of the spirit that might enable them to emancipate themselves from the workhouse. *The Nation* asserted that workhouse dietaries weakened bodies to such an extent that the pauperised young permanently lost the strength needed to labour.[35]

Despite the Commissioners' refusal to assume responsibility for Cork workhouse conditions, they did implement changes in the following year. The Commissioners justified their new position by suggesting that older workhouse dietary arrangements were now out-dated given the profound shifts that had occurred in communal dietary behaviour since the Famine. As the physical condition of able-bodied labourers had seemingly improved, the standard of workhouse diets now needed to be raised.[36] Yet this action was also undoubtedly a response to widespread public criticism and a heightened sensitivity to the welfare of the rising post-Famine generation in institutional contexts. Workhouse diets did not necessarily become universally appealing or nutritionally richer from the 1860s, but managers made some improvements as the public now expected them to demonstrate sensitivity to nutritional health issues. This adjustment can be interpreted as an important outcome of broader debates about how best to govern institutionalised bodies, negotiate health and produce individuals, through bodily regulation, who might leave the institution reformed and socially productive. It also served as a reminder of public feeling about the young and concern over the potentially detrimental impact of institutional life on Irish socio-economic development. Although Boards of Guardians and institutional managers intended workhouses to act as deterrent sites, one of their other key functions was to advance society by maximising labouring potential by combating idleness. Food-related concerns often surfaced when the public saw this improving potential as being threatened by overly harsh and inappropriate dietary regimes. This allowed Poor Law critics to brand state policy and the workhouse system as responsible for wearing down the health of Ireland's rising generation rather than ensuring its vitality. In that way, critics brought the validity of state-sponsored improving strategies into question. Nonetheless, despite the ongoing existence of dissatisfaction with the Irish Poor Law system in the 1860s and 1870s, particularly among Catholic communities who fought with the Irish landed elite to reform the system, it was only in the 1880s that truly significant improvements began to be made.[37]

Prison feeding controversies

The post-Famine prison was a further site enveloped by public concern over the long-term effects of innutritious feeding. Diet played a formative role in prisoner experiences. Unappealing meals were integral to institutional programmes of adjusting, correcting and rectifying deviant moral behaviour. Between 1835 and 1845, state bodies rebuilt or improved county prisons across the British Isles.[38] Correspondingly, changes were made to the experience of prison life that made confinement lonelier and less bearable – a step taken to ensure improved prisoner management. Prison meals now consisted of monotonous combinations of bread and water, forming part of a wider plethora of recently introduced psychological punishments that included the silent system and the treadmill.[39] Michael Ignatieff describes these measures as 'micro-punishments' that mostly replaced increasingly unacceptable punitive techniques such as whipping and chaining.[40]

The Famine saw further prison dietary reductions, intensifying the sense of discipline and punishment endured by prisoners. Until 1849, the officially recommended prison dietary in Ireland consisted of a breakfast of eight ounces of meal made into stirabout and served with a pint of milk, followed by a pound of bread and a pint of new milk for dinner.[41] The Famine encouraged a sudden rethinking of this arrangement once the Inspectors-General of Prisons in Ireland, Frederic B. Long and James Galway, became convinced that the impoverished were purposefully committing crimes to become imprisoned and secure prison food.[42] In response, Long and Galway sanctioned a lower dietary scale in 1849.[43] As Table 3.2 demonstrates, this marked a notable drop in quantity.

Table 3.2 Recommended Irish prison dietaries in 1850.

	Class 1: males	*Class 2: females*	*Class 3 under 10*
Breakfast	8 oz. meal in stirabout ½ pint of new-milk	7 oz. meal in stirabout ½ pint of new milk	5 oz. meal in stirabout ½ pint of new milk
Dinner	14 oz. bread 1 pint of new milk	12 oz. bread ¾ pint of new milk	½ pint of new milk
Supper	———	———	4 oz. bread 1 ½ naggin of new milk

This striking reduction heightened public concern about prisoner well-being. Public unease deepened in the 1850s as long-term imprisonment instead of transportation became gradually more central to Irish penal codes. Australia no longer needed convict labour.[44] In response, the creation of the Irish Convict System in 1853 established a national system of corrective incarceration.[45] As magistrates began to prescribe lengthier prison sentences for individuals who would once have been transported, fears mounted about the potential implications of under-feeding prisoners for a number of months, if not years. Just a year after they reduced prison diets, the Inspectors-General conceded that convicts tended to 'flag in spirits' and become predisposed to disease due to subsisting on a low diet. However, they partly ascribed this problem to the weakening effect of famine conditions that had caused individuals to arrive at prisons already 'physically debased, and unable to bear up against any severe disease if attacked'.[46]

Problematically, as longer sentences became more common, it seemed increasingly plausible that prisoner health could only be sustained through healthy feeding.[47] This stance was ideologically challenging. It demanded that those most in need of punishment should be given superior quantities and qualities of food than offered to workhouse paupers and which, in many instances, was superior to the food typically consumed by the non-institutionalised poor. Importantly, those in favour of improving prison dietaries bolstered their arguments by stressing the long-term social value that might ensue. These individuals were not, on the surface, openly invested in prisoner welfare. Nonetheless, they chose to question the social value and moral logic of returning physically incapacitated prisoners to Irish society. In doing so, they successfully reinforced the notion that prisons were meant to be sites in which institutional managers reformed personal character rather than engage in its degradation and demoralisation.

This perspective was evident in barrister Edward Gibson's defence of the penal system penned in 1863. Responding to public criticism of prison meat provision, Gibson observed that 'the humble fare of our agricultural population is also, with some bitterness, contrasted with the dietary of our criminals; it is objected that the latter are well fed, healthy and wicked, while the former are poor, hungry and upright'.[48] Yet Gibson warned that reducing food provision below the bodily limits of health was uneconomical as prisoners would only end up hospitalised and consequently further dependent on public expenditure. He emotively warned that 'it should also be remembered, that if the system of starving crime into surrender is adopted, criminals on their discharge may become a burden on the rates, having with the spirit to rob been deprived of the strength to work'.[49] In his *Life among Convicts*, published in 1863, Charles Bernard Gibson, chaplain in the convict system, also raised vociferous objections to Irish prison feeding arrangements. Gibson was particularly concerned with the permanent undermining of the constitutions of prisoners. Like Edward Gibson, he warned that restricted feeding produced only degraded and demoralised individuals who were destined to continue being social burdens needing care in workhouses and hospitals. 'To make prison dietary penal', he argued, 'is a great mistake, and bad economy.'[50]

Theoretically, food restriction was an obvious, perhaps effective, punitive technique. Yet to some, the sustained weakening of prisoner bodies extended beyond acceptable moral and humane boundaries. Nonetheless, individuals such as Gibson voiced their concerns in an increasingly unsympathetic era. In the 1860s, prison managers took steps to considerably lower prison diets in Britain to the minimum quantity and quality of food which medical scientists believed it was possible for humans to subsist upon without starving to death.[51] In 1863, British prison medical superintendent and semi-government advisor William Guy suggested that individual dietary classification based upon the needs of different age groups was impractical as prison medical officers were unpaid and therefore unwilling to devote their time to personalising dietary regimes.[52] In sharp contrast to advocates of fuller prison feeding, Guy asserted that 'as they [the prisoners] are maintained at the cost of the community which they have injured and impoverished, it [diet] ought to be as economical as possible'.[53] He added that prison mangers had provided too much food in light of their exaggerated estimate of the depressing physical and mental effect of imprisonment.[54] Five years later, British chemist and Public Health Officer Henry Letheby concurred that the most suitable prison diet was one consisting of the minimum amount of food required by the body to avoid illness which, in his view, consisted of two pounds of dry, solid material and five and a half pints of water per day.[55] Controversially, the setting of this new minimum standard of food intake ominously demonstrated that prison dietaries in Ireland – reduced considerably during the Famine – were in fact lower than those recommended by Letheby. As Table 3.2 demonstrates, the Inspectors-General of Prisons recommended only twenty ounces (or 1.25 pounds) of solid food and one and a half pints of liquid for male adult prisoners in Ireland.

Leading medical figures entered into these debates by producing empirical evidence on the physically debilitating nature of Irish prison life. In 1867, John Blake, MP for Waterford, announced to the House of Commons that recent changes in Irish prison discipline had a 'wearing effect' upon prisoner bodies. Long-term prisoners, he insisted, needed fuller, more nutritious food allocations.[56] Inspired by Blake's remarks, English surgeon and naturalist Edwin Lankester entered into the dispute. In the pages of the *British Medical Journal*, Lankester argued that the daily cost of food supplied in Irish prisons was an average of just two-and-a-half pence per day. As an alternative, he advocated a system based on food quality, not quantity. Rebuking administrators who had devised dietary regimes based on cost and weight, Lankester asserted that prison managers needed to redesign their dietaries in light of the advances made in knowledge of nutrition. Citing the nitrogenous contents of vegetables and meats, the digestibility of various substances, the manner by which the stomach disposes of vegetables, the role of heat in the body, the physiological function of salt, and so on, he called for a restructuring of the principles underlying prison feeding, advocating the importance of health above discipline. Dismissing published dietary tables on the basis that descriptions of gruels, Irish stews and stirabouts gave little indication of what was in reality being served, he personally visited gaols in Co. Fermanagh and Co. Cork. In the former, Lankester observed a deficiency in flesh-forming constituents including meat, a foodstuff thought to encourage healthily digestion. He continued by castigating the Cork County Prison dietary for being 'an eminently starvation dietary' that rendered prisoners vulnerable to physical and mental illness. Lankester concluded that 'it is forgotten that an underfed body is often the worst possible machine to operate upon morally and that one of the first conditions of a sound mind is a sound body'.[57]

Following an official investigation in 1868, the Inspectors adjusted Irish prison diets. In their responses to the questionnaires distributed as part of this enquiry, thirty-two out of thirty-nine prison governors and thirty-seven out of thirty-nine prison surgeons, agreed that food provision for those serving sentences of hard labour was insufficient, impeding any prospects of prisoners securing employment upon release.[58] Thirty-six governors recommended an additional supper meal.[59] The report that followed supported the allocation of meat and vegetable soups, and also tea. Its authors stressed the importance of ensuring quality and recommended the adoption of milk-testing techniques and the purchasing of lactometers. They disallowed the substitution of gruel for milk on the basis that science had confirmed the latter to be more nutritious. Finally, they recommended replacing small portions of meal with bulkier supplies as prisoner tended not to enjoy eating meal, causing a 'falling away in the condition of the prison inmates, coupled with an ineptitude to labour'.[60]

Prison diets remained undeniably unappealing even after the Inspectors implemented these changes. However, fears of starvation and nutritional decline became less pronounced after the late 1860s. In her study of late nineteenth-century prison diets, Ciara Breathnach even contends that after around 1870 prisoners in Ireland in fact tended to gain weight while imprisoned.[61]

Evidently, food provision was seen as crucial to the physical and moral reform of imprisoned criminals. As a practice, it needed complex negotiation if it was to serve its dual purposes of ensuring health and improving the imprisoned self. Furthermore, the increasingly pervasive scientific language of nutrition – coupled with mounting fears that a persistent exposure to an innutritious diet produced long-term physical harm – added new dimensions to ideas on how this improvement could be realised. Between around 1850 and 1870, resistance to prison practices arose most distinctly when dietary regimes were seen as failing to serve socially ameliorative purposes. Prison feeding evolved into a controversial topic precisely because ostensibly trivial matters such as what to feed prisoners were publicly seen as intimately connected to social well-being and the future moral development of Irish society.

Juvenile criminality and the Irish body

Concern about the welfare of the imprisoned young escalated in the 1850s. Mirroring debates on workhouse children, critics of the Irish prison system began to cast doubt on the suitability of imprisonment for juvenile criminals. Reformers began to assert that child criminals needed to be segregated from imprisoned adults.[62] This perspective gained currency in a decade marked by deep concern over orphaned and destitute children, many of whom, surviving without the positive moral influence of parental guidance due to having lost family members in the Famine, were feared to have fallen into the company of adult prison offenders from whom they learnt criminal ways.[63] In 1851, the Inspectors-General of the General State of Prisons in Ireland warned of the 'great social peril' likely to arise from the 'corruption of the rising generation' and made a case for age-specific institutionalisation to ensure that the younger generation never became 'a moral pest and a burden on the public purse'.[64]

Many prison reformers saw the rearing of children in criminal settings as a catastrophic impediment to physical, mental and moral growth.[65] In the 1840s, British social reformer Henry Mayhew had influentially portrayed physical, mental and moral degradation as a product of hardship and outlined a social sub-stratum whom he termed 'the dangerous classes' – a brutish tribe-like group prone to engage in crime.[66] Mayhew portrayed juvenile criminals as physically and mentally distinguishable from the more respectable classes.[67] They were physically degenerate, he insisted; often suffering from physical ailments such as scrofula while their psychological malfunctions were symptomatic of their lack of moral control.[68] Accordingly, the institutional techniques devised to tackle this problem emphasised reforming the bodies and minds of the young, the aim being to arrest further descent into permanent physical, mental and moral degradation.

In the 1850s, juvenile delinquency was often understood in an organic framework; as a quasi-disease entity whose aetiological origins lay in the moral contagion created by childhood association with adult criminals. In this model, crime was a problem whose seeds were planted in early life leaving permanent physical, psychological and moral imprints. Accordingly, the Inspectors-General proposed the construction of separate institutions for the young.[69] This system was intended to emphasise the regulation of physical and psychological health to restore nurturing influences. The work of English educationalist and social reformer Mary Carpenter offered a suitable guide.[70] For Carpenter, to be in a 'perishing' or 'dangerous' condition meant to suffer from a 'grievous moral disease' needing treatment in what she termed a 'moral hospital'.[71] Carpenter depicted children as physically and mentally immature; as a group whose muscles, bones and brain were in an incomplete state of growth. In contrast, however, Carpenter asserted that the muscular and mental powers of the 'perishing' child had prematurely developed as juvenile delinquents had adopted an overly active and independent role unsuited to their age.[72] By pathologising juvenile criminality in this manner, Carpenter promoted a model of institutional reform that was particularly attentive to the physical and psychological needs of the young.[73]

The Irish reformatory and industrial school system fused notions of individual, personal reform with broader improving strategies. In 1858, Dublin barrister Patrick Joseph Murray argued that 'by the reformation of the young offender, the country will be relieved from the cost of repeated convictions, from the expense of his prison support; from the evil of his corrupting example, and from the loss which his habits of plundering inflict on the community'.[74] When social reformer and philanthropist James Haughton spoke to the Statistical Society of Dublin on the matter in 1857, he argued that better education of the young would stem the early planting of the seeds of criminality and also socially and morally elevate the Irish population.[75]

The state established reformatory schools in Ireland in 1858 and industrial schools in 1868.[76] Reformatories housed convicted children aged under sixteen while industrial schools specifically catered for neglected, orphaned or abandoned children viewed as having high potential to turn to crime.[77] The underlying organic framework that underpinned contemporary thought on juvenile crime meant that diet proved central to the management of these institutions. Prominent Dublin-born physician John Lentaigne was appointed as inspector of Irish reformatories in 1868 and later as inspector of industrial schools. Lentaigne's medical background ensured that the institutions under his inspection came to serve quasi-medical purposes. Lentaigne reflected this imperative in his recommended dietary regimes designed to tackle some of the diet-related diseases prevalent among the pauperised and imprisoned young. He considered scrofula, ophthalmia, consumption and epilepsy to result from imperfect nurturing in early life.[78] In his view, if the young were underfed then their tendencies to pursue immoral lifestyles increased. On one occasion, he asserted that 'the experience of my life satisfies me that scrofula and crime are intimately connected'.[79] Accordingly, Lentaigne recommended fuller dietary provisions in reformatories and industrial schools than offered in workhouses and prisons. For Lentaigne, good feeding would arrest the development of crippling chronic illness, restore normative processes of childhood growth and fulfil the important goal of achieving bodily, psychological and moral salvation. In the 1870s, Lentaigne openly drew from the research of German internist physician Felix von Niemeyer who had recently pioneered a high protein, low carbohydrate diet. Niemeyer had argued that coarse diets containing little nutriment increased childhood susceptibility to scrofula as the tender organs of infants failed to assimilate appropriate levels of nutriment. Niemeyer argued that this caused impoverished and vitiated circulation meaning that children were reared with impaired nervous powers, devoid of energy or vigour and deficient in self-control and self-reliance.[80] He overtly linked scrofula to the personality traits then often associated with crime.[81]

These organic perspectives on criminality justified the provision of healthy, varied and generous food supplies in Irish reformatories and industrial schools. In his annual reports, Lentaigne routinely lambasted managers who fed their residents with insufficient amounts of bread, milk, stirabout and Indian meal.[82] In the face of public criticism, he insisted that, unlike workhouses, industrial schools were not intended to rescue people from starvation but instead to act in *loco parentis* to children by preparing them for a healthy future existence. Lentaigne openly referred to the latest medical thought on food to add weight to this claim. When high incidence rates of ophthalmia struck various industrial schools and reformatories, Lentaigne drew the attention of managers to research undertaken by prominent British physician and ophthalmic surgeon Robert Brudenall Carter who, in his influential *Diseases of the Eye* penned in 1876, argued that ophthalmic conditions among 'street Arabs' and orphans directly resulted from insufficient feeding. Lentaigne referred to this as further proof of the value of generous feeding.[83] Some industrial schools even evolved into sites where childhood blindness could be managed. In the 1870s, Lentaigne supported the dispatchment of blind workhouse girls to Merrion Industrial School for Roman Catholic Girls, Co. Dublin where visually able girls were trained to nurse and administer to the needs of the blind.[84]

Reformatories, and particularly industrial schools, clearly offered alternative forms of bodily regulation and their dietary regimes contrasted sharply with those of prisons and workhouses. There, diet formed a more explicit part of a broader programme of bodily reform and regeneration that simultaneously sought to tackle the social problem of juvenile criminality and to prepare problematic youths for a morally secure future. As such, they served as sites where day-to-day matters of eating carried meanings that extended beyond the purely physical. Healthy childhood feeding, at least according to Lentaigne, was an essential precursor of socio-national improvement. It would protect the rising generation from harmful social forces with potentially enduring implications for the future of Ireland. In that sense, reformatories and industrial schools in many ways epitomised contemporary views on how Irish institutions could be used in a way that fulfilled the rhetoric of development that underpinned their existence. Notably, the management of reformatories and industrial schools prompted relatively little public antagonism, more divorced as it was from accusations of harsh bodily discipline, starvation and physical weakening.

Conclusion

This chapter demonstrates the myriad uses of food in the post-Famine institution and the ways in which seemingly trivial matters of feeding came to be connected to far broader social concerns: specifically crime and poverty. In an era of mounting concern about national decline, institutional life offered a context where strict bodily regimes could be instigated, and dietary restrictions used, to modify and regulate physical and moral behaviour. This process was not always straightforward. The ethos of prisons, workhouses, reformatories and industrial schools ostensibly focused on restoring improved individuals to society. Between the Famine and around 1870, dietary regulation was crucial to institutional strategies and the critiques formed of them because the public understood food as deeply connected to bodily strength, moral well-being and psychological health. Good eating encouraged a healthy moral existence. In contrast, innutritious eating fostered disease, demoralisation and physical degeneration. In fact, as the examples of workhouses and prisons suggest, in relation to food institutional management came under fire precisely when it was seen as not fully engaging with a broader national project of producing healthy, reformed citizens. However, as the next chapter demonstrates, the concerns over the feeding of the institutionalised that prevailed between 1850 and 1870 were soon complemented by a more far-reaching alarm over the extent of under-nourishment and inappropriate feeding in the community across Ireland following the Famine.

Notes

1 For a classic critical interpretation of this trend, see M. Foucault, *Madness and Civilisation* (London: Tavistock, 1967). In response, Porter identified the nineteenth century as the period of a 'great confinement' in R. Porter, *Madmen: A Social History of Madhouses, Mad-Doctors and Lunatics* (Stroud: Tempus, 1987), pp. 12–28.

2 O. Macdonagh, 'Ideas and institutions 1830–45', in Vaughan (ed.), A *New History of Ireland V*, p. 195.

3 Ibid., p. 206.

4 M. Finnane, *Insanity and the Insane in Post-Famine Ireland* (London: Croom Helm, 1981), pp. 14–18.

5 P. Gray, 'Irish social thought and the relief of poverty, 1847–1880', *Transactions of the Royal Historical Society*, 20 (December 2010), 141–56 on p. 142.

6 Ibid., pp. 146–7.

7 M. J. D. Roberts, *Making English Morals: Voluntary Associations and Moral Reform in England*

1787–1886 (Cambridge: Cambridge University Press, 2004).

8 A. Clark, 'Wild workhouse girls and the liberal imperial state in mid-nineteenth century Ireland', *Journal of Social History*, 39:2 (Winter 2005), 389–409 on p. 389.

9 See E. M. Crawford, 'The Irish workhouse diet 1840–90', in C. Geissler and D. Oddy (eds), *Food, Diet and Economic Change Past and Present* (Leicester and New York: Leicester University Press, 1993).

10 For the development of the Irish workhouse system, see P. Gray, *The Making of the Irish Poor Law 1815–43* (Manchester: Manchester University Press, 2009); H. Burke, *The People and the Poor Law in Nineteenth Century Ireland* (Dublin: Women's Education Bureau, 1987).

11 G. C. Lewis, *Remarks on the Third Report of the Irish Poor Inquiry Commissioners* (London: W. Clowes, 1837), p. 9.

12 *Appendix to Sixth Annual Report of the Poor Law Commissioners*, H. C. 1840 [253] xvii.447, pp. 238–41; *Appendices B to F to the Eighth Annual Report of the Poor Law Commissioners*, H. C. 1842 [399] xix.119, p. 152; J. O'Connor, *The Workhouses of Ireland: the Fate of Ireland's Poor* (Dublin: Anvil Books, 1995), pp. 98–101, pp. 238–41.

13 Crossman, *Poor Law in Ireland*, p. 14.

14 Clark, 'Wild workhouse girls', p. 389.

15 'Life and Death in Irish Poorhouses', *Freeman's Journal* (6 March 1851), p. 3.

16 S. G. Osborne, *Gleanings in the West of Ireland* (London: T. and W. Boone, 1850), pp. 147–55.

17 'The Dietary of the Kilrush Union', *Freeman's Journal* (29 April 1851), p. 1.

18 'The Workhouse Slaughter: Medical Inquiry in Clare', *Freeman's Journal* (10 July 1851), p. 2.

19 V. Crossman, 'Cribbed, contained, and confined? The care of children under the Irish Poor Law, 1850–1920', *Éire-Ireland*, 1 & 2 (Spring/Summer 2009), 37–61.

20 B. Philips, *Scrofula: Its Nature, its Causes, its Prevalence and the Principles of Treatment* (Philadelphia: Lea and Blanchard, 1846), pp. 158–62.

21 *Fourth Annual Report of the Commissioners for Administering the Laws for Relief of the Poor in Ireland*, H. C. 1851 [1381] xxvi.547, p. 183; P. Gorey, 'Childhood ophthalmia in Irish workhouses, 1849–1861', in A. Mac Lellan and A. Mauger (eds), *Growing Pains: Childhood Illness in Ireland, 1750–1950* (Dublin: Irish Academic Press, 2013).

22 D. McLoughlin, 'Pauper children in Ireland, 1840–70', in B. Ó Conaire (ed.), *The Famine Lectures – Léachtai an Ghorta* (Boyle: Roscommon Herald, 1997).

23 Crossman, 'Cribbled, contained and confined?', p. 43; C. O Mahony, *Cork's Poor Law Palace: Workhouse Life 1838–1980* (Cork: Rosmathún Press, 2005), pp. 184–90.

24 J. Arnott, *The Investigation into the Condition of the Children in the Cork Workhouse* (Cork: Guy Brothers, 1859), pp. 6–7.

25 Ibid., pp. 9–10.

26 Ibid., pp. 18–19.

27 Ibid., p. ii.

28 Ibid., p. 22.

29 Ibid., pp. 28–30.

30 Ibid., p. 34.

31 Ibid.

32 Ibid., p. 37.

33 Ibid., p. 38.

34 'Cork Poorhouse Investigation', *Freeman's Journal* (18 May 1859), p. 5.

35 'The Workhouse System', *Nation* (21 May 1859), p. 9.

36 M. Doyle, *The Agricultural Labourer viewed in his Moral, Intellectual and Physical Conditions*

(London: Groombridge and Sons, 1855), p. 31.
37 See V. Crossman, 'Facts notorious to the whole country: the political battle over Irish poor law reform in the 1860s', *Transactions of the Royal Historical Society*, 20 (December 2010), 157–69.
38 P. Carroll-Burke, *Colonial Discipline: The Making of the Irish Convict System* (Dublin: Four Courts Press, 2000), p. 211.
39 M. Ignatieff, *A Just Measure of Pain: The Penitentiary in the Industrial Revolution 1750–1850* (London: Macmillan Press, 1978), pp. 175–9.
40 Ibid., p. 198.
41 *Twenty-Eighth Report of the Inspectors-General on the General State of Prisons in Ireland*, H. C. 1850 [1229] xxix, p. 22.
42 Ibid., p. viii.
43 Ibid., p. ix.
44 Carroll-Burke, *Colonial Discipline*, pp. 31–3.
45 Ibid., p. 19.
46 *Twenty-Eighth Report of Inspectors-General*, p. 77.
47 H. Phibbs, *A System of Penal Discipline* (London: Longman, Brown, Green and Longmans, 1850), p. 15.
48 E. Gibson, 'Penal servitude and tickets of leave', *Journal of the Statistical and Social Inquiry Society of Ireland*, 3 (April 1863), 332–43 on p. 334.
49 Ibid., p. 335.
50 C. B. Gibson, *Life Among Convicts* (London: Hurst and Blackett, 1863), p. 55.
51 M. J. Weiner, 'The health of prisoners and the two faces of Benthanism', in R. Creese, W. F. Bynum and J. Bearn (eds), *The Health of Prisoners: Historical Essays* (Amsterdam: Rodopi, 1995) pp. 52–5; A. Hardy, 'Development of the prison medical service', in Creese, Bynum and Bearn (eds), *The Health of Prisoners*, pp. 64–8.
52 *Forty-Fourth Report of the Inspectors-General on the General State of the Prisons of Ireland, 1865*, H. C. 1866 [3690] xxxiv.235, pp. lx.
53 W. A. Guy, 'On sufficient and insufficient dietaries, with especial reference to the dietaries of prisoners', *Journal of the Statistical Society of London*, 26 (September 1863), 239–81 on pp. 239–41.
54 Ibid., pp. 279–80.
55 'Dr. Letheby's third lecture on food', *Medical Press and Circular*, 5 (25 March 1868), 257–60 on pp. 257–9. See also K. J. Carpenter, 'Nutritional studies in Victorian prisons', *Journal of Nutrition*, 136:1 (January 2006), 1–8.
56 'Ireland: dietary in county prisons, resolution', *House of Commons Debates*, 26 July 1867, 189, cc. 173–80.
57 E. Lankester, 'On prison and workhouse dietaries', *British Medical Journal*, ii:357 (2 November 1867), 380–2.
58 *Report of the Committee appointed by His Excellency the Lord Lieutenant to inquire into the Dietaries of County and Borough Gaols in Ireland (1867–8)*, H. C. 1868 [3981] xxxv.665, p. 15.
59 Ibid., p. 17.
60 *Prison Dietaries (Ireland)*, H. C. 1867–8 [131] lvii.533.
61 C. Breathnach, 'Malnutrition, malingering and weight gain in Irish prisons, 1885–1900'. Workshop presentation delivered at Deviance in Modern Irish History Conference, University of Limerick, 31 March 2012.
62 For fuller analysis, see I. Miller, 'Constructing moral hospitals: childhood health in Irish reformatories and industrial schools, c.1851–90', in Mac Lellan and Mauger (eds), *Growing Pains*.

63 *Twenty-Ninth Report of the Inspectors-General on the General State of the Prisons in Ireland*, H. C. 1851 [1364] xxviii.357, p. xix.
64 Ibid., p. xx.
65 M. May, 'Innocence and experience: the evolution of the concept of juvenile delinquency in the mid-nineteenth century', *Victorian Studies*, 17:1 (September 1973), 7–29 on pp. 21–2.
66 G. Himmelfarb, *The Idea of Poverty: England in the Early Industrial Age* (London and Boston: Faber and Faber, 1984), pp. 326–7, p. 367, p. 395; D. Taylor, 'Beyond the bounds of respectable society: the "dangerous classes" in Victorian and Edwardian England', in J. Rowbotham and K. Stevenson (eds), *Criminal Conversations: Victorian Crimes, Social Panic and Moral Outrage* (Ohio: Ohio State University, 2005).
67 M. Weiner, *Reconstructing the Criminal: Culture, Law and Policy in England, 1830–1914* (Cambridge: Cambridge University Press, 1990), pp. 33–5.
68 Ibid., pp. 26–36; D. Pick, *Faces of Degeneration: A European Disorder* (Cambridge: Cambridge University Press, 1989) pp. 176–203.
69 *Thirty-fifth Report of the Inspectors-General on the General State of the Prisons in Ireland*, H. C. 1857 [2236] xxii.173, p. xxxviii.
70 e.g. *Second Report of the Inspector Appointed to Visit the Reformatory Schools of Ireland*, H. C. 1863 [3194] xxiv.623, pp. 14–18.
71 M. Carpenter, *Juvenile Delinquents: Their Condition and Treatment* (London: W. And F. G. Cash, 1853), p. 15.
72 Ibid., pp. 293–4.
73 Ibid., p. 163.
74 P. J. Murray, *Reformatories in Ireland, and for Dublin in Particular* (Dublin: W. B. Kelly, 1858), p. 1, p. xlvi.
75 J. Haughton, 'The social and moral elevation of our people', *Journal of the Dublin Statistical Society*, 3 (July 1857), 63–72 on p. 65.
76 Reformatory Schools (Ireland) Act, 1858 (21 & 22 Vict.), C.A.P. ciii; Industrial Schools Act (Ireland), 1868 (31 & 32 Vict.) C.A.P. xxv.
77 *Commission to Inquire into Child Abuse Volume 1* (Dublin: Stationery Office, 2009), p. 36.
78 *Fourteenth Report of the Inspector appointed to visit the Reformatory and Industrial Schools of Ireland*, H. C. 1876 [C.1494] xxxiv.777, p. 22.
79 *Tenth Report of the Inspector appointed to visit the Reformatory and Industrial Schools of Ireland*, H. C. 1872 [C.671] xxx.661, p. 71.
80 *Fourteenth Report of the Inspector*, p. 22; F. von Niemeyer, trans. G. H. Humphreys and C. E. Hackley, *A Text-book of Practical Medicine, with Particular Reference to Physiology and Pathological Anatomy* (New York: D. Appleton and Co., 1869), p. 745.
81 *Tenth Report of the Inspector*, p. 45.
82 *Eleventh Report of the Inspector appointed to visit the Reformatory and Industrial Schools of Ireland*, H. C. 1873 [C.858] xxxi.739, p. 20.
83 R. B. Carter, *A Practical Treatise on Diseases of the Eye* (London: Macmillan and Co., 1875), p. 216; *Fourteenth Report of the Inspector*, p. 108.
84 *Eighteenth Report of the Inspector appointed to visit the Reformatory and Industrial Schools of Ireland*, H. C. 1880 [C.2692] xxxvii.373, p. 70.

4

The decaying post-Famine body: tea, bread and nutritional decline

Did Irish diet improve following the Famine? This culturally charged question troubled many late nineteenth-century contemporaries who referred back to the pre-Famine era as one when the Irish populace had enjoyed fuller nutritional health. In contrast, for critical observers, the poor had since existed in an unremitting condition of physical and psychological decay that seemed to be perpetually worsening. National dietary habits significantly realigned following the Famine. In their *Feast and Famine*, Clarkson and Crawford trace the gradually declining dominance of the potato, a crop superseded by Indian meal and oatmeal, bread, dairy produce, tea, meat, fish and eggs. Contemporaneously, from the 1860s the numbers of people employed in food retailing grew rapidly, as did the number of grocers per head.[1] Expanding railway and road networks encouraged commercial activity to spread, widening access to new foodstuffs even in remote regions.[2] However, the commercialised economic system that evolved differed profoundly from that predicted in the sanguine hopes of political economists and scientists who had idyllically envisioned a self-sufficient post-Famine population producing and consuming vegetables, meat and crops to attain the high levels of nutrition once obtained from the potato.

This chapter identifies ongoing concern about food consumption and posits that physicians and other actors continued to deeply problematise the Irish body through the lens of dietary intake long after the Famine. Rather than ushering in an age of national advancement, the decline of Ireland's monocrop culture produced new sets of food discourses that, like their pre-Famine equivalents, were drawn upon to explain a lack of socio-economic development. This chapter also demonstrates that physicians, journalists and social commentators in Ireland identified a new national condition of adverse physical and psychological health after the Famine, the root cause of which they stereotypically found in the rising popularity of tea drinking among the poor. Helen O'Connell identifies excessive tea drinking as a problem associated with poverty in the pre-Famine period, an argument that demonstrates that the ability to purchase a luxury good was not necessarily a sign of wealth.[3] This chapter adds to this debate by maintaining that an emphasis on excess was complemented after the Famine with a refined food discourse that placed emphasis on nutritional needs. Medical and lay critics of excessive tea drinking framed their opinions in terms of nervousness and under-nutrition. Moreover, the issue of excessive tea drinking contributed to, if not exemplified, a foreboding sense of national physical and mental decline first made evident in mid-century discussion of institutional feeding. In this way, personal food intake continued to be linked to – and often blamed for – a persistent lack of socio-economic advancement.

Reforming diet

Ireland's transition to a healthier dietetic modernity was far less stable than pre-Famine political economists had predicted. In the 1850s, an anticipated nationwide dietary revolution continued to be greeted confidently by those who felt assured that displacing the potato would protect against major future famines and simultaneously modernise food production. Yet paternalistic mechanisms that might have guided the population in its dietary choices failed to emerge, a challenging scenario given that the products cheaply available in a consumerist culture were often not the most nutritious. Although medical scientists with expertise in food continued to take on public roles after the Famine, they often involved themselves in matters such as institutional feeding and food adulteration rather than intervene in communal consumption habits seemingly beyond their control. Accordingly, most physicians adopted a descriptive, non-interventionist, role: diagnosing faults in post-Famine diets and, by extension, the Irish body.

The visibility of nutritional science rose during the Famine when its advocates attempted to apply their doctrines to outline suitable replacements for the potato. Above all, they recommended variety and nutritional balance. Yet, ironically, this new knowledge of food had inadvertently identified the long-condemned potato as highly nutritious. Widened access to new foodstuffs from the 1850s certainly precipitated variety. But was that variety synonymous with nutritional well-being? An array of late century actors concurred that it was not, a stance exemplified in the provocative evidence given to the Select Committee on Irish Industries by President of Queen's College Cork and Fellow of the Royal College of Science, Thomas Sullivan in 1884. The Committee questioned Sullivan as follows:

> Are not the people able to buy both clothes and a better class of food, and what may be called the comparative luxuries of tea, sugar, and everything of that kind, in a very different proportion from what they were in 1848? – Undoubtedly; but I should demur at the same time to tea and sugar being considered the measure of prosperity in this country.
>
> But you would admit they are able to consume a better class of bread? – I could not say 'a better class of bread'; as a chemist, I say the old system of food when I was a boy in a country place was better than it is now. I speak only of the South, and of when I was a boy; and I have not the slightest hesitation in saying that the food of the people has deteriorated, and that their food was superior when I was a boy.[4]

In his responses, Sullivan insisted that food variety had failed to promote nutritional health. Sullivan's argument was not entirely nostalgic. As Cormac Ó Gráda's historical analysis of height and stature demonstrates, pre-Famine Irishmen were considerably taller and often healthier than their English counterparts, a likely outcome of a potato-rich diet.[5] Although consumption patterns certainly reorganised after the Famine, the optimism with which such a change would have been greeted in the 1840s had mostly receded some four decades later. In its place stood cultural pessimism about the corporeal well-being of the Irish body, unease about the disintegration of older ways of life and wistful memories of an earlier era when diet was monotonous but citizens were healthier.

Where had it all gone wrong? According to the doctrines of mid-century political economists and their supporters, food reform should have reinvigorated Ireland. During the Famine, the *Dublin University Magazine* made concerted efforts to associate the potato with 'habits of filth'; a connection exemplified in derogative depictions of the peasant's dunghill and his unclean pig residing with him in his cottage. Implicit in this powerful representation were commonplace images of social primitivism and cultural backwardness, coupled with underlying assumptions that consuming alternative foodstuffs would foster civilised habits and new psychological mindsets. Forcing the peasant to seek out new foodstuffs meant transplanting him from a subsistence lifestyle and obliging him to interact with modern trading systems – actions predicted to transform him into a modern economic being. The *Magazine* speculated that subsistence lifestyles closed Irish peasants off from mercantile and social worlds, being a solitary form of existence requiring minimum assistance from others. Modern civilisation, however, was understood to have advanced only through mutual dependence and labour division. On that matter, the magazine exclaimed: 'What lessons of prudence were to be learned! What habits of frugality to be acquired in the solitary monotony of this unsocial existence! The very fact that throughout the whole process, the man might subsist without ever handling a coin was enough to account for his knowing but little of the value of either industry or money.'[6]

Various writers with an interest in Irish migrant and emigrant labourers also linked diet to economic productivity. In his *A Tour of Ireland* penned in 1844, James Johnson remarked that when fed on potatoes with their 'bone' in them in Ireland, the children of cottiers looked 'chubby' and 'the people healthy'. But when Irish labourers arrived in Britain seeking employment, their poor physical strength made them unfit for work until fed for a number of days on a rich diet of bacon, bread and potatoes. Johnson metaphorically portrayed Irish labourers as 'like horses taken from grass, and incapable of hard labour till fed for a time on hay and corn'.[7] His claims reflected a commonly held belief that the potato diet suited only the light forms of agricultural work characteristic of pre-Famine society. Meeting the physical demands imposed by more sophisticated forms of labour seemed to depend upon the consumption of a fuller diet which, in turn, improved economic productivity. In this model, the Irish body was presented as a malleable, adjustable entity that could be moulded, through food intake, to suit economic ends.

The mass emigration that accompanied the Famine fortified these ideas on Irish labouring potential. Many labourers emigrated to urban-industrial centres in America, Canada and Britain where they often secured employment in low-paid, backbreaking jobs as they lacked capital and skills.[8] They also tended to enter and leave work on a seasonal basis, being employed as harvesters or railway navvies.[9] In 1852, land agent William Bullock Webster reported that Irish emigrants who had arrived in Canada, although typically larger than French Canadian labourers, were inferior farm labourers. Webster observed that Canadian labourers ate a breakfast of bread and milk, a lunch of *soupe aux pois*, bread and onions, followed by an evening meal of meat and vegetables. It was only when the Irish emigrant emulated this diet that he worked efficiently, suggested Webster, a step that also served to 'raise him to a higher standard as a social being'.[10] Webster's statement further demonstrates how contemporaries linked dietary intake to broader socio-economic agendas. In Webster's account, food was more than simply digestible matter. Instead, it was something that shaped and defined the health of social and economic domains.

Nonetheless, the potato proved resilient in Ireland as detailed by popular Belfast novelist Charlotte Riddell in 1866. Having resided in Carrickfergus, Co. Antrim until 1855, Riddell would have been personally acquainted with the social impact of the Famine and the shifting dietary habits that followed the catastrophe. In a conversation in her novel *Maxwell Druit*, a group of her characters hold the following conversation:

> 'The famine must have taught the Irish not to depend on potatoes,' interrupted Mr. Gyton. 'Would a murrain teach the English not to depend on beef and mutton?' demanded Mr. Drewitt. 'Certainly not; but beef and mutton are not potatoes, are they?' 'Potatoes were beef and mutton to the Irish,' answered the owner of the Headlands. 'And, good heavens! How can you expect a country to prosper whose people are satisfied with that cursed root, as Cobbett called the potato?' asked Mr. Gyton. 'The people here are not at all averse to butchers' meat,' Maxwell replied, coolly, 'only it is sometimes true philosophy to be satisfied with what one can get.'[11]

Riddell's text demonstrates that she understood the potato as a deeply ingrained component of Irish culture; a resonant emblem of national and individual identity.[12] As Riddell suggested, although a broad consensus existed on the need to abandon a mono-crop existence, the means by which this could be achieved and, indeed, the extent to which it could be achieved, remained uncertain.

If the durable popularity of the potato was to be conquered and food reform implemented, then persuasive mechanisms needed to be set in place to guide the population in an appropriate direction. But did these exist? Following the Famine, state bodies mostly retreated from assuming direct responsibility for Irish dietary behaviour. Perhaps they hoped that forces operating in Ireland would spearhead this drive. Occasional reports certainly surfaced of landlords harnessing scientific expertise to maximise output by introducing labourers to new foodstuffs. In the 1860s, commercial farmer Alan Pollok of Co. Galway began supplying his labourers with peas and beans in accordance with the scientific precept that a pound of peas formed the equivalent amount of muscle as fifteen pounds of potatoes. Pollok also considered peas to be rich in lime and phosphoric acids that fed the locomotive organs and the brain.[13] However, reports such as these were unsurprisingly rare given that the landlord class was notoriously characterised by absenteeism and disinterest in fostering tenant development.[14]

Moreover, cynicism to nutritional science endured long after the Famine. Sceptics insisted that natural – rather than scientifically guided – dietary adaption would occur. They assumed that the forging of a new national diet would be instinctual, just as decisions made to consume potatoes prior to the Famine had, in their view, emanated from an instinctive awareness of the crop's high nutritional value, as scientifically confirmed during the Famine. Tensions between knowledge and instinct were eloquently articulated in 1861 by an anonymous contributor to the *Dublin University Magazine* who strongly opposed medico-scientific intervention in culinary practice. 'Only the Devil', the author insisted, 'could have suggested to Soyer the horror of a red-herring pie, or potatoes mashed with cod-liver oil . . . and, surely, it must have been the Devil – if not Moloch himself – who put into Liebig's head the horrible notion of extracting the juices of raw beef and mutton, by cold muriatic acid and calling the product "soup".' For the author, nutritional science was a 'Satanic influence'.[15]

Continuing his diatribe, the author rebuked chemists who analysed the biological consistency of crops and meats and then upheld certain foods as healthier than others. In his view, emotionally detached research conducted in chemical laboratories resoundingly failed to make sense of important matters such as taste and appetite or, in the author's words 'holy instincts which reason could not comprehend'.[16] He marked out taste as particularly incomprehensible to laboratory analysis and regretted the activities of scientists who, he believed, had failed to advocate new foodstuffs for Irish labourers that were as palatable as the potato once had been and who had disconnected consumption from its individual and cultural dimensions. Scientific discourse seemed to have dislodged and misplaced the human experience of ingestion despite the fact that these indicators provided a crucial index of public food choice. The author concluded by asserting that knowledge was formed in the kitchen, not the laboratory.[17] Female intuition, he insisted, offered the most suitable guide for culinary regeneration, not cookbooks and scientific regimes of knowledge. The author portrayed female cooks as having a higher dietetic authority than either Liebig or Soyer, declaring that:

> A woman cook has no business to reason, because she is a woman. She should implicitly follow prescription; heeding what has come to her by tradition, and not striving to go beyond it . . . cookery to her should be a veritable culture – a religion – a belief reposing on faith, not to be reasoned upon without danger or departed from without heresy.[18]

In this account, dietary regeneration rested in the authority of instinct, not science. Of course, this stance relied upon assumptions that a female family member did indeed possess an instinctive awareness of the nutritional value of particular foodstuffs; that she had the means and knowledge to prepare nutritious food; and that she needed little guidance from external sources. These presumptions were equally flawed. Just seven years earlier, another anonymous contributor to the *Dublin University Magazine* had asserted that 'the modern Irish, compared with other nations in a similar state of advancement in all other respects, were, and perhaps are the most uneducated in the culinary art of any people under the sun' and that 'the great bulk of the peasantry in the remote rural districts of Ireland, especially the south and west, could not dress food of any other description than potatoes and eggs'.[19]

In what ways, then, did the Irish diet actually evolve after the Famine? An official inquiry undertaken by Edward Smith in the 1860s investigated the food purchasing behaviour of agricultural labourers. Smith acquired an impressive reputation in the 1850s for his research into human nutrition. This included influential experiments into prison diets that challenged some of Liebig's fundamental concepts. Smith also established a minimum standard of nutritional intake: 4,300 grains of carbon and 200 grains of nitrogen per day. In doing so, he sought to empirically define the boundaries between nutritional sufficiency and insufficiency. In the early 1860s, he served as Medical Officer for the Privy Council. As part of his duties in this role, the Council dispatched him to investigate eating patterns in North-West England during the Lancashire Cotton Famine.[20] A second dietary survey conducted by Smith, recorded in the 1864 report of the Medical Officer of the Privy Council, was more extensive and investigated consumption patterns throughout the entire British Isles, including Ireland.[21] It focused on agricultural labourers with relatively small earnings and whose conditions reflected the average living standards for that social grouping. Accordingly, the eating habits of social groupings unable to work, such as the sick, remained unrecorded. Geographically, Smith's investigations in Ireland primarily targeted western regions, although a quarter of his Irish samples originated from southern and northern regions. Overall, he enquired into fifty-two families in Ireland: a sample of 269 people, 236 of whom were adults.

Smith's results offered a complex portrait of post-Famine dietary change, as indicated in Table 4.1. They highlighted the resilience of the potato as well as the widespread purchasing of alternative foodstuffs. Smith determined that 44 per cent of his interviewees consumed at least five pounds of potatoes per week, particularly in the harvest season. His interviewees only ate Indian meal and oatmeal when potato supplies ran low. When explaining the ongoing appeal of the potato, Smith's interviewees explained their ongoing attraction to the potato as being due to the potato's low cost rather than faith in, or knowledge of, its nutritional properties.[22] As anticipated during the Famine, Indian meal maintained a notable presence in Irish dietary customs, providing a dietary staple for 92 per cent of interviewees. However, the labourers with whom Smith corresponded ascribed this neither to a trust in its nutritional value nor to a

Table 4.1 Irish rural diets in the early 1860s compiled by Edward Smith.

Food item	*Proportion of population who consumed it (%)*	*Quantity consumed per adult weekly (lbs)*
Milk*	98	6.75
Indian meal (used for puddings, stirabout and cakes)	92	10.5
Sugar (consumed with Indian meal, tea and coffee)	80	4.75
Wheaten flour (used for cakes)	68	2.5
Tea	57	0.25
Meat (70% of which was bacon)	57	4.5
Potatoes*	44	5.75
Fats (e.g. dripping, lard, suet, butter)	40	1.25
Fish (consumed with potatoes)	31	Not recorded
Bread	26	3.75
Coffee	24	Not recorded
Eggs	20	Not recorded

* Seasonal usage only.

preference for its taste. Instead, when potato supplies ran low, meal seemed to grant the largest amount of nourishment rather than nutrition. Recalling the disparaging opinions on meal that he encountered, Smith asserted that 'it would scarcely be an exaggeration to say that it is universally disliked, while at the same time it is held in high estimation as a temporary food until better times come, and is universally admitted to have been and still is of the greatest service to the labouring classes'. Reiterating this point, he remarked that 'Indian corn is as universally courted as it is disliked'.[23] Importantly, Smith noted that although the educated classes believed that Irish labourers laboured more efficiently when fed on meal rather than potatoes, labourers themselves held contrasting views, perceiving meal as a food that decreased their efficiency.[24] Notably, many of Smith's interviewees desired more meat in their diets although they did not understand meat as valuable for building bodily health and strength.[25] Cultural preferences and dietary traditions clearly dictated the interactions between new and old dietary customs. Smith's findings also demonstrated that day-to-day issues such as cost and availability primarily dictated consumer choice and that Irish consumers cared little for the doctrines of nutritional science.

One of the most surprising outcomes of Smith's survey was its confirmation that Irish rural diets appeared favourable to health and, in many ways, were even superior to those of English agricultural labourers. To a certain extent, this interpretation can be situated in broader trends in scientific literature on diet that glorified the simple dietary arrangements of rural communities – a common thread in British medical critiques of modern, consumerist urban diets.[26] Smith went so far as to announce that 'throughout the country I found them a fine, well-built, and often athletic race, with children sufficiently fleshy and rosy, and bearing all the marks of health. The wife, however, was usually more robust and healthy looking than is observed in England.'[27] He attributed this to a simple, unvaried diet and concluded that analysis of Irish dietaries implied that food variety might not necessarily be an essential component of health after all.[28] Intriguingly, Smith's findings implied that Irish agricultural poverty did not necessarily mean poor nutrition. Conversely, the perseverance of poverty also demonstrated that physical health was clearly not an essential prerequisite for economic advancement and social progression. On the contrary, bodies could be healthy even when residing in economically backward and relatively unsophisticated agricultural locations.

However, if Smith's investigations had demonstrated that labourers typically made consumption choices on the basis of cost and availability instead of nutritional value or natural physiological instinct, then what was to happen once new, consumer products became available? Ominously, Smith identified 'a general longing after the so-called luxuries of their brethren in England'.[29] The popularity of luxury goods such as tea and coffee had recently risen, warned Smith. Yet he added that these substances contained less nutritional value than milk whose usage they threatened to displace.[30] Smith's research therefore complicated many of the key assumptions about, and stereotypes of, Irish dietary customs and, in many ways, exposed profound differences between improving discourses, medico-scientific rhetoric and day-to-day realities.

'The pleasures of the tea-pot'

Despite the lingering nature of potato consumption, faith in dietary change as a signifier of physical, social and economic improvement was high in the immediate post-Famine period. The agricultural prosperity of the 1860s – stimulated by rising prices during the Crimean War and years of good weather that bolstered crop yields – fostered optimism.[31] For some, the healthiness of the post-Famine Irish body appeared certain. Conservative Irish landlord Henry Bruce, speaking in the House of Commons in 1870, announced that the increased consumption of white bread was a symbolic marker of Ireland's social progression away from a problematic mono-crop existence. Yet Bruce's claim formed part of a wider defence of the resident landlord, being intended to emphasise the social achievements of that class in reforming and rejuvenating Ireland.[32]

Many late century commentators interpreted a shift towards consumerism more critically. Liam Kennedy observes that a national network of rural retailing extended after the Famine as farm incomes rose and a consumer consciousness developed.[33] The poor increasingly relied upon purchasing food from shopkeepers. However, many local communities detested shopkeepers who encouraged reliance upon their services by accumulating customer debt.[34] Nonetheless, shopkeepers came to play a significant role in agrarian communities, sometimes rivalling landowners as wielders of local power and patronage and enjoying a relationship with the rural population that Samuel Clark compares to that enjoyed by the parish priest.[35] For reasons such as these, shopkeepers found themselves subject to intense public opprobrium, to such a degree that the nationalist United Irish League conducted organised protests against them in the 1890s.[36] Importantly, the extension of shopkeeping played a formative role in shaping post-Famine dietary readjustment, albeit in an unforeseen direction.

Ireland's socio-economic landscape changed dramatically after the Famine. Ireland integrated more firmly into a free trade area but also exposed herself to the vagaries of that system. In consequence, the country's inhabitants now found themselves vulnerable to international patterns of economic downturn instead of disruptions in potato production. Agricultural depressions created widespread poverty and distress in rural communities, even having a knock-on effect in Dublin where wealth depended heavily upon exporting agricultural produce. The early 1860s witnessed severe agricultural depression while the late 1870s saw the commencement of a remarkably sustained economic downturn that created deep levels of endemic urban and rural poverty that persisted until well into the following century.[37]

These mitigating factors shaped post-Famine constructions of the Irish body. Enquiries made by the Congested Districts Board in the 1890s indicated that Irish rural dietaries had diverged dramatically from the ideals laid out by pre-Famine improvers, as well as the more positive trends identified in Smith's dietary surveys of the 1860s. The Board was established in 1891 as a form of Constructive Unionism – a Conservative strategy that aimed to pacify Irish agrarian unrest and reduce demands for Home Rule by relieving poverty or, as sceptics suspected, to 'kill Home Rule with kindness'.[38] Constructive Unionism was particularly intent on tackling rural poverty, partly because political unrest was most acute in rural Ireland. Unlike Smith's more positive rendering of rural dietary health, the Board's annual reports portrayed rural poverty and dietary customs negatively; as problems requiring urgent resolution. Even in a good year, so the Board's first report claimed, the community is 'little more than free from the dread of hunger'. The Board portrayed inadequate living standards and insufficient diets as common in even the more prosperous districts of the west of Ireland.[39]

Leslie Clarkson's analysis of the investigative reports that preceded the Board's establishment reveals the popularity of bread in seventy-eight analysed districts, tea in seventy, Indian meal in fifty-eight and bacon in twenty-three, with milk, fish, eggs, oatmeal, butter, sugar, cabbage and meat being consumed to lesser degrees. Although labourers still ate potatoes, it seemed clear that rural food consumption had diversified by the 1890s.[40] Clarkson identifies tea and bread as dominant forces in rural consumption patterns in this period.[41] Similarly, as Ciara Breathnach notes, the poor often bartered food items such as eggs to purchase foodstuffs containing less nutritional value.[42] Technological innovation, too, contributed to dietary anxieties. The nutritional quality of the bread being bought by the poor waned in the late nineteenth century. Bakeries had played a relatively limited role in pre-Famine consumption, but following the Famine, mass production methods cheapened the cost of bread.[43] From the 1880s, gradual reduction roller milling steadily replaced traditional flour-milling practices. New processing methods displaced the traditional use of millstones to grind grain and cruder sieving and separating techniques. However, this had a discernible downside in that processed white bread was less nutritious than unprocessed bread.[44]

Prominent Belfast surgeon William MacCormac was among the first medical figures in Ireland to comment on the deficiencies of late nineteenth-century diets. MacCormac actively campaigned to improve the physical condition of Belfast's poor. In the 1860s, he confronted the issue of working-class diet, writing in the *Belfast Newsletter* that:

> I would have tracts to urge the preparation of wheatmeal bread; for white bread, with weak tea, used three times a day, is not azotised enough, is quite unfitted for exclusive sustenance, impairs in this town yearly the health of thousands. I would have tracts to point out the confection of wholesome stews and wholesome nutriment. For how are working people to know these things unless through printed tracts or spoken words? The art of cooking and of keeping garments clean and comfortable should be taught in every school ... everything in short, ought to be done, not to degrade, but to elevate; not to confine the aspirations to this life, but to lead them to the reasonable hope and expectancy of a yet more elevated life to come.[45]

MacCormac identified ongoing problems in Irish dietary behaviour and argued that these needed to be pedagogically resolved. He fortified this argument by referring to chemical analysis that had demonstrated that the fine, white flour used to manufacture white bread contained less nutritious value than unbolted flour. MacCormac warned that producers removed the most nutritious ingredients of the grain – wheat phosphates and gluten – to obtain the whiteness desired by customers. As an alternative, he promoted wholemeal bread prepared with bran phosphates, a chemical constituent thought to nurture the flesh and bones.[46] Despite these concerns, the impact of large city bakeries in provincial centres in Ulster strengthened from the 1880s. In the same decade, Dublin evolved into a major baking centre.[47]

Changing exportation patterns also influenced concern about post-Famine dietary readjustment. After the Famine, graziers exported Irish-produced meat to Britain at ever-rising levels to cater for an expanding urban market in that country.[48] This development had an important knock-on effect in Ireland where the poor began to become over reliant on consuming cheap, imported goods instead of locally produced food.[49] Above all foodstuffs, tea dominated criticism of post-Famine diets and provided an exemplary culprit among an array of modernising forces seen to be impacting detrimentally on Irish well-being. Unlike bread, tea was imported. Generally considered a luxury item prior to the Famine, the poor increasingly relied upon tea as a dietary staple in the last half of the century, a development facilitated, and encouraged, by its ever decreasing cost. According to evidence given to the Royal Commission on Labour of 1894, between 1873 and 1893 the price of tea dropped from 3 s. 1 d. to 2 s. per pound in Castlereagh, Co. Roscommon.[50] In 1863, Smith calculated that rural households consumed 1.25 oz. of tea in an average week. Yet towards the end of the century, concerned members of the Congested Districts Board warned that the typical family purchased as much as a pound per week in some regions of Connaught.[51] Clarkson and Crawford also note a startling rise, estimating that by 1904, family tea consumption in rural districts averaged nine ounces a week and close to twelve ounces in urban centres.[52]

Tea tended to be shop-bought. However, as Breathnach observes, the poor often purchased cheap quality black Assam tea.[53] Tea could also be procured from a group known as 'tea-men' who travelled around the country. Oral history evidence later collected in Carrowmenagh, Co. Donegal, discloses the unpopularity of these figures. According to one interviewee, 'these taymen began to pervade the countryside and torment the people' and were 'worse than leprosy'.[54] Correspondingly, milk became less popular. Graziers reared ever-larger numbers of animals for exportation as meat. This ultimately placed limitations on local access to milk in Ireland as the cattle reared for meat tended not to be the strongest milkers.[55] Critics also blamed the expansion of the Irish creamery system for having encouraged excessive tea drinking. Small farmers dispatched fresh milk to these establishments where it was separated. Creamery managers returned skimmed milk to these farmers. Yet its taste was unfavourable, meaning that labourers chose to feed it to their livestock rather than consume it themselves.[56] At the creamery, elements of the milk were extracted, leaving a less palatable and appetising fat content. As the Bishop of Ross later claimed, 'it would seem to me as if there had been a sort of molecular disintegration of the milk itself'.[57]

Physicians demonised tea in much the same way that they had once castigated the potato, allowing for a renewed problematisation of the Irish body. In Britain, tea was a marker of middle-class social civility and an index of polite society.[58] Yet anxieties about its over-use in working-class communities proliferated, allowing the substance to occupy a highly ambiguous space in the late Victorian social terrain.[59] In fact, the boundaries between tea as a safe or unsafe substance were remarkably unstable.[60] Commentary on Irish tea-drinking habits surfaced alongside corresponding discussion in Britain.[61] In 1872, for instance, one lady reported to the *Freeman's Journal* that:

> Taking shelter in a cottage, near Banbridge, County Down, some time ago, during a shower of rain, and noticing the teapot on the hob, I observed that tea stewed in that way did a great deal of harm. The woman who lived in the cottage at once admitted that the parish doctor had said, 'the folks were killing themselves with tea', and that it caused him more trouble than anything else. A few days ago

> a gentleman, just come up to town, was mentioning that the poor people in his neighbourhood suffered dreadfully from 'tic'. I replied that this was a disease often caused, I believed, by excessive tea-drinking. 'Indeed', he answered; 'well I must say, they do take immense quantities of tea'.[62]

The apparent evils of excessive tea drinking evolved into a topic of lively debate after the non-conformist Dean of Bangor, Henry Thomas Edwards, made a remarkably erudite public condemnation of the practice in Wales in 1883. Edwards was best known for his efforts to incorporate denominationalism into the national education system. Just a year prior to his unfortunate suicide, Edwards made his feelings known at a public meeting on education by asserting that schools' managers needed to incorporate cooking and nutrition into their syllabuses. In his announcement, Edwards asserted that:

> Excessive tea-drinking creates a generation of nervous, hysterical, discontented people, always complaining of the existing order of the universe, scolding their neighbours, and sighing after the impossible. Good cooking of more solid substances would, I firmly believe, enable them to take far happier and more correct views of existence. In fact I suspect that overmuch tea drinking, by destroying the calmness of the nerves, is acting as a dangerous revolutionary force among us.

The Irish press heavily publicised and debated the Dean's speech because parallel concerns prevailed in Ireland. The *Irish Times* insisted that the Dean's outburst contained important warnings for the country. Tea, so the newspaper informed its readers, was an unsuitable dietary staple for adults and proved physically harmful to children subsisting upon nothing else, as suspected to be the case among the Irish poor. 'Tea-making to excess among this class is a form of laziness which produces – there can be no doubt about it – mischievous results', explained the newspaper. The *Irish Times* insisted that the humbler classes should consume oatmeal and milk – foodstuffs that calmed the nerves and encouraged endurance. Continuing, the editorial argued that 'his [the Dean of Bangor] gloomy forebodings predict little less than our general physical and moral decadence as a people and nation if we persevere in our addiction to the pleasures of the tea pot'.[63]

The Dean's statements and their subsequent journalistic reports were loaded with cultural resonance. They framed tea drinking in terms of nervousness by portraying the drink as a stimulant rather than a suitable source of nourishment. When drunk excessively, tea generated nervous excitability and over-stimulated bodies and minds rather than building bodily strength. Suggestions such as these stemmed from fashionable medical theories developed internationally by, among others, American neurologist George Miller Beard, who had delineated relationships between diet, nervous exhaustion and the weakening nature of modern life.[64] In Irish medical and journalistic commentary on tea, the substance was highlighted as being excessively consumed for the purpose of sensory stimulation alone; a custom denounced for depleting nervous energy supplies and impacting adversely on physical stamina.

This apprehension arose in a period when the Irish housewife was being exalted as a figure whose domestic work was critical to ensuring a healthy society, as Joanna Bourke persuasively outlines.[65] More so than ever, housewives were expected to nurture, feed and preserve the health of family members. Those who failed to do so risked public castigation, especially if seen as not fulfilling their nurturing responsibilities due to spending their days intoxicated with tea. Emotive journalistic accounts proliferated of washerwomen, kitchen girls and mothers filling the out-patient departments of hospitals complaining of headache, nausea, loss of appetite, physical distress after eating and chronic dizziness. In 1887, the *Belfast Newsletter* depicted a cycle of events where the tea-obsessed housewife gradually lost her appetite, slowly came to loathe food and eventually sought solace in the tea-cup, although this final step ultimately intensified her condition. Once addicted, she turned to methods of tea preparation that allowed her to secure as much tannin (or tannic acid) as possible to quell her ever-intensifying physical cravings. Ultimately, she became afflicted with a damaging array of nervous complaints. The root of the problem, according to this journalistic account, lay in the female practice of keeping a pot of tea stewing on the stove throughout the day and drinking from it continuously.[66]

Many physicians linked excessive tea drinking with chronic dyspepsia (or indigestion). They identified dyspepsia as a chief disease of modernity most likely to manifest in those who had succumbed to the demoralising sway of modern life. In Britain and America, medical authors blamed consumerism for rising incidences of chronic dyspepsia. According to mainstream dietetic thought, the stomach was a rich epicentre of nerves. The ingestion of unsuitable substances had a detrimental nervous influence that spread from the stomach throughout the body via the nervous system.[67] Accordingly, authors on digestion warned that the exposure of the nervous system to harmful, weakening – often foreign – foodstuffs presented problems not only for the stomach but also for the entire body. In his *Causes and Treatment of Imperfect Digestion* published in 1860, Wexford-born physician Arthur Leared made use of an elaborate physiological model of digestion that presented nature as having placed certain foodstuffs in particular geographical regions that were suited to the constitutions of the particular races who resided there. Leared described regional and national groups such as the British, Italian and Eskimo races as having once consumed locally sourced food that suited their unique constitutions. For Leared, international communication and the development of global transportation systems had created an 'unnatural' global spread of foodstuffs. Dietary articles were now entering stomachs that they were unintended for. According to Leared, 'the mere circumstance of confounding together many articles of diet, the products of opposite climates, appears to me a very probable source of dyspepsia in those otherwise predisposed'.[68] This context allowed physicians to present tea as a deleterious foreign substance unsuited to the Irish constitution.

Contemporary medical authors also understood nervousness as a symptom of national degeneration and decline. During the late nineteenth century, medical and psychiatric writers penned pessimistic accounts of how modernity had impacted negatively on individual and national health. They argued that physical and mental weaknesses replicated themselves through hereditary factors, meaning that both personal and national vitality could perpetually worsen if defects were passed on to future generations. Authors on degeneration often blamed the poor, a social grouping seen as prone to reproducing in large numbers and passing on physical and mental defects to their offspring.[69] Irish tea discourse mirrored this fashionable intellectual trend by identifying excessive tea drinking and its resultant nervousness as bearing national ramifications. This rhetoric also, perhaps inadvertently, destabilised pre-Famine suggestions that dietary change and integration into a capitalist economy could not fail to guarantee physical strength and economic productivity.

Medical literature, newspapers, official inquiries and government commissions all explored these apparent connections between tea and nervousness, indicating that a diverse range of actors understood tea drinking as a root cause of physical and national decline. The theme punctuated evidence given to the Royal Commission on Labour of 1893–4. At this, Mr Lynch, a labourer from Delvin, Co. Westmeath, insisted that 'the children are spoilt in their youth from not having milk. The people are killing themselves with tea. The men don't work so well in consequence. Stirabout and milk used to be a grand thing for them.'[70] In similar fashion, a farmer named Mr Ramage maintained that, 'I think the modern food is deteriorating the men's strength.'[71] Mr L. Ward, a ploughman, stated that 'they were stronger men in the old days. Now they are more prone to heart disease and other ills which I believe is owing to the modern diet.'[72] Another witness claimed that when recruiting men to construct a railway in the west of Ireland, he found that local men were too weak to labour.[73] Embedded in these debates was a pressing sense that nutritional health had been compromised as the popularity of the potato diminished. By the 1890s, a distinctive image of the post-Famine Irish body was in play: one characterised by weak physical calibre and that dangerously threatened to perpetually reproduce, tarnishing the physical vitality of future generations.

Psychiatric authors also understood mental complaints as replicable through reproduction. In fact, the psychiatric dimensions of tea drinking were a remarkably fruitful source of post-Famine apprehension. This allowed psychiatrists to partake in debates on Irish dietary change. If the stomach was indeed the epicentre of the human nervous system, then it made sense that dietary intake could impact upon the mind. Leared, for instance, depicted individuals suffering from nervous temperaments as especially prone to morbidly acute and over-sensitive mental impressions. On this, he argued that:

> The patient feels undue anxiety on every subject, is absurdly alive to the slightest touch of ridicule, and finds insult where none was meant. He is constantly apprehensive of danger; and if his mind dwells on religion, he sees in it nothing but dark threatening unrelieved by a gleam of hope.

For authors such as Leared, excessive tea drinking did not directly cause insanity. However, dyspepsia stimulated by excessive tea consumption certainly caused nervous excitement that, in turn, caused psychological decline in those seen as predisposed to the condition – particularly women.[74] This concept permeated expert and lay literature on tea drinking. In 1872, the *Freeman's Journal* reported on a thirty-two-year-old servant girl who, despite having enjoyed good health for years, had recently become irritable, suffered from laughing and crying fits and had 'got into a state of great weakness'. She had tried to conceal these problems from her mistress by continuing work as usual, but one day, when trying to clean a grate, had collapsed speechless and senseless before having several hysterical fits. Subsequent medical examination revealed how she had become addicted to tea over a number of years, now caring for little else so long as she procured her favourite substance.[75]

Concern about excessive tea drinking crescendoed in the 1890s upon the publication of an official investigation by the Irish Inspectors of Lunatics, George Plunkett O'Farrell and E. Maziere Courtenay, into a nationwide rise in asylum admissions. In their investigations, O'Farrell and Courtenay agreed upon the indigestibility of shop-bought tea as an explanatory factor for rising incidences of insanity. They noted that in Armagh, the annual number of first admissions had increased by a figure of eighty-two in a period of just five years.[76] O'Farrell and Courtenay established that the industrialised regions surrounding Belfast had also witnessed rising admissions between 1883 and 1892 despite the region's population having remained fairly constant.[77] The Inspectors ascribed these rising asylum admissions to the inability of the poorer classes to buy nutritious food; heightened levels of vexation caused by adverse economic conditions; and an inter-related derangement of physical and mental functions. They pinpointed the withdrawal of the support of family life due to emigration, hereditary predisposition and alcoholism as further contributory factors. In certain districts including Ballinasloe, O'Farrell and Courtenay noted that few admissions could be ascribed to excessive alcohol consumption due to the remarkable effectiveness of the temperance movement in that area.[78] Instead, the Inspectors blamed rising admissions on the widespread consumption of Indian tea of inferior quality there, stewed rather than infused. Diet, they suggested, had unquestionably contributed to increasing insanity levels meaning that large numbers of asylum patients now bore the scars of scant, improper food: 'the insanity of malnutrition'.[79] The Inspectors cited one case where a severely restricted diet had caused epileptic seizures and mania, although psychiatrists had rapidly cured this problem with a period of asylum rest and nutritious feeding.[80] O'Farrell and Courtenay did find some evidence which complicated their discussion of the adverse psychological capacity of tea. Although a steady rise in admissions had occurred in Clonmel, the authors noted that excessive tea drinking was less common in that area. Furthermore, they determined that asylums in Cork had not seen a notable increase in admission rates despite excessive tea consumption being a problem in that city. Despite this sometimes contradictory evidence, the Inspectors concluded that the innutritious dietary of poorer populations had caused widespread anaemia and constitutional weakness, rendering citizens vulnerable to scrofulous and neurotic disease. The ill-effects of decocted tea when used as a dietary staple, they maintained, had created high communal levels of dyspepsia which then facilitated neurotic disturbance, mental depression and psychological decline.[81] By 1895, terms such as 'tea drunkards' had entered popular discourse in Ireland, as had so-called 'tea mania', the symptoms of which included headache, vertigo, insomnia, palpitation of the heart, mental confusion, nightmare, nausea, hallucinations, morbid depression of spirits and even suicidal impulses.

An article published in the *Journal of Mental Science* on the subject in 1894 by Thomas Drapes, leading Irish psychiatrist and resident medical superintendent at Enniscorthy District Asylum, further reveals how tea captured psychiatric attention in this period. For Drapes, what was most puzzling and worrying about the apparent national increase of insanity was that cases of committals had risen despite the population of the country having rapidly declined due to emigration. He confirmed that nearly all Irish asylums' superintendents blamed tea for its detrimental impact on Irish mental well-being, particularly when consumed as a substitute for nutritious food. In an era marked by mounting public alarm about national decline and future vitality, Drapes warned that 'we see its effects in the number of pale-faced children, who are brought up on it instead of the old time-honoured, but now nearly abandoned, porridge and milk'.[82] His arguments pointed to a new crisis in Irish dietary customs, one that he saw as having stemmed from interacting with modern economic systems rather than from an aversion to engaging with those systems. The threat seemingly posed by tea resonated with broader concerns about the post-Famine direction of Ireland. The discussion that it provoked also expressed contemporary apprehension about the loss of the nutritious potato. This emotive rhetoric helped to explain the bodily problems then associated with poverty and economic under-development that pervaded post-Famine discussion of the Irish condition.

Although contemporary medical authors were concerned about various aspects of the post-Famine diet, the problematic habit of consuming tea with a few slices of processed bread seemed to present the worst possible outcome of Irish engagement with consumerism. This custom formed a key element of post-Famine food discourse as it rendered visible the socially and individually detrimental ramifications of removing consumers from their food source and of replacing the potato with cheap, imported products. Of course, processed bread and rising imports of cheap American ham also probably affected the nutritional health of the Irish populace. Yet tea evolved into an exemplary target of dietary criticism as its innutritious nature was easier to establish. Moreover, the habit of subsisting upon tea virtually alone appeared particularly alien given Ireland's historical reliance upon consuming home-grown food. Tea was a foreign substance, seemingly being ingested to excess. For some, it symbolised the most negative aspects of Irish encounters with social and economic modernity. Tea-based anxieties also perpetuated a sense of the Irish poor being irrational, hedonistic beings whose behaviour still required governance and regulation.

Conclusion

Evidently, dietary reform was not a straightforward process. For many, it failed to live up to the high aspirations laid out in pre-Famine improvement discourses. In fact, its path of development allowed those narratives to be deconstructed. Although reliance on the potato had clearly receded, as many had once hoped it would, food anxieties continued to surface after the Famine, partly due to an acknowledgement that the potato had in fact contained enough nutritional value to guarantee bodily health. The nature of post-Famine dietary readjustment allowed physicians, as well as psychiatrists, to define the country's engagement with modernity as potentially unhealthy and pathological in nature. Firm mechanisms to guide Irish food consumption habits had not been set in place following the Famine and the state, medicine, science and landlords demonstrated relatively little influence in this area. They detailed how the populace had failed to replace the potato with alternative crops and foodstuffs of high nutritional value. They also found new ways to perpetuate a sense that social groupings continued to exist in Ireland whose bodies needed closer governing. However, dietary regulation was remarkably more difficult in the community than in institutional settings. If anything, food reform had created dietary problems that seemed resoundingly worse and harder to manage and resolve than those associated with the potato diet. Excessive tea drinking became particularly portrayed as having compromised the strength of an Irish body that had long remained shielded from weakening external influences. Commentators used these observations to explain a continuing lack of socio-economic progression. In response, a profound sense developed that food was better in the 'old days'.

Notes

1 Clarkson and Crawford, *Feast and Famine*, p. 89.
2 R. V. Comerford, 'Ideas and institutions, 1830–45', in Vaughan (ed.), *A New History of Ireland V*, pp. 378–9.
3 H. O'Connell, '"A raking pot of tea": consumption and excess in early nineteenth-century Ireland', *Literature and History*, 21:2 (Autumn 2012), 32–47.
4 *Report from the Select Committee on Industries (Ireland)*, H. C. 1884–5 [Cmd.288] ix.1, p. 7.
5 C. Ó Gráda, 'The height of Clonmel prisoners 1845–9: some dietary implications', *Irish Economic and Social History*, 28 (1991), 24–33. For regional variation, see D. Oxley, 'Living standards of women in pre-Famine Ireland', *Social Science History*, 28:2 (Summer 2004), 271–95.
6 'The famine in the land: what has been done and what is to be done', *Dublin University Magazine*, 29 (April 1847), 501–40 on p. 522.
7 Johnson, *Tour in Ireland*, p. 314.

8 K. A. Miller, *Emigrants and Exiles: Ireland and the Irish Exodus to North America* (Oxford and New York: Oxford University Press, 1985), pp. 315–18.
9 G. Davis, 'The Irish in Britain, 1815–1939', in A. Bielenberg (ed.), *The Irish Diaspora* (Harlow: Pearson Education Limited, 2000), p. 23.
10 W. B. Webster, *Ireland Considered as a Field for Investment or Residence* (Dublin: Hodges and Smith, 1852), p. 89.
11 F. G. Trafford, *Maxwell Drewitt* (New York: Harper and Brothers, 1866), p. 78.
12 Ibid.
13 'Letters from Dr W. N. Cote: diet of laborers in Ireland', *Medical and Surgical Reporter*, 11:2 (9 January 1864), 40. See also P. G. Lane, 'An attempt at commercial farming in Ireland after the Famine', *Studies: An Irish Quarterly Review*, 61:1 (Spring 1972), 54–66.
14 K. H. Connell, *Irish Peasant Society: Four Historical Essays* (Dublin: Irish Academic Press, 1996 [1968]), p. 130.
15 'Ministers of the devil', *Dublin University Magazine*, 57 (June 1861), 696–709 on p. 696.
16 Ibid. p. 698.
17 Ibid., p. 699.
18 Ibid, pp. 700–1.
19 'The food of the Irish', *Dublin University Magazine*, 43 (February 1854), 127–46 on p. 127.
20 For more on Smith's dietary surveys, see T. C. Barker, D. J. Oddy and J. Yudkin, *The Dietary Surveys of Dr Edward Smith 1862–3* (London, 1970).
21 *Sixth Report of the Medical Officer of the Privy Council*, H. C. 1863 [3416] xxviii, p. 216.
22 Ibid., p. 286.
23 Ibid., p. 285.
24 Ibid.
25 Ibid., p. 288.
26 Miller, *Modern History of Stomach*, pp. 11–38.
27 *Sixth Report of the Medical Officer of the Privy Council*, p. 283.
28 Ibid., p. 290.
29 Ibid., p. 284.
30 Ibid., p. 290.
31 Turner, *After the Famine*, pp. 104–9.
32 'Sir Frederick Heygate on the Irish Land Bill', *Belfast Newsletter* (10 March 1870), p. 4.
33 L. Kennedy, 'Traders in the Irish rural economy, 1880–1914', *Economic History Review*, 32:2 (May 1979), 201–10.
34 Clark, *Social Origins of the Irish Land War*, p. 126.
35 Ibid., p. 128.
36 M. D. Higgins and J. P. Gibbons, 'Shopkeeper-graziers and land agitation in Ireland, 1895–1900', in P. J. Drudy, *Ireland: Land, Politics, and People* (Cambridge: Cambridge University Press, 1982).
37 For the relationship between economic cycles, and agrarian and urban economies, see M. Daly, *Dublin: The Deposed Capital* (Cork: Cork University Press, 1984), pp. 53–64.
38 Breathnach, *Congested Districts Board*, pp. 38–9.
39 *First Annual Report of the Congested Districts Board for Ireland*, H. C. 1893–4 [C.6908] lxxi.525, pp. 8–10.
40 L. Clarkson, 'The modernisation of Irish diet', in J. Davis, *Rural Change in Ireland* (Belfast: Institute of Irish Studies, Queen's University Belfast, 1999).
41 See P. Lysaght, 'When I makes tea, I makes tea', *Ulster Folklife*, 33 (1987), 44–71.
42 Breathnach, *Congested Districts Board*, pp. 38–9.
43 Clarkson and Crawford, *Feast and Famine*, pp. 99–101.

44 G. Jones, 'The introduction and establishment of roller milling in Ireland', in A. Bielenberg (ed.), *Irish Flour Milling: A History, 600–2000* (Dublin: Lilliput Press, 2003).
45 H. M'Cormac, 'To the Millowners, House Proprietors, Employers and Others of the Town of Belfast', *Belfast Newsletter* (31 January 1863), p. 3.
46 'Wholemeal bread', *Boston Journal of Chemistry*, 3:2 (1 August 1868), 27.
47 Bielenberg, *Ireland and the Industrial Revolution*, pp. 71–2.
48 Turner, *After the Famine*, p. 58.
49 Clarkson and Crawford, *Feast and Famine*, pp. 103–5.
50 Royal Commission on Labour. The Agricultural Labourer. Vol. IV. Ireland. Part IV, H. C. 1893–4 [C.6894–xxi] xxxvii Pt.1.341, p. 98.
51 Breathnach, *Congested Districts Board*, p. 40.
52 Clarkson and Crawford, *Feast and Famine*, p. 103.
53 Breathnach, *Congested Districts Board*, p. 42.
54 National Folklore Commission, lml.l.8344, pp. 174–8.
55 Turner, *After the Famine*, p. 49.
56 *Royal Commission on Congestion in Ireland: Appendix to the Sixth Report*, H. C. 1908 [Cd.3748] xxxix.701, p. 40.
57 *Minutes of Evidence taken before the Inter-Departmental Committee on Physical Deterioration Volume II*, H. C. 1904 [Cd.2201] xxxii.45, p. 412.
58 J. Fromer, *A Necessary Luxury: Tea in Victorian England* (Athens, OH: Ohio University Press, 2008).
59 I. Miller, '"A dangerous revolutionary force amongst us": conceptualising working-class tea drinking in the British Isles, c.1860–1900', *Cultural and Social History* 10:3 (September 2013), 419–38.
60 T. Ketabgian, 'Foreign tastes and "Manchester tea-parties": eating and drinking with the Victorian lower orders', in T. S. Wagner and N. Hassan (eds), *Consuming Culture in the Long Nineteenth Century: Narratives of Consumption, 1700–1900* (Lanham, MD: Lexington Books, 2007).
61 See, for instance, 'Tea-drinking', *British Medical Journal*, i (1888), 812; 'Insanity and tea-drinking', *Lancet*, 138 (1891), 302.
62 'A Cup of Tea', *Freeman's Journal* (4 June 1872), p. 8.
63 *Irish Times* (20 October 1883), p. 3.
64 G. M. Beard, *A Practical Treatise on Nervous Exhaustion (Neurasthenia): Its Symptoms, Nature, Sequences, Treatment* (New York: William Wood, 1880), p. 150.
65 J. Bourke, *Husbandry to Housewifery: Women, Economic Change, and Housework in Ireland, 1890–1914* (Oxford and New York: Oxford University Press, 1993).
66 'The Abuse of Tea', *Belfast Newsletter* (27 September 1887), p. 6.
67 Miller, *Modern History of the Stomach*, pp. 11–38.
68 A. Leared, *The Causes and Treatment of Imperfect Digestion* (London: John Churchill, 1860), pp. 31–3.
69 See, for instance Pick, *Faces of Degeneration*.
70 *Royal Commission on Labour Part IV*, p. 126
71 Ibid., p.140.
72 Ibid., p. 141.
73 *Royal Commission on Labour. The Agricultural Labourer. Vol. IV. Ireland. Part III*, H. C. 1893–4 [C.6894–xx] xxxvii Pt.1.265, p. 20.
74 Leared, *Causes and Treatment of Imperfect Digestion*, pp. 77–8.
75 'Short Sanitary Sermons', *Freeman's Journal* (14 September 1872), p. 6.
76 *Alleged Increasing Prevalence of Insanity in Ireland: Special Report from the Inspectors of Lunatics to*

the Chief Secretary, H. C. 1894 [C.7331] xliii.647, p. 4.

77 Ibid., p. 5.

78 See P. A. Townend, *Father Mathew, Temperance and Irish Identity* (Dublin: Irish Academic Press, 2002).

79 *Alleged Increasing Prevalence of Insanity in Ireland*, pp. 4–5.

80 Ibid., pp. 5–6, p. 9.

81 Ibid., p. 16.

82 T. Drapes, 'On the alleged increase of insanity in Ireland', *Journal of Mental Science*, 40 (October 1894), 519–48 on pp. 535–6.

5

Purity, adulteration and national economic decline

In 1860, Denis Moylan, the newly appointed Lord Mayor of Dublin, instigated a campaign to clamp down on butchers who knowingly sold contaminated meat. Moylan's crusade garnered considerable support from the *Irish Times* – a newspaper that, in subsequent years, tirelessly vilified butchers, warning on one occasion that 'the poor are plundered in every conceivable manner and to an unconceivable degree'.[1] The newspaper's numerous editorials on the subject portrayed Dublin's poorest residents as daily exposed to fraudulent meat transactions.[2] That same year, new state legislation provided for the appointment of city analysts across Ireland through the implementation of the Act for Preventing the Adulteration of Food or Drink.[3] These analysts were to be scientific men: individuals able to empirically disentangle the constitutive chemical elements of meat, milk, butter, coffee and sugars to reveal deleterious – sometimes poisonous – substances knowingly or inadvertently added. Their services were primarily used to identify food adulteration, although analysts did occasionally investigate fears of poisoning and even love potions.[4]

Evidently, in the 1860s public attention was being drawn to the potential hazards lurking in food, a development reinforced by state bodies having implemented interventionist legislation. Combined, these mutually reinforcing developments sought to tackle a burgeoning anxiety about deleterious food production practices by upholding purity as a new safety standard. These activities coincided with the post-Famine evolution of a consumerist culture outlined in previous chapters. Accordingly, this chapter demonstrates that the advance of consumerism in Ireland was met with new forms of scientific engagement with consumers and producers that encouraged food quality to be considered in new ways. The type of 'quality' endorsed in this rhetoric of purity differed profoundly from the 'quality' identified in mid-century nutritional discourse. Rather than outlining which foodstuffs were healthy or unhealthy for the human system, as mid-century nutritional scientists had done, those concerned about the retail of diseased meat and adulterated food pinpointed biological threats in foodstuffs that were otherwise nutritious and healthy. This step encouraged producers and consumers to internalise further new ways of knowing food, and of appreciating the microscopial content of foodstuffs. In light of this, from the 1860s physicians and public health officials made concerted efforts to delineate the boundaries between purity and impurity and to impose relevant legal standards. This chapter suggests that this war on impure food was fought on various fronts ranging from cattle raising to butchering and dairy production. Moreover, it maintains that advocates of food purity cast purity as an ideal which, if realised, could not fail to bolster physical, moral, economic and national well-being. Irish moral life was to be enhanced as decadent practices became disallowed, economic life was to advance in line with the production of superior foodstuffs and communal health was to be safeguarded. In that sense, food continued to form an important part of broader post-Famine improving regimes.

In addition to outlining post-Famine interventions in food purity, this chapter investigates public resistance to the morally enhancing, scientifically grounded discourses of purity. Resistance played out on two interconnected levels. Firstly, producers contested the need for scientific standards of purity because these threatened to displace long-standing butchering and food production practices. Secondly, resistance emerged in the fraught context of late nineteenth-century Anglo-Irish economic relations. Food adulteration legislation, coupled with an absence of policies to protect the Irish economy, allowed Irish traders and politicians to openly question whether state legislation pertaining to food production was truly benefiting Irish economic life. This pessimistic narrative reflected concern over the economic implications of British rule. Overall, this chapter suggests that the pervasive concept of purity impacted significantly on post-Famine social relations, particularly those between consumers and producers, animals and humans, science and the public and, ultimately, Ireland and Britain. Food purity was an elusive ideal that mutated from a moral concern into an issue of national importance. These debates about economic decline ran in tangent with anxieties about declining physical and psychological well-being. Combined, these mutually reinforcing narratives contributed to a profound cultural pessimism about the trajectory of post-Famine physical, social and economic life. Throughout the period under examination, food continued to offer an important lens through which this perceived decline could be observed, explained and understood.

Implementing adulteration legislation

In 1860, legislation was implemented in Ireland to tackle the retail of diseased meat and adulterated foodstuffs. However, the system initiated suffered from various problems. In 1864, sixty-five people were prosecuted nationwide for food-related offences; a figure that rose to 130 in 1874, 305 in 1884 and as high as 995 in 1894.[5] Although this rise can be partly attributed to a proportionate increase in traders, it also demonstrates the existence of a sustained and reasonably effective effort to tackle rogue food traders. Nonetheless, of the total prosecutions recorded between 1864 and 1894, 46 per cent were made in Leinster (which incorporated Dublin) and 31 per cent in Ulster (incorporating

Belfast). The predominantly rural regions of Connaught and Munster accounted between them for just 23 per cent, with a significant proportion of these prosecutions occurring in the city of Cork.[6] This scenario can be partly accounted for by the uneven dispersion of analysts across Ireland. By 1874, just five had been appointed: John Hodges (Co. Antrim), Cornelius O'Keefe (Co. Cork), Thomas Woods (King's Co.), John Leebody (Co. Londonderry), and Charles Cameron. Although based in Dublin, Cameron's duties stretched far beyond the capital as he was simultaneously appointed in areas including Galway, Carlow and Tipperary.[7] Fifteen counties were left unprovided for, a problem that led Cameron on one occasion to retrospectively conclude that the 1860 Act 'proved to be a dead letter everywhere save in Dublin'.[8] In practice, adulteration regulation was essentially urban-centric. It was in urban arenas that public health officials made concerted efforts to engineer public space into a sanitised site.

Even despite this uneven dispersion, the adulteration Acts had various practical limitations. Figure 5.1 demonstrates that nationwide prosecutions for adulteration rose steadily from the 1860s, and then particularly sharply in the 1890s. The Adulteration of Food and Drink Act of 1860 played an important role in the initial phase although, as Cameron later bemoaned, the punishments issued under it were often inadequate. The Act determined the term 'adulteration' somewhat vaguely. For instance, used tea-leaves that had been re-dried and then re-sold could not be dealt with as that particular practice involved no additions, despite it being very clearly viewed as fraudulent and deceitful.[9] Furthermore, the Act stipulated that traders needed to be given advance notice before their food was taken away for analysis, meaning that an analysis could not take place without the knowledge of the vendor. Vendors could even witness

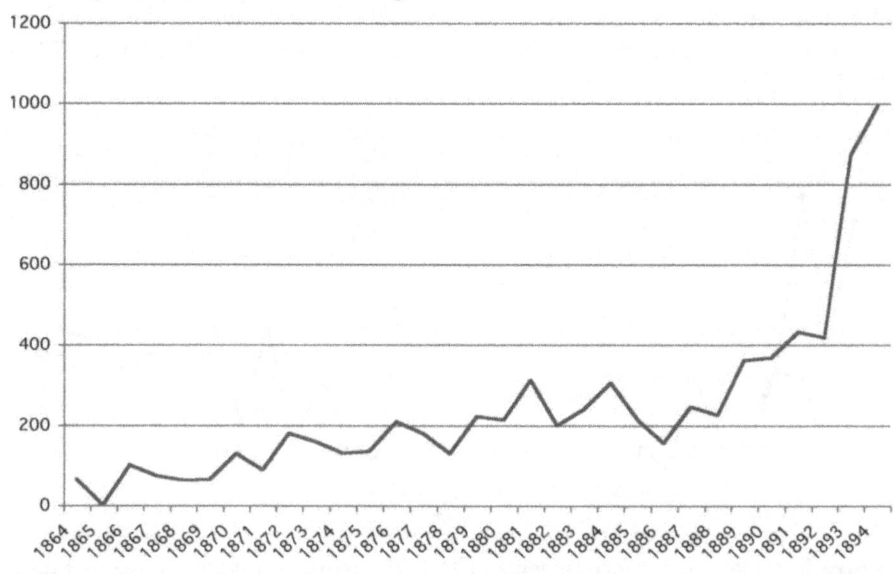

Figure 5.1 Successful prosecutions relating to food adulteration in Ireland, 1864–94.

the analysis if they wished, a scenario that led Cameron to complain that the crowds of angry dairymen and upset wives present at many of his analyses was obstructing his work. In addition, the power to seize food remained confined to a small number of officials. This meant that Dublin's sanitary officers were easily recognised, an issue that reduced the likelihood of vendors handing adulterated samples to them. By 1872, Cameron was able to sardonically claim that 'if I want good cream, I have only to tell an inspector to go and buy some milk for the purpose of analysis, and he gets good cream at the rate of milk'. At worst, inspectors were abused and assaulted.[10] Evidently, legislation that regulated food production had practical limitations.

A further important point is that prosecution levels were disproportionately weighted to incidences concerning non-meat products. Figure 5.2 suggests that a relatively small number of traders in diseased meat were successfully prosecuted in Dublin. In fact, numbers decreased from thirty-five per year in 1873 to below five in the mid-1880s. This is despite, in 1883 alone, some 2,640 slaughterhouse inspections having taken place in the city.[11] Rising prosecution levels from the late 1880s onward can perhaps be accounted for by Cameron having increased the number of civilian sanitary officers operating in Dublin to twelve in 1884. This coincided with a distinct rise in prosecution levels.[12] In addition, the Dairies, Cow Sheds and Milk Shops (Ireland) Order of 1886 demanded that all Dublin-based cow-keeping, dairy and milk businesses register with the Public Health Committee. This Order also stipulated that cow sheds needed to be well lit, ventilated and cleansed; that they must be fitted with asphalted, flagged or bricked floors; that manure be kept separately; and that milk from diseased cows should not be retailed as human food.[13] The impact of these measures was palpable in the steadily rising numbers of prosecutions from the following year. Notably, this rise corresponded with a decline in the pounds of meat confiscated; a figure that almost halved from a total of 120,286 in 1883 to 69,331 in 1893.[14]

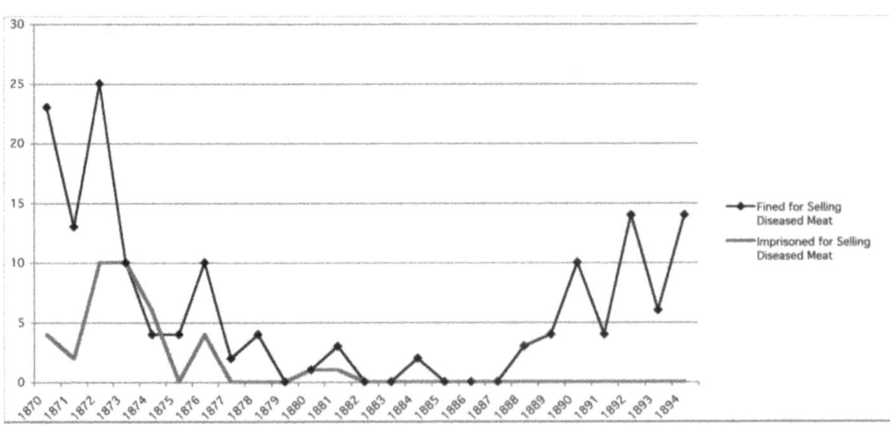

Figure 5.2 Fines and imprisonments in Dublin relating to trading in diseased meat, 1870–94.

Nonetheless, prosecutions for trading in diseased meat remained remarkably low in comparison to other types of adulteration. These low levels of meat-related prosecutions are in many ways surprising given that Dublin boasted an extremely lively meat trade. Juliana Adelman depicts post-Famine Dublin as an 'animal city', a reference to the high visibility of animal life (particularly cattle) intersecting with human existence.[15] The majority of Irish cattle passed through Dublin prior to being shipped alive to England. This coincided with the reorientation of Irish agriculture to cattle output. A vibrant English market existed for Irish meat, encouraged by Ireland's exclusion from the legislative stipulation that producers needed to slaughter animals outside of territorial waters before meat entered British markets.[16] An organised system of managing food quality was established in post-Famine Ireland that sought to tackle problems relating to food purity. Yet its implementation was uneven and met public resistance due to an array of mitigating factors.

'Perfect torpedoes': cattle and urban improvement

From the 1860s onward, shifting ideas on disease epidemiology helped to create an escalating moral panic about the consumption of diseased meat. In that decade, apprehension about meat consumption mounted as the public gradually accepted that infectious diseases could pass from animals to humans. This conceptual development emerged in a period when cattle production acquired importance to the Irish economy. The concept of inter-special disease transmission was nascent and, for that reason, liable to contestation.[17] In fact, it was a highly controversial idea that required considerable cultural and intellectual readjustment for both scientists and the public alike.[18] Consuming diseased flesh had certainly been deplored in earlier periods, but on the basis that the flesh of sick animals seemed to decay quicker than the flesh of healthier animals.[19] In contrast, in the 1860s scientists and public health officials began to suggest that consuming diseased flesh could directly transmit disease from animals to humans.[20] This novel and controversial suggestion threatened to blur the established boundaries between human and non-human life. Simultaneously, it demanded changes in the regulation of animal behaviour to safeguard human existence. Importantly, the idea of animal–human disease transmission engendered new dynamics in Irish food production, although the task of convincing farmers and retailers of the apparent dangers in selling diseased meat was fraught with difficulties.

In the 1860s, Ireland's meat trade suffered from recurrent outbreaks of cattle disease.[21] At worst, critics in England derogatively portrayed Ireland as a nursery and hotbed of pleuro-pneumonia (inflammation of the pleura and lungs).[22] In reality, the country was relatively free from outbreaks in the first half of the decade whereas other regions of the British Isles were struck repeatedly.[23] When Irish incidences did increase in 1866, public health officials implemented legislative measures that demanded the slaughtering and burial of infected animals, as well as those deemed liable to infection.[24] Those involved in debates on this matter raised contentious questions about accountability and whether Irish farmers should be held responsible for the spread of disease. When Professor John Gamgee, principal of the Veterinary College of Edinburgh, read a paper on Irish cattle mortality to the Royal Dublin Society in 1862, he insisted that compensation should be paid to farmers suffering financial losses. In Gamgee's view, an absence of compensatory provision was forcing farmers to retail diseased meat to butchers who, in turn, sold it to the public. Gamgee adopted a compassionate approach by portraying farmers as forced to sell diseased stock to pay rents. He presented the sale of diseased meat as a by-product of uncontrollable epidemiological events. In contrast, Moylan remained unsympathetic, insisting that farmers did not deserve compensation as they had a public responsibility to stem disease propagation. In Moylan's view, negligent farmers should suffer the financial consequences of their own negligence and adopt a sanitary mentality.[25]

Diseased meat continued to enter the public market. Yet the capacity to scientifically detect diseased meat lagged far behind the production of theoretical knowledge on animal–human disease transmission. Keir Waddington argues that, in Britain, meat inspection remained chaotic throughout the late nineteenth century and that practical improvement occurred slowly. This argument is borne out in the Irish context.[26] Even if a meat sample had been analysed and designated as unsound, the intent of the butcher in having *knowingly* retailed it still needed to be legally established. In addition, it proved persistently difficult to empirically confirm whether a meat sample was diseased or not. This problem became evident during the proceedings of a poisoning trial in Newtonwards, Co. Down in 1865 that followed a series of deaths seemingly connected to the consumption of diseased calf meat. According to sworn medical evidence, the meat samples procured differed little in appearance from their disease-free equivalents. Analysts failed to detect poisonous chemicals despite the somewhat obvious connections between the meat consumption and subsequent deaths.[27]

Despite these theoretical and analytical limitations, mounting concern over meat quality resulted in a sustained assault on traditional meat production practices. This impacted most forcefully on urban butchers. Dublin's public health officials and the *Irish Times* aligned themselves with the view that diseased meat was a potential vector of cross-special disease when consumed.[28] This concept, after all, fortified their stance on the need to stamp out the trade in diseased meat.[29] Throughout the remainder of the century, campaigns against urban butchers persisted and proved pivotal to a lively, often emotive, journalistic discussion of public health and sanitation. In 1876, the *Irish Times* warned its readers:

> Look closely at that innocent looking cart leaving the door of a dairy yard with a load of hay late at night, and under that load of hay you will find the leg of a dead cow, the victim of pleuro-pneumonia on her way not to her burial, but to some cheap butcher, who, in all probability, will retail her flesh in some poor neighbourhood as sound beef; or to some army contractor, who will pass the meat into the

> barracks under the nose of some intelligent 'control' officer as contract beef. Look at these lean cows on their way to the store market in Dublin, as they are driven very slowly and gently towards it. Observe the melancholy expression of their eye, the yellow appearance of their skin, and the rough and unwholesome look of their hair. They are driven past the veterinary inspector, who says nothing, and does not object to their entering the market. These cows are perfect torpedoes, charged with destruction.[30]

This powerful indictment reminded readers of the lax procedures in place to stop diseased animals passing through urban space to be eventually consumed by unsuspecting customers. As such, it pointed to the existence of obstacles, and apathy, to food inspection and regulation.

In Dublin, meat inspection was placed under the control of Cameron, an individual appointed as city analyst in 1862 and who held the position until his death in 1921. Throughout his entire period of service, Cameron was remarkably active in identifying and prosecuting traders of unsafe foods. Lydia Carroll has produced an in-depth biography of Cameron, although her study fails to fully investigate the forms of medico-scientific knowledge that informed his activities or public responses to them.[31] Analysis of these imperatives is crucial to understanding the historical regulation of Dublin's food supplies and subsequent public reactions, as well as the further extension of medical authority into day-to-day matters of consumption. Importantly, Cameron openly supported theoretical suppositions that zymotic diseases (acute infectious maladies) and epizootic disease (acute infectious animal maladies) could pass between species via flesh consumption. In one public lecture, he insisted that the consumption of diseased meat passed cow-pox poisons and lung distemper to humans and added his knowledge of a remarkably dangerous parasite known as *trichina spiralis*: a small worm whose movement caused agonising pain as it passed through the human system before ultimately causing an excruciating death.[32] Despite these emotive public warnings, Cameron feared that Dublin's citizens were reluctant to relinquish meat even despite its potentially fatal bodily threats. In response, he initiated a system of market inspection with police assistance. Newly appointed inspectors kept a close watch on markets, slaughterhouses, railway stations, steam-packet offices and other places where butchers prepared or deposited meat. The inspectors immediately dispatched meat that appeared diseased or putrid to Cameron for examination who, upon pronouncing it unfit, would request a magistrate's order for its destruction. Publicly, Cameron remained confident about the efficacy of these measures, later proclaiming that 'I believe that in no other city in the United Kingdom, there have been such large quantities of unsound food detected or so many persons engaged in the diseased meat traffic convicted.'[33]

This concerted assault on retailers of diseased meat held important consequences for urban butchers who found themselves subject to sustained public demonisation. Journalists and public health officials now presented urban slaughterhouses as unhealthy spaces of miasmic disease and urban pollution; sites where unregulated production activity threatened communal health. Their ideas drew from medical thought that understood disease as spread by bad air and insanitary conditions and was increasingly complemented by an awareness of the potential dangers of germs. Urban meat establishments were typically small. Many butchers resided above, or next to, their slaughterhouses.[34] As in many major international cities, Dublin's slaughterhouses became designated as public nuisances as a new sanitary ethos gained currency.[35] Public health officials characterised them as sites of demoralisation, putridity and disease; as spaces where unhealthy and insanitary influences threatened to spill out into the dense residential dwellings with which they co-existed. In these slaughterhouses, so critics asserted, butchers cruelly packed animals together with no ventilation or light where they waited to be converted into food in yards littered with putrefying dung and layers of fresh and dried blood. Slaughterhouses also transmitted immorality, so critics suggested, as the minds of passing children could be vitiated by the sight of ill-treated and slaughtered animals.

Public health officials also condemned slaughterhouses as locus points of infectious diseases ready to spread into public arenas. Disease was omnipresent in butchering establishments, so they insisted. In 1876, a committee of local residents and staff from Cork Street Fever Hospital, Dublin, attributed thirty-three cases of scarlet fever to the decomposed blood present in a nearby newly built slaughterhouse. On the subject of this outbreak, the *Irish Times* declared that 'the storage of gunpowder is less dangerous to the well-being of a city than the establishment of a slaughter-house in the midst of a dense population'.[36] Journalists and other authors invoked key medical texts such as British epidemiologist William Farr's *Vital Statistics* to fortify these arguments. *Vital Statistics* was an influential text that had identified urban butchers as prone to short life expectancy in consequence of exposure to the odour and stench of dead meat, working in sites with limited ventilation and resting on low-lying ground that failed to carry away blood, leaving a residuum of miasma ready to pollute urban environments. Farr had juxtaposed this scenario to the working conditions of the rural meat producer, idyllically depicted as owning vast agricultural space where his cattle roamed freely, air circulated healthily and where trading took place at large country fairs rather than cramped urban market stalls.[37]

Legislation was not always smoothly implemented. At worst, public health and private enterprise interests profoundly clashed as the institutionalisation of public health signalled significant structural changes to traditional butchering practices. The Dublin Improvement Act of 1849 had set out to halt the further construction of private slaughterhouses although trade pressure had forced an additional stipulation to be added that pre-existing owners would not be required to surrender their premises.[38] However, the presence of ever-ageing older establishments in itself did little to improve the public reputation of urban butchering. A series of bills proposed in the 1860s requested that inspectors be granted greater powers to inspect and seize unwholesome meat found in markets and fairs, close existing slaughterhouses and better regulate unhygienic markets.[39] These proved unsuccessful, despite mounting pressure from organisations such as the Dublin Sanitary Association. Like many concerned contemporaries, the Association depicted vulnerable citizens as not only forced to buy meat in Dublin's complex web of private slaughterhouses hidden away in back-street slums, but as also compelled to live beside insanitary business premises. They portrayed the complex geographical outlay of the butchering business as a distinct obstacle to efficient hygienic supervision.[40]

Public and scientific condemnation of centrally located private slaughterhouses encouraged the planning of a large public abattoir at the city outskirts. In his 1861 pamphlet, Michael Cahill, High Sheriff of Kilkenny, proposed that this could be built in the open fields behind Smithfield Market. The land there was high enough to allow for adequate drainage, he maintained, while the nearby Royal Canal would provide an abundant supply of water for cleansing.[41] It was not until 1882 that Dublin's public abattoir finally opened. However, the establishment was built so far outside the city that it fell outside its boundaries, meaning that the city boundaries needed to be extended to incorporate it.[42] The abattoir was essentially built to banish urban butchers from the sanitised public realm of the modern city and exile them from public view.[43] Its presence antagonised private butchers because, as Adelman also discusses, it signalled the deconstruction of long-standing traditions in urban food production.[44]

The Dublin Victuallers Association represented urban butchering interests. Upon the opening of the public abattoir, its members complained that butchers lost the revenue accumulated from manure, offal and blood as these were not returned to them at the public abattoir. Its members also claimed that slaughtering and dressing meat in the abattoir would double expenses as butchers now needed to convey meat to and from Dublin's outskirts before being able to retail their goods at city centre market stalls. This inconvenience, they warned, would force price rises and ultimately damage the national economy by encouraging consumers to buy cheaper imported meat. The Association then accused the Dublin Corporation of seeking to establish a monopoly in the sale of animals by deliberately tarnishing the reputation of butchers.[45] Importantly, its members also strove to undermine the theoretical building blocks of public health legislation. Fully aware of the uncertain nature of expert knowledge on the links between meat and human disease, they pointed to a lack of decisive evidence that slaughterhouses posed a danger to communal health. Dublin's butchers, the Association also reminded its critics, did not seem particularly prone to contracting epidemic disease.[46]

The Association immediately initiated a boycott of the public abattoir other than in cases of absolute necessity. Figure 5.3 indicates a gradual increase in the number of animals slaughtered in the establishment following its opening that then dwindled particularly sharply from 1888. Butchers had the support of prominent cattle dealer William Field, MP for St Patrick's district and member of the Dublin Corporation.[47] The abattoir's limited success in sanitising the meat trade, as demonstrated by the data in Figure 5.3, ultimately led to the transfer of its custody from the Public Health Committee to the Market Committee in 1892.[48] Evidently, a profound clash of ideas existed on who held authority over urban meat production: official, expert or business bodies. Those

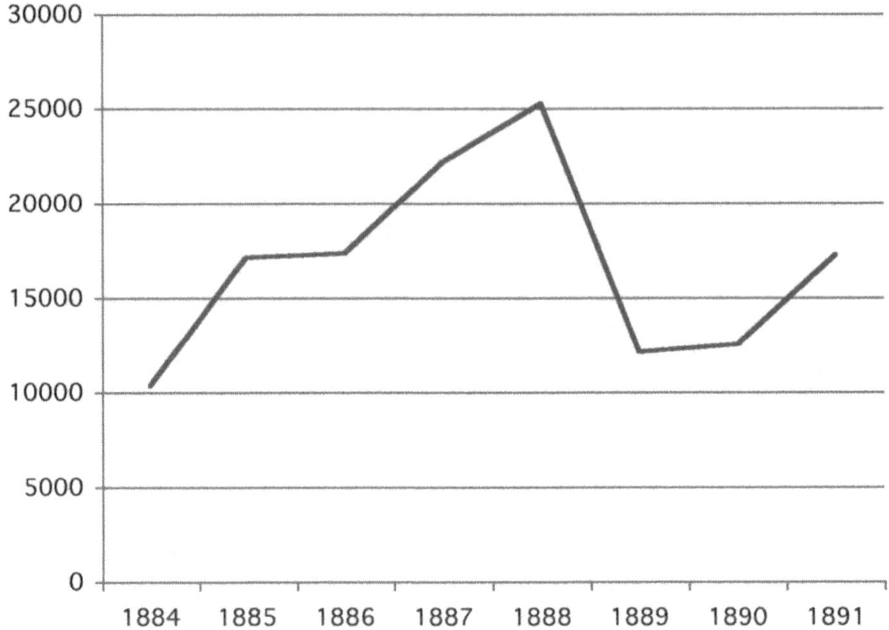

Figure 5.3 Number of animals slaughtered at Dublin's public abattoir, 1884–91.

opposed to public slaughterhouses presented idyllic visions of clean, sanitary and healthy cities. For them, the removal of butchers from the city would modernise, improve and reform the consistency of urban life itself. This rhetoric – grounded in new forms of sanitary science – antagonised traders who rebelled against their public demonisation and rallied against the penetrative scientific ideologies that underpinned their social castigation.

Similar debates surfaced in Belfast. Concern over diseased meat consumption mounted in the late 1890s. Then, only meat produced in Belfast was liable for inspection in the city. However, rising demand encouraged butchers to retail meat purchased from further afield. This made regulation more difficult. Objections to the city's public abattoir persisted and were, perhaps, not entirely unjustified given an ongoing absence of conclusive evidence about the dangers of urban butchering. At a meeting of the Belfast Corporation in 1895, Councillor Masterson argued that scientific alarmists were 'frightening poor, timid people' and insisted that they should moderate their ideas. In contrast, Councillor O'Neill maintained that scientists were not alarmists and, if anything, more meat inspections should be undertaken.[49] This illustrative example reveals a continuing diversity of attitudes to the apparent dangers of meat. Whether or not hygienic science was a socially protective force or a false form of knowledge continued to be heavily debated.

Nonetheless, in October 1900 the Belfast Corporation initiated a policy of inspecting all meat killed outside the city to be sold at Belfast's markets, imposing a sharp fine of up to 40 s. on offenders.[50] This resulted in a declining usage of private slaughterhouses external to the city and an increase in the numbers of cattle being processed in the public abattoir – a dramatic rise from 35,273 in 1904 to 59,003 in 1906. In 1909, local authorities proposed that Belfast's abattoir should be extended to accommodate this demand and fitted with up-to-date technologies and a stomach cleaning depot. This new design allowed up to 200 cattle to be converted into food every ten hours while animals could be killed, bled and dressed in forty-five minutes. An inquiry in 1909 allowed producers to express their objections. At this, Samuel Carson, president of the Belfast Masters Butcher Association, complained that the site rested on top of a disused sewage works and had been built next to a chemical works. In consequence, Carson asserted, he had not once used the abattoir in the previous seventeen years and would be less inclined to do so in light of the proposed modifications. Carson also objected to the fact that butchers had to kill animals consecutively in the new abattoir. Tradition and business practicalities dictated that three days of killing per week was appropriate at the start of the week so that trading could take place at weekend market days.[51]

Public abattoirs emblematised new, modern and 'improved' modes of food production, although private butchers (correctly) interpreted these sites as a conceptual and practical threat to traditional, small-scale operations. Private slaughterhouses remained in operation as trade alliances formed to protect the interests of smaller butchers and their right to slaughter cattle on private premises. These alliances vigorously objected to the reformist tendencies of bureaucrats and public health authorities and openly questioned the validity and empirical basis of medico-scientific ideologies.[52] The science itself, they claimed, was dubious.

Negotiating adulteration

Meat was not the only foodstuff that fell under the scientific gaze of the food analyst. In 1863, the clerk of the South Dublin Union dispatched two sugar samples to Cameron for analysis. The Board of Guardians feared that suppliers were mixing workhouse sugar with sand and adding water to sugar bins to add weight and increase its cost. Cameron's subsequent analysis confirmed that the sugar was indeed damp and that it contained treacle, sporules of fungus, particles of cane, albumen and starch granules. A more alarming discovery was an estimated 100,000 minute beetles in each pound of the sugar 'closely resembling in appearance and nature the insect which, by burrowing into the skin, produces the itch [scabies]'.[53] On the subject of this unearthing, the *Irish Times* asserted that 'the child that swallowed ten grains of that sugar swallowed 500 living, burrowing beetles! Is it any wonder that the young droop and fade away in the workhouse? Need we be surprised that so many young creatures die of illness that we cannot account for?'. The newspaper warned that traders were probably supplying similar concoctions of sugar to the public. 'This is a public question', asserted the *Irish Times*, 'and one not confined to the inmates of the poorhouse.

Sugars of this horrible description may be commonly sold, and the only way to stop the sale of them is by prosecuting those who sell them.'[54] Expressing similar revulsion, the *Dublin Medical Press* also wondered if the analysed sugar samples represented the quality of public supplies.[55] In all probability, Irish citizens had unknowingly consumed harmless mites for centuries. What was radically different about the situation in 1863 was that microscopial analysis could now identify previously unknown additions in food supplies and proclaim them unfit for human consumption. It was, perhaps, not the case that Dublin's sugar supplies were worsening but instead that the analytical gaze of medical science was rendering its sometimes disturbing content visible for the first time. These new analytical strategies helped to further refine ideas of what constituted 'pure' and 'impure' food and activated new forms of social intervention.

In Britain, prominent food reformer Arthur Hill Hassall had recently spearheaded a successful anti-adulteration campaign.[56] A corresponding crusade had yet to emerge in Ireland, a situation lamented in a *Dublin Medical Press* editorial published in 1856 that warned that Dublin's bakers and grocers daily dispensed 'alumed bread and poisonous potations'.[57] Characteristically, the nationalist press blamed discoveries of adulterated food in Ireland entirely on British influence – a tactic that added weight to political agendas of abstaining from trade with Britain but which achieved little in the way of seriously tackling adulteration. In the late 1850s, *The Nation* printed numerous editorials with provocative titles such as 'How we are Poisoned by Civilised and Enlightened British Merchants'.[58] In 1867, the publication conceded that some Irish traders adulterated but insisted that they never stooped to English levels of adding powdered glass to snuff, sawdust to cayenne pepper and red lead to curry powder, although they might, admittedly, add a little water to milk or alum to bread dough from time to time. These claims, they hoped, would increase trade among Irish businessmen.[59]

Despite *The Nation*'s efforts to distinguish between national standards of food morality, it seemed increasingly apparent that traders were adulterating food supplies in Ireland. Furthermore, Irish adulteration practices often involved adding far more than harmless substances such as water and alum. In 1870, the Dublin Public Health Committee accused Paul Willock, a vendor on South George's Street, Dublin, of adding mineral poisons to his confectionary and selling sweets to impoverished children as luxury items. Local physicians had noticed high incidences of stomach complaints among the children of that area and reported Willock. Cameron's subsequent investigations revealed that vermillion and mercury had been added to lozenges and sugar sticks and that sugared almonds were packed with chromate of lead, a substance believed to cause diarrhoea and wasting even when ingested in small doses. At the legal proceedings that ensued, Willock was ordered to pay a fine of three guineas although, revealingly, the judge who prosecuted him described the Adulteration of Food and Drinks Act as 'about as stupid an Act of Parliament as ever was passed, as it included in the same category adulteration by means of harmless ingredients and adulteration by the aid of poisonous substances'.[60]

Poisoned sweets were the most clear-cut example of dangerous adulteration and were undeniably integral to anti-adulteration rhetoric. James Dunne of the Royal College of Surgeons in Ireland wrote frequently to the *Freeman's Journal* on the matter. In 1873, he argued:

> No wonder that the children of trades people and the poor are sickly, and frequently of immature development, when, besides all the other evils of a crowded city, they are beset on all sides of the street by unripe or rotten fruit, unwholesomely prepared sweets, and advocates of plaster of Paris as a juvenile luxury.[61]

On another occasion, he emotively asserted:

> With the echo of cholera rolling over the seas to us, with the Liffey sending forth night and day its pestilential breath, with the adulteration of food, and through the great heat now the danger of tainted meat, heaven knows the poor have enough to contend against without permitting their children to be poisoned wholesale by 'lime' dipped in sugar-water and peppermint, rotten fruit, and horrible mixtures called 'taffy'.[62]

As with discussion of diseased meat, public representations of food adulteration emphasised working-class vulnerability and were framed in terms of social improvement. Few could deny that arsenic or lead should not be added to children's sweets. Insects were also unwanted additions, although journalists tended to attribute their discovery to carelessness rather than deliberate intent. However, regardless of the frequent publication of stories of children succumbing to the deadly effects of poisonous sweets and insect-ridden sugar supplies, the majority of samples investigated by city analysts were less provocative and newsworthy, focusing as they did on more trivial matters such as the amount of water in milk or salt in butter. From a total of 882 analyses made by Cameron in 1884, 788 were of milk, buttermilk or sweetmilk (or fresh milk). In that year, he examined thirty-one butter samples while the remaining sixty-three were coffee, mustard, pepper, ginger, flour, oatmeal or drugs.[63] Despite the existence of a sensationalised public rhetoric on adulteration, Cameron's work mostly focused on regulating dairy production.

In many ways, the addition of non-toxic substances to dairy produce was a thornier problem. Water was not a poisonous addition (presuming it was knowingly free from water-borne disease). Furthermore, water was traditionally used in milk and butter production. In these instances, the boundaries between what did or did not constitute adulteration were relatively fluid. Late nineteenth-century analysts were armed with an ability to separate dairy products into their constitutive elements to precisely reveal percentages of solid substances, fats and water. They evaporated milk to reveal its fat content and solidity, and ignited it to reveal its ash content.[64] They dried and weighed butter to determine its water content, and burnt its fat in capsules, or dissolved it with pure ether, to reveal ash content.[65] They optimistically upheld these analytical techniques as a key to ending shameful production practices. One anonymous letter published in the *Freeman's Journal* in 1863 confidently claimed that 'chemical science and law combined will be found, if only availed of by the public, to be more than a match for the roguish dairyman, and will compel him, for his own sake, to abandon his dishonest practices'.[66]

After the Famine, milk was increasingly consumed by urban communities.[67] The unwelcome practice of watering down urban milk supplies captured public attention from the 1860s, generating fears that traders were depriving unsuspecting consumers of nutrition. Prosecutions mostly resulted in a fine, the amount of which was relative to the quantity of water introduced into the product. Analysis of fines awarded in Dublin in 1881 reveals that judges typically ruled that those found guilty of adulterating milk with a water content of 12 per cent pay a fine of £2, 20 per cent of £3, 50 per cent of £9 and 100 per cent of £19.[68] Yet even as late as 1887 the *Irish Times* could be found publishing accounts of a Dublin 'milk-ring': a system of over a thousand dairies in which producers adulterated milk with as much water as possible before selling it to the unsuspecting poor.[69] The enduring nature of this problem suggests that dairy producers easily met the cost of fines or that they perceived the chances of being caught by the law to be so slim that they continued to adulterate.

Although milk traders failed to systematically organise themselves against adulteration laws, localised agitation was common, particularly when the sanitising ethos of medical science and public health was seen to have impinged upon traditional rural practices. In 1879, the *Belfast Evening News* argued that the Food and Drugs Act of 1875 was harsh on rural farmers. On this subject, the newspaper asserted that 'we have no hesitation in saying that if the milk in most farmhouses in the country where no milk is sold all being used by the family were analysed during the winter season, it would be condemned by some analysts'. The editorial insisted that producers found it necessary to add water when separating butter to make buttermilk. Yet the adulteration Acts had imposed new standards that effectively prohibited this traditional custom. The newspaper also suggested that the expert opinion of the analyst – intent on uncovering unscrupulous trading practices – almost always over-ruled pleas of lack of intention made by dairy producers.

The *Belfast Evening News* penned its condemnation shortly after the trial of John M'Keown, of Newtonbreds, Co. Down. Prior to M'Keown's trial, samples of his milk had been dispatched to Cameron in Dublin who determined it to be adulterated with 16 per cent water and Hodges in Belfast who independently concluded that the sample was unadulterated. Ultimately, a judge dismissed the case on the basis that that the transit to Dublin seemed to have affected the sample.[70] Nonetheless, controversies such as these undermined public faith in new standards of purity and the legislation in place to enforce them.[71] In the same year, a group of farmers met in Holywood, Co. Down, to discuss how to protect their businesses from the analysts. At this meeting, Capt. William Graham of Ballydavey asserted that farmers were now able to add only 10 per cent water if they were to avoid prosecution, despite that amount being inadequate to properly churn milk. Moreover, Graham insisted that a reduced water content resulted in the production of inferior butter that failed to stay fresh for long, a problem already being noticed by English butter dealers who had objected to the declining quality of Irish dairy produce. A pledge to stop delivering milk to urban centres 'until justice was delivered to Holywood' was agreed upon.[72] The boundaries between purity and impurity were undeniably more fragile in relation to dairy produce than poisoned sweets and sugar supplies. Echoing corresponding debates on diseased meat, those opposed to adulteration legislation for practical and financial reasons framed scientific knowledge as a threat to commercial interests and openly challenged the validity of its investigative techniques. Water was a traditional element of milk and butter production and, in any case, could not easily be depicted as particularly harmful. This confusion complicated definitions of adulteration and purity and sparked considerable tension between public and scientific realms.

High water content was not the only problem identified in milk supplies in the late nineteenth century. In the 1870s, as Jacob Steere-Williams convincingly demonstrates, the issue of milk quality evolved from a moral and economic anxiety into a major public health concern, once medical scientists began to suspect that diseases such as typhoid might transmit through liquids.[73] Tuberculosis, too, came under suspicion of being spread through milk consumption. This shift in emphasis reflected changing ideas about disease specificity and the gradual acceptance of ideas that many diseases had specific bacteriological or pathogenic causes. Medical scientists were now identifying germs as omnipresent and responsible for many illnesses. This reductionist perspective created new food-related concerns.[74] In Dublin, Cameron was at the forefront of investigations into these potential links. In 1878, he speculated that an outbreak of typhoid fever in suburban Pembroke could be traced to unhygienic local milk supplies. Several typhoid cases had surfaced during the Christmas period and Cameron later confirmed that the affected households had all bought milk from the same dairy. Cameron inspected the dairy yard, observing its relative cleanliness. Yet he noted that the site did not have a latrine and that the cow manure, situated close to the cows, was also used to deposit human faeces. Suspicious, Cameron speculated that polluted water must have entered the milk supplies during an illegal act of watering down milk. He fortified his hypothesis with a shrewd observation that a third of the cows at the dairy yard were not giving milk, despite the vendor having supplied an impressive forty households with milk. Cameron used this discovery to posit that the milk supply had acted as a vector of typhoid.[75]

Cameron's report also cited dust and dirt as potential causative factors of typhoid by suggesting that morbid material had blown into the milk. Drawing from the recently published ideas of prominent Irish physicist John Tyndall, he argued that the air teemed with solid particles of mineral, vegetable and animal matter that could infiltrate milk supplies should care not be taken.[76] His further microscopial analysis identified that that the muslin that had been used for filtering during milking was covered with cow hairs, epithelial debris, cow dung, straw, hay, vegetable fibres, soot, clay, ash, wool, linen and cotton. Cameron depicted a microcosmic world, invisible to the human eye, that, once revealed by the techniques of modern analytical science, could be cleansed and sanitised to eradicate noxious influences from public space.[77] His ideas were highly speculative. In fact, the existence and nature of this microscopic realm was a minefield of debate, speculation and counter-arguments.[78] Ultimately, Cameron's views on typhoid and milk remained mostly forgotten until British Medical Officer of Health Arthur Newsholme investigated links between sewage-polluted oysters and typhoid over ten years later.[79] At the time, the Royal College of Physicians of Ireland dismissed Cameron's opinions for the reason that typhoid had been present in other regions of Dublin not supplied with milk from the dairy yard in question.[80]

In the face of scepticism, Cameron persistently and vigorously reiterated his views on how germs and bacteria might spread through food. In 1882, he traced an outbreak of abdominal problems in Dublin to the presence of particles of cow's hair, straw, organic debris and bacteria in milk supplies that had been rendered visible microscopically.[81] Two years later, in the *Dublin Journal of Medical Science*, he recorded that he had traced the aetiological origins of certain gastric illnesses to the consumption of unobservable moulds in bread, animal flesh infected with parasitical disease, worms entering the body with unclean salads and vegetables, and microscopic mushrooms – creatures on the borderline between animal and vegetable.[82] Cameron's somewhat apocalyptic vision of Irish urban food supplies implied that nature itself was contaminated and impure but could be cleansed and purified through human agency.

At worst, medical science's ever-expanding recommendations on food safety came to be perceived by the public as offering only bewildering, sometimes contradictory, advice. In 1873, the *Freeman's Journal* complained that:

> The perusal of those warnings which are now daily given by learned members of scientific bodies is calculated to have a very depressing effect on the constitution of plain men and women. We must not drink milk lest we should get typhus, nor water lest we should get typhoid, nor whiskey lest we should tempt cholera, nor tea lest we should be poisoned outright. There are very few eatables in the world worth talking about – at least there are so many ingredients in our common foods that one's dinner is becoming a matter of serious thought.[83]

Evidently, public health officials radically reconsidered food content in the late nineteenth century. Although adulteration through deliberate human activity was a pivotal focal point of concern in the 1860s, this extended to matters of cleanliness and disease management as scientists discerned links between germs, food and disease. Food was no longer considered solely in terms of its chemical influence in the body. Public health officials rethought food in terms of its potential bacterial content and the potentially harmful influences of previously unknown organisms in the human body. This development spawned new encounters between man and the natural world, consumers and producers, and science and the public. Adulteration legislation was relatively effective in Dublin although the new food discourses that it engendered, mirroring contemporaneous discussion of meat, caused tension between traditional and modern modes of producing food.

Purity and national economic decline

Towards the close of the century, the shifting biologically grounded public health imperatives that had manifested in the form of a vigorous anti-adulteration campaign became gradually entangled with debates on the Anglo-Irish economy. This was acutely palpable in discussion of Irish dairy production. Food purity elevated into a topic with national implications as fears escalated about the declining condition of the post-Famine food economy. Since the Famine, merchants in the south of Ireland had profited from a rising demand for Irish butter in Britain – a fortunate outcome of geographical proximity. The Cork Butter Exchange boosted Ireland's agricultural economy.[84] Yet, from the 1870s, Irish butter prices steadily collapsed in the face of foreign competition from Scandinavian countries, particularly Denmark. Butter imports, meanwhile, rose from £500,382 in 1860 to £1,172,732 in 1870 and £1,561,233 in 1880.[85] This rise was striking, even if inflation is taken into account. The domestic butter industry was also adversely affected by the fraudulent retail of butterine (a watered-down variety of butter later renamed margarine) as butter.[86]

In the 1880s, something seemed to be fundamentally wrong with Irish butter production and its international reputation. Evidence given to the Select Committee on Industries (Ireland) by Manchester butter trader J. B. Dowdall in 1884 ascribed declining international interest in Irish butter to its 'irregularity in quality, to the unsightly packages – the old brown firkin being the ugliest and dirtiest seen in England – to the adulteration of salt and water, and to the Cork branding system, driving the large wholesale dealers on to foreign and American butter'. He evocatively asserted that in Cork he had observed 'butter so packed that, whilst it was fresh in the centre, the whole circumference was lined an inch or two thick, like the bark of a tree, with old, tallow-lie butter of the previous season', while 'some first corks contained ten and eleven per cent of water'. Dowdall warned: 'let anyone try to imagine the wrath of the English buyer when every now and then he is treated to a specimen like this of our national manufacture, and how he will anathematise all things Irish'. In Dowdall's view, the 'roguery' of adulteration bore damaging long-term implications for the Irish butter industry.[87]

These debates mirrored, and in many ways reinforced, a persistent cultural pessimism about national well-being. They coincided, after all, with growing apprehension about the Irish poor descending into a chronic condition of tea-driven degeneration. These interlocked concerns strengthened arguments that post-Famine food reform had failed to deliver its promises of national regeneration and improvement. In these debates, traditional, perhaps more careless, Irish production techniques came to be deeply problematised and identified as requiring improvement. In 1882, Charles F. Bastable, professor of Political

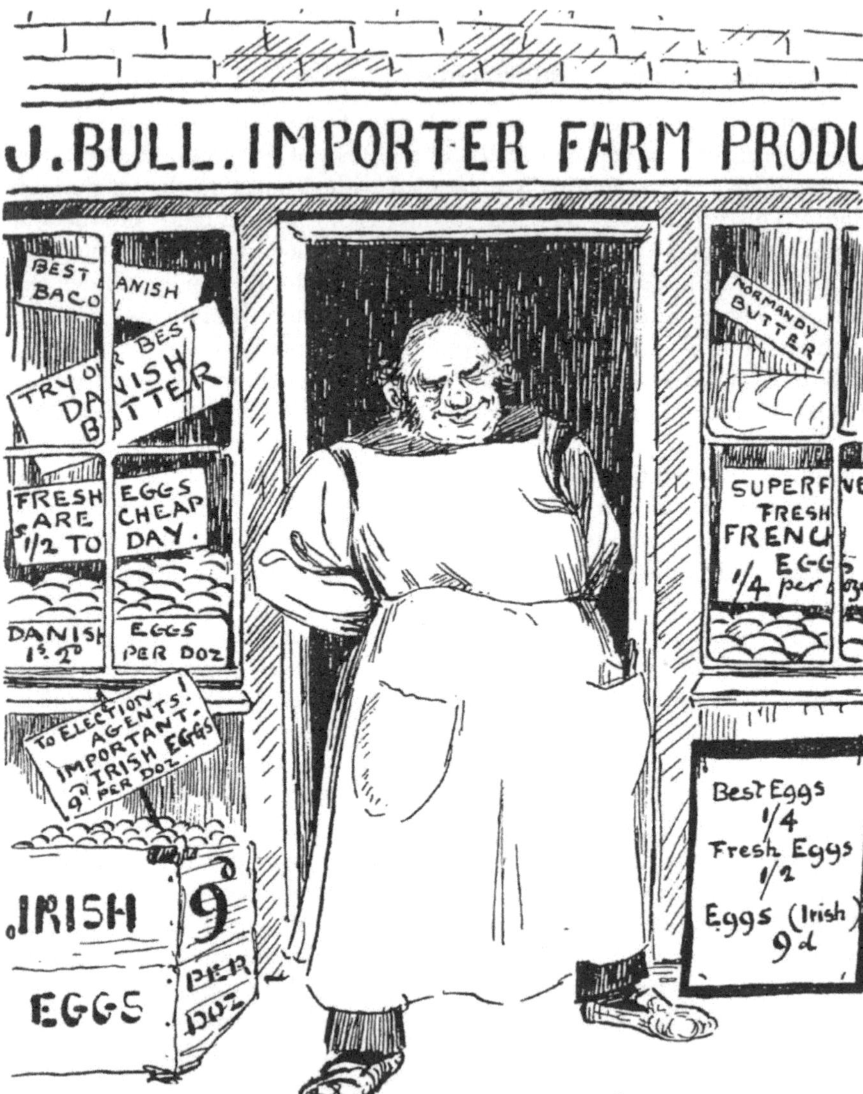
J. BULL. IMPORTER FARM PROD
NORMANDY BUTTER
FRESH ARE 1/2 TO
EGGS CHEAP DAY.
DANISH 1s. 2d
EGGS PER DOZ
TO ELECTION AGENTS! IMPORTANT. IRISH EGGS 9d. PER DOZ
IRISH EGGS 9d PER DOZ
Best Eggs 1/4
Fresh Eggs 1/2
Eggs (Irish) 9d

JOHN BULL'S BREAKFAST.

Figure 5.4 'John Bull's Breakfast', *Irish Homestead*, 1896.

Economy at the University of Dublin, spoke to the Statistical and Social Inquiry Society of Ireland on the subject. He stressed that Irish butter was being manufactured in undesirable conditions that rendered it unappealing to English customers. Butter makers produced it in old-fashioned casks, he argued, allowing dirt to infiltrate butter. These casks compared unfavourably to the clean modern cases used in Scandinavia that had a more inviting appearance. Bastable also regretted that practices of adulterating with water and salt to secure maximum profit had tainted foreign perceptions of Irish butter. In his view, the problem was not entirely the fault of small Irish producers whom he depicted as either unaware of modern, improved production techniques or too poor to buy the modern appliances used in Scandinavia.[88]

Bastable was a proponent of free trade. His proposed solutions naturally gravitated towards securing improvements in butter production without interfering with *laissez-faire* principles of free trade.[89] Constitutional nationalists framed the problem as an inevitable outcome of ineffective central legislation rather than careless or fraudulent economic behaviour. Their intervention helped to politicise the issue of purity. At the Select Committee on Irish Industries of 1884, William John Lane, Irish Parliamentary Party (IPP) politician and member of the Cork Corporation, insisted that the matter was now a national question as butter was crucial to Irish prosperity.[90] Lane asserted:

> To discuss the question of the Irish butter industry from either the farmer's or trader's point of view would be an inexcusable mistake. Its national importance could hardly be over-estimated. The manufacture of butter is the staple industry of Ireland, and any close student of what is going on in other countries must recognise that the future agricultural prosperity of Ireland largely depends on the full development of its dairy industries.

Lane continued by implicating free trade as detrimental to Irish national interests. Ireland, he insisted, was a country whose natural resources favoured butter manufacturing and whose geographical position placed it in an advantageous position in terms of trading with Britain.[91] Lane's perspective implied inertia on the part of the state to adequately encourage Irish industry, allowing him to form a critique of Anglo-Irish economic relations. Why, he asked, had the state failed to provide systematic dairy education in the way that Danish state bodies had done? Why had it not yet established agricultural schools that might revive Irish dairy farming and counter Danish competition?[92]

Questions such as these added new layers to ongoing debates about purity. For some decades, anti-adulteration rhetoric had overtly targeted the moral standing of producers and traders who engaged in fraudulent transactions. On the contrary, Lane's perspective insisted that adulteration stemmed from deficient knowledge and expertise rather than solely from a lack of moral restraint. He called upon the state to rectify this situation by asserting that political inaction had determined the conditions now retarding Irish economic advancement. Not everyone shared his views. When Cameron discussed the matter at a meeting of the Society of Public Analysts in 1893, he argued that the root of the problem rested in the ignorance of farmers in the art of making good butter. Cameron maintained that producers needed to elevate the Irish butter industry to a level of perfection on a par with Denmark where a scientifically advised government had intervened and expanded the butter market. Yet prominent chemist and analyst for Co. Longford, Charles Robert Tichborne, although acquiescing on the need for education, asserted that many small farmers were far from ignorant and knew precisely what they were doing when adding water to their produce, creating a false economy.[93]

Public concern mounted in 1893 when analysts prosecuted a group of Irish butter traders in Manchester; a development that captured the attention of the Irish Butter Association who feared that the publicity surrounding the prosecution was further tarnishing the international reputation of Irish butter. Working-class communities in the north-west of England preferred the salty taste of Irish butter to its Danish equivalent.[94] The saltiness of Irish butter was suited to the atmosphere of industrial factories as it kept fresh for longer.[95] However, in Ireland, analysts defined high quantities of salt as a fraudulent addition. The Manchester legal proceedings visibly demonstrated ongoing tensions between butter-making traditions and the new demands placed upon them by public health officials. Traditional production forms threatened the integrity of Irish trade but, for some, modern trade devalued the quality and taste of Irish produce, ensuring that it lost its distinctive qualities of Irishness.[96] Problematically, city analysts in Manchester and Salford – highly important cities for the Cork butter industry – were particularly efficient prosecutors.[97] Soon afterwards, the Irish Dairy Association was formed, a group who, in 1895, argued that if Ireland was independent, appropriate legislation would have been passed to protect Irish dairy producers. The Association also evocatively cited a lack of education combined with widespread economic depression as having led to the 'starving of Ireland'.[98]

The unresolved question of what precisely constituted an unadulterated dairy product was at the heart of public debate on dairy produce and the flailing Irish economy. The reputation of food analysis suffered when traders and judges condemned it as an unwelcome, intrusive part of a bureaucratic system and a hindrance to trade. Public opinion was often sympathetic to dairy producers. When Judge Adams reversed the decision of a Co. Limerick prosecution where a fine of ten shillings had been inflicted upon a producer manufacturing butter with 19 per cent water content, he joked that only analysts believed 16 per cent to be the largest permissible quantity, adding that some of the best Irish butters contained 22 per cent. This provoked Cameron who promptly wrote an angry letter to the *Freeman's Journal*, in which he asserted that:

> Those who utter rubbish about twenty or thirty per cent of water in butter not being adulteration are doing their best to kill the Irish butter trade, and the judges who accept such trash as reliable evidence stand in just as much need of the excess of water being kneeded out of the gruel they call their brains. But if judges and butter dealers alike are satisfied to see Ireland's remaining industry destroyed,

> they are entitled, we suppose, to do what they please with their own. Well they are doing it, and for middle-headed, blind, reckless rushing to ruin their conduct has no parallel in any other trade.[99]

In some legal proceedings, judges entirely rejected the authority of analysts. In September 1894, a judge fined a farmer in Nenagh, Co. Tipperary for producing butter with an 18 per cent water content. That same day, magistrates in Mitchelstown, Co. Cork, refused to impose a fine on a farmer whose butter had a 20 per cent water content. In response, the *Freeman's Journal* portrayed farmers as persecuted individuals who lacked access to the resources needed to raise their butter quality to the standards insisted upon by food analysts. The newspaper asserted:

> To set up such a chemist's notion as the law, and punish as criminals those who fail to realise it, is the height of stupidity, as well as the height of tyranny. Let the question be determined once and for all, and determined according to the common sense of the manufacturers, merchants and consumers, and not according to the idiosyncrasies of scientific gentlemen in their laboratories. Meantime, we hope that the magistrates will be careful not to punish innocent and industrious people who do their best, and who are making an article that is bought for what it is by the general consumer, who much prefers his own taste to Sir Charles Cameron's.[100]

Conclusion

Apprehension about national bodily well-being increased after the Famine, creating a powerful discourse of national degeneration that castigated excessive tea drinking among the poor. Ireland also seemed to be entering into a simultaneous condition of economic decline. To a large extent, the amelioration of stagnation in food production hinged upon issues of purity and adulteration. Initially, those concerned about food quality targeted immoral trading practices. Public health officials offered solutions by constructing new definitions of food quality and legally imposing new standards. They also sought to redefine food production as a scientifically defined sphere of activity. Although initially framed as a measure to protect working-class health, purity control gradually evolved into an important economic and national matter. A lack of adherence to new food standards became identified as having tarnished Ireland's international reputation and as stifling economic vitality. Although the terms of the debates over food purity shifted dramatically throughout the late nineteenth century, the accuracy of the science that had underpinned the new demands placed on producers often seemed precarious and, at worst, seemed to threaten traditional production methods. Purity persisted as a national issue, prompting questions about the accountability of dairy producers and the extent to which they could be persuaded, or educated, to modernise and reform their practices. Simultaneously, food production evolved into a highly politicised issue that served as a prism through which British influence in Ireland was, for some, being rendered visible and assessed. Issues such as these, as demonstrated in the following chapter, were to play a formative role in the development of new educational techniques.

Notes

1 *Irish Times* (26 December 1862), p. 2.
2 'The Lord Mayor's Court Yesterday', *Irish Times* (11 April 1863), p. 3.
3 An Act for Preventing the Adulteration of Articles of Food or Drink (23 & 24 Vict.) C. A. O. LXXXIV.
4 C. A. Cameron, *Reminiscences of Sir Charles A. Cameron* (Dublin: Hodges and Figgis, 1913), p. 161.
5 *Judicial Statistics Ireland,* Command Papers, Accounts and Papers, Commons, 1865 [3563], lii.657; 1875 [c.1295], lxxxi.259; 1884–5 [c.4554], lxxxvi.243; 1895 [c.7799], cviii.323.
6 Ibid.
7 *Returns of All Counties in Ireland in which Public Analysts have been Appointed, with Names, Dates of Appointment, and Salaries*, H. C. 1874 [C.410] lvi.861.
8 C. A. Cameron, 'Note on the operation in Dublin of the Acts relating to adulteration', *Analyst,* 10 (October 1885), 175–9.
9 C. A. Cameron, 'Half-yearly report on public health', *Dublin Journal of Medical Science*, 3 (1 May 1872), 394–425 on pp. 409–10.
10 *Report from the Select Committee on Adulteration of Food*, H. C. 1856 [379] viii.1, pp. 226–7.
11 Royal College of Physicians in Ireland (hereafter RCPI). *Report on the State of Public Health in Dublin* (1883), pp. 44–5.
12 RCPI, *Report on the State of Public Health in Dublin* (1883), p. 50.
13 RCPI, *Report on the State of Public Health in Dublin* (1886), p. 69.
14 RCPI, *Report on the State of Public Health in Dublin* (1883–1893).
15 J. Adelman, *Animal City* (forthcoming).
16 Turner, *After the Famine*, p. 157.
17 M. Worboys, 'Germ theories of disease and British veterinary medicine, 1860–1890', *Medical History*, 35 (July 1991), 308–27.
18 A. Hardy, "Animals, disease and man: making connections', *Perspectives in Biology and Medicine*, 46:2 (Spring 2003), 200–15 on p. 203.
19 A. Hardy, 'Pioneers in the Victorian provinces: veterinarians, public health and the urban animal economy', *Urban History*, 29:3 (December 2002), 372–87 on p. 376.
20 K. Waddington, *The Bovine Scourge: Meat, Tuberculosis and Public Health, 1850–1914* (Woodbridge: The Boydell Press, 2006), p. 6.
21 See Adelman, *Animal City*, chapter two; A. W. Foot, *Symptoms and Treatment of the Cattle Plague* (Dublin and London: McGlashan and Gill, 1866).
22 *Farmer's Magazine*, 36 (July 1869), 55.
23 J. Gamgee, *The Cattle Plague* (London: R. Harwicke, 1866), p. 273.
24 Cattle Disease Act (Ireland), 1866 (29 & 30 Vict.) A. P. IV.
25 'Royal Dublin Society', *Irish Times* (15 December 1862), p. 4.
26 Waddington, *Bovine Scourge*, p. 9.
27 'Diseased Meat in Dublin', *Irish Times* (23 October 1866), p. 4.
28 G. Jones, *'Captain of all these Men of Death': The History of Tuberculosis in Nineteenth and Twentieth-Century Ireland* (Amsterdam: Rodopi, 2001), pp. 102–3.
29 See also A. Hardy, 'John Bull's beef: meat hygiene and veterinary public health in England in the twentieth century', *Review of Agricultural and Environmental Studies*, 91:4

(2010), 369–92 on p. 379.
30 'The Dairy System in Dublin', *Weekly Irish Times* (4 November 1876), p. 2.
31 L. Carroll, *Champion of the Poor: Sir Charles Cameron, Medical Officer of Health, 1862–1921* (Dublin: A. & A. Farmar, 2010).
32 C. A. Cameron, 'Our Sanitary Commission No. XII: On Diseased and Unsound Food', *Freeman's Journal* (26 September 1873), p. 2.
33 Ibid.
34 M. J. Winstanley, *The Shopkeeper's World, 1830–1914* (Manchester: Manchester University Press, 1993), p. 140; I. MacLachlan, 'A bloody offal nuisance: the persistence of private slaughter-houses in nineteenth-century London', *Urban History*, 34:2 (2007), 227–54 on p. 227.
35 Prunty, *Dublin Slums*, pp. 91–6.
36 *Irish Times* (10 April 1876), p. 4.
37 *Irish Times* (30 March 1876), p. 4; W. Farr, *Vital Statistics, or, the Statistics of Health, Sickness, Diseases and Death* (London, 1837).
38 An Act for the Improvement of the City of Dublin (12 & 13 Vict.) C A P.XCVII.
39 *Markets and Fairs (Ireland). A Bill for the Better Regulation of Markets and Fairs, and to Abolish Local and Customary Denominations of Weight, and Regulate the Mode of Weighing Articles Sold, in Ireland* (1862).
40 'Dublin Sanitary Association and the Slaughter-houses', *Irish Times* (10 January 1880), p. 3.
41 M. Cahill, *Remarks on the Present State of Dublin with Suggestions for the Improvement of Smithfield and the Erection of a General Abattoir and Carcase Market* (Dublin: Hodges, Smith & Co., 1861), p. 21.
42 Prunty, *Dublin Slums*, p. 93.
43 P. Y. Lee (ed.), *Meat, Modernity, and the Rise of the Slaughterhouse* (Durham, NH: University of New Hampshire Press, 2008), p. 2.
44 Adelman, *Animal City*, chapter two.
45 Association of Victuallers, *A Defence of the Dublin Victuallers* (Dublin: R. D. Webb and Son, 1882).
46 'The Butchers' Trade and the Abbatoir Question', *Freeman's Journal* (20 December 1879), p. 7.
47 Daly, *Dublin: The Deposed Capital*, p. 262.
48 RCPI, *Thirty-second Annual Report on the State of Public Health in Dublin* (1893).
49 'Belfast Corporation', *Belfast Newsletter* (2 May 1895), p. 5.
50 'Meat inspection in Belfast', *Belfast Health Journal*, 3:4 (21 March 1905), 69.
51 Public Records Office of Northern Ireland (hereafter PRONI), LA/7/3/JA/25, Bound Typescript of the Proceedings of a Sworn Inquiry held by a Local Government Board Inspector into an Application by Belfast Corporation for … Alteration to the New Abattoir (November 1909).
52 MacLachlan, 'A bloody offal nuisance', p. 230.
53 *Irish Times* (30 May 1863), p. 2.
54 Ibid.
55 'The sugar contract for the North Dublin Union', *Dublin Medical Press* (8 July 1863), p. 256.
56 B. Wilson, *Swindled: From Poison Sweets to Counterfeit Coffee, the Dark History of the Food Cheats* (London: John Murray, 2008), pp. 93–150.
57 'The adulteration question', *Dublin Medical Press* (9 April 1856), p. 235.
58 'How We Are Poisoned by Civilised and Enlightened British Merchants', *Nation* (10

October 1857), p. 5.

59 'Adulteration for the Farmer', *Nation* (30 March 1867), p. 11.

60 'Important Prosecution of Vendors of Poisonous Confectionary', *Irish Times* (30 December 1870), p. 5.

61 J. Dunne, 'Bitter Sweets', *Irish Times* (28 January 1873), p. 5.

62 J. Dunne, 'Sweets', *Irish Times* (23 July 1873), p. 5.

63 RCPI, *Report on the State of Public Health in Dublin* (1885).

64 Bound volume recording the analysis made on drugs from various dispensaries in Cos Antrim, Armagh, Down and Londonderry (8 November 1899–23 September 1899), PRONI, D2682/1/1, pp. 59–65.

65 Ibid., pp. 71–87.

66 'The Adulteration of Milk', *Freeman's Journal* (22 September 1863), p. 3.

67 Clarkson and Crawford, *Feast and Famine*, p. 102.

68 RCPI, *Report on the State of Public Health in Dublin* (1882).

69 'The "Milk-Ring" in Dublin', *Irish Times* (25 March 1887), p. 3

70 *Belfast Evening News* (8 March 1879), p. 5.

71 See also C. Otter, 'The vital city: public analysis, dairies and slaughterhouses in nineteenth-century Britain', *Cultural Geographies*, 13 (October 2006), 517–37 on pp. 522–6.

72 'Holywood: The Adulteration of Buttermilk', *Belfast Newsletter* (11 August 1879), p. 8.

73 J. Steere-Williams, 'The perfect food and the filth disease: milk-borne typhoid and epidemiological practice in late-Victorian Britain', *Journal of the History of Medicine and Allied Sciences*, 65:4 (October 2010), 514–45.

74 C. Hamlin, *A Science of Impurity: Water Analysis in the Nineteenth Century* (Bristol: Adam Hilger, 1990), pp. 130–1.

75 C. A. Cameron, 'On an epidemic of fever caused by infected milk', *Dublin Journal of Medical Science*, 91 (1 July 1879), 1–23.

76 See J. Tyndall, 'On dust and disease', *Proceedings of the Royal Institution of Great Britain*, 6 (1870), 1–14.

77 Cameron, 'On an epidemic of fever', p. 13.

78 See M. Worboys, *Spreading Germs: Diseases, Theories and Medical Practice in Britain, 1865–1900* (Cambridge and New York: Cambridge University Press, 2000).

79 J. M. Eyler, *Sir Arthur Newsholme and State Medicine, 1865–1935* (Cambridge: Cambridge University Press, 1997), p. 120.

80 'Discussion of Dr Cameron's paper "On an epidemic of fever caused by infected milk"', *Dublin Journal of Medical Science*, 91 (1 July 1879), 66–85.

81 C. A. Cameron, 'Report on public health', *Dublin Journal of Medical Science*, 73 (2 January 1882), 112–29 on p. 114.

82 C. A. Cameron, 'On micro-organisms and alkaloids which render food poisonous', *Dublin Journal of Medical Science*, 78 (1 December 1884), 473–90.

83 'The Adulteration of Tea', *Freeman's Journal* (25 October 1873), p. 6.

84 J. S. Donnelly Jr., 'Cork Market: its role in the nineteenth-century Irish butter trade', *Studia Hibernica*, 11 (1971), 130–63 on p. 130.

85 *Select Committees on Industries (Ireland)*, p. 738.

86 'The Irish Pure Butter Trade Protection Association', *Weekly Irish Times* (1 October 1887), p. 7. For debates on butterine, see M. French and J. Philips, *Cheated not Poisoned? Food Regulation in the United Kingdom, 1875–1938* (Manchester and New York: Manchester University Press, 2000), pp. 58–65.

87 'The Irish Butter Question', *Freeman's Journal* (7 March 1884), p. 2.

88 C. F. Bastable, 'The Irish export trade in butter, with special reference to the regulations

of the Cork Market', *Journal of the Statistical and Social Inquiry Society of Ireland*, 8:60 (August 1882), 331–9.
89 C. F. Bastable, *The Commerce of Nations* (London: Methuen and Co., 1892).
90 *Select Committee on Industries (Ireland)*, p. 195.
91 Ibid., p. 727.
92 Ibid., p. 220.
93 'The Society of Public Analysts', *Irish Times* (19 July 1893), p. 6.
94 *Select Committee on Industries (Ireland)*, p. 220.
95 'Butter Adulteration', *Freeman's Journal* (17 September 1894), p. 2.
96 *Committee on Butter Regulations: Minutes of Evidence*, H. C. 1902 [Cd.944] xx.123, p. 1.
97 'The Irish Butter Trade: What is Adulteration?', *Belfast Newsletter* (4 January 1894), p. 5.
98 'Irish Dairy Association Conference', *Irish Times* (7 February 1895), p. 3.
99 'Water in Butter', *Freeman's Journal* (5 November 1894), p. 5.
100 'Butter Adulteration', *Freeman's Journal* (17 September 1894), p. 2.

6

Reforming Irish domestic and agricultural education

In 1900 it seemed to many contemporaries that post-Famine Ireland was in an unremitting condition of physical, social and economic decline. Ireland's food economy remained hindered by an inability to modernise while the poor seemed chronically underfed. This chapter argues that turn-of-the-century educational reformers attempted to harness the Irish school system to ensure that teachers offered practical (rather than theoretical) agricultural and domestic training, a step taken to address and resolve pressing post-Famine food concerns. Their intervention formed part of an ambitious social reform programme implemented in this period under the aegis of constructive unionism: a form of political intervention that promised to lay the foundations of a stable, prosperous Irish society.[1] This chapter explores the reconfiguration of Irish agricultural and domestic education in 1900 and identifies the motivations that underpinned this radical overhaul. Reformers advocated adjustment in both agricultural and domestic instruction as they saw these as complementary and mutually reinforcing elements of the broader project of improving the nation. This mindset allowed reformers to focus on, and attempt to intervene in, two key decaying sites: the agricultural workplace and the home.

The need for educational reform

In the late nineteenth century, the limitations of the pre-existing agricultural and domestic education system seemed increasingly apparent. The menace of foreign economic competition evident from the 1880s onward resulted in public criticism of the outmoded and overly theoretical nature of Irish agricultural education. Towards the end of the century, educational reformers vehemently derided school agricultural instruction as impractical and denounced it for having failed to keep pace with shifting economic circumstances. In his evidence given to the 1884 Select Committee on Industries, a Mr Woodall sardonically observed that 'the [National School] teachers have always gone to the institution at Glasnevin; but in my time they went there on a Saturday afternoon; they walked there and back again; they looked over the farm, and saw the animals, and felt them, I suppose; they looked round, and went back, and they had an agricultural education'.[2] In relation to National School instruction, head school inspector W. O'B. Neill asserted in 1890 that 'the children took little interest in the text book, and what answers they did give came from memory, and not from a practical and intelligent knowledge of the subject'. To affirm this, Neill insisted that pupils could respond correctly to questions about crops that they had never even seen (and probably never would) such as celery, spinach, lettuce, broccoli and rhubarb. Neill insisted that National School textbooks needed to be rewritten to suit agricultural practicalities.[3] Similarly, in 1895, District Inspector of Education for Dublin W. P. Headen lamented that 'the phraseology and general treatment of the subject in the text book in use are too difficult, so that teachers are in many cases tempted into the use of catechisms', adding that teachers rarely referred pupils to 'the processes going on beneath their very eyes in the farms and gardens around them'.[4] Likewise, in 1896, J. S. Oussen, district school inspector of Ballymena, Co. Antrim, pessimistically dismissed agricultural instruction via textbooks as 'hopeless' and 'of little value'.[5]

Thomas Baldwin's *An Introduction to Practical Farming* was under fire in these critiques; it was a textbook that was indeed technical and dry. For instance, the author of the 1877 edition discussed milk production as follows:

> Milk newly drawn from the cow has a temperature of about ninety degrees Fahrenheit, which is reduced before it reaches the dairy. It has almost always a slightly alkaline taste, which it gradually loses on exposure to air. It contains, in every 100 parts, about eighty-seven parts of water, four parts of fatty matter or butter, five parts of a peculiar kind of sugar called milked sugar, three and a quarter parts of cheesy matter or curd, and three-quarters of a part of mineral water.[6]

A revised textbook distributed from 1898 contrasted sharply in tone. It was written by Thomas Carroll, then manager of Glasnevin, in consultation with Charles Cameron, Edmund M'Weeney, a Catholic University of Ireland bacteriologist, and Frederick Moore of the Botanical School of Trinity College, Dublin. The authors made use of an observably simpler, more pragmatic tone. For instance, they described milk production as follows:

> The parts of milk that have interest for the farmer are its fat, its curd and its ash. These are the parts of milk that build up the bodies of young animals.
>
> The fat of milk is butter. This portion of the milk serves to supply fat to the animal and to keep it warm.
>
> The curd of milk is the part from which cheese is made. It is that part of the milk that is turned into muscle or lean meat in the animal.
>
> The ash of milk which is obtained by drying up milk, and burning the small quantity of matter that remains, is the part of milk that goes to make up the bones and the mineral portion of the bodies of animals.
>
> The ash of milk contains a very rich matter that is taken up from the land by the cattle feeding upon it. The farmer is interested in this, because the removal of this matter by the selling of milk from the farm will impoverish the farm, as there is only a limited quantity of the substance – called phosphorus – in soils.[7]

Nationalist MP William O'Malley of Connemara, Co. Galway, complained in the House of Commons that even the revised text was 'very difficult'.[8] Yet as demonstrated by the example of milk production, and as emphasised in Chief Secretary Gerald Balfour's subsequent reply to O'Malley, the revised edition contained shorter sentences, practical overviews of information split into concise sentences and, overall, a clearer and more accessible elucidation of agricultural matters still grounded in theory but presented pragmatically. Notably, the introduction of the new textbook preceded a gradual improvement in examination passes that rose from 60.9 in 1893 to 68.3 in 1897.[9] Nonetheless, the revision of a textbook alone could hardly transform agriculture into a practical classroom subject.

Similar concerns permeated discussion of cookery instruction. Some private initiatives emerged in the late nineteenth century including a model school in Belfast, established in 1878 by Miss Charters. This contained a room specifically designated for practical cookery instruction. Charters admitted senior girls from National Schools and offered evening classes to the wives and daughters of artisans at a slightly higher rate.[10] Dublin boasted a National Training School for Cookery, the impetus for which stemmed from similar projects in operation in London that, like their new Irish counterparts, purported to be socially enhancing.[11] The school managers adopted an agenda of training teachers who, upon qualifying, would teach cookery across Ireland so that 'in time throughout the length and breadth of the country a knowledge of the proper preparation of food will be spread among the industrial classes – a knowledge which will add materially to their comfort'. Because the institution was intended as a site to spark improvement among the rural poor, its kitchens were fitted with appliances commonly found in small farming communities. Its syllabuses instructed on how to prepare bread, soups, eggs, tea, coffee and vegetables – foods consumed by rural labouring families.[12] 120 girls attended in 1890.[13] However, the institution continued to rely upon voluntary contributions meaning that only relatively short courses could be offered rather than intensive prolonged training.[14]

Until 1900, National School cookery instruction provision remained limited. It was offered as an extra, optional subject from 1855. Yet in 1874, just six schools offered cookery classes nationwide. In that year, teachers examined sixty-eight pupils but only twenty-six passed. A decade later, only fourteen schools offered cookery options. By 1894, this figure had risen dramatically to fifty-five. Pass rates also increased significantly in this period. In 1884, only 371 out of 896 pupils passed their examinations, a disappointing total of 41 per cent. A decade later, 1,251 out of 1,289 examinees passed, a more impressive total of 97 per cent.[15] It should be borne in mind, however, that these decades witnessed a programme of intensive school building that partially accounts for this rise. As T. J. McElligott demonstrates, the number of National Schools nearly doubled from a count of 1,873 to 3,990 between 1870 and 1900.[16]

Problematically, the availability of cooking facilities failed to equal this ever-rising demand. The rising popularity of cookery instruction placed considerable demands on many schools, a problem compounded by limited financial support. When headmistress Mrs Ffrench requested permission from the Commissioners of National Education to establish cookery instruction at her Belfast school, the Commissioners made plans to convert a first floor kitchen into a classroom, the most significant expense incurred being the installation of a gas stove.[17] Smaller schools tended not to have the same luxuries of space or spare classrooms, a scenario lamented by numerous Irish headmistresses. When Miss Coulter of Carrickfergus Model School, Co. Antrim, applied to the Commissioners for a building grant to cater for rising demand in 1899, she pleaded that cookery:

> Should be taught in a separate room in which I could make preparations before the lesson begins without disturbing the working of the school, such as laying out ingredients, utensils, etc ... We hold the classes at present in a small gallery, which cannot be ventilated during the lesson without causing a draught. Owing to the burning and smell of gas, and the large number present in the room, the temperature is, as a rule, too high, and the fresh air soon becomes exhausted. While the cookery classes are in operation the smell pervades the whole department. As this school is worked on the Tripartite System, and there is only one small gallery, I cannot dispense with it so, as soon as the cookery lessons are over, it must be used for the ordinary English classes. This is unhealthy for the pupils and myself.[18]

The headmistress of Newry District Model School also applied for a building grant as she believed that cookery needed to be taught in facilities separate from other classrooms if her school was to run efficiently. Although the Commissioners suggested adding a new door to a pre-existing schoolroom, and shelving to store utensils, the headmistress retorted by insisting that using that room for cookery would make it unsuitable for teaching other subjects. In 1898, a surveyor's report concluded that the construction of a new specialist room would require encroaching upon the girls' playground at a cost of approximately £450. Eventually, the Commissioners decided that a small scullery could be attached to the pre-existing room to end the carrying of coal, water, slops and waste through the school building.[19]

Due to limited space and resources, cookery instruction remained predominantly theoretical which was a major concern in an era marked by unease about the pitiful cookery skills of the poor. In 1892, Unionist MP for South Tyrone Thomas Wallace Russell vociferously declared in the House of Commons that the Irish education system 'wants to be taken to pieces and re-modelled'. Russell particularly lamented the limited importance being awarded to cookery in the school system given that, in his view, 'in Dublin, Limerick and Cork the people are not fed, and they are not fed because their wives and daughters do not know anything of cookery'.[20] Likewise, in 1895 one school inspector insisted that 'in many parts of Connaught the people are exceedingly poor, and it seemed strange to see grown girls fairly advanced in grammar, geography, and arithmetic but left wholly unacquainted with plain cookery, management of poultry, dairy management, &c'.[21] Similarly, the

Commissioners asserted in 1893 that 'it is a matter for surprise that this most useful subject is not more generally taken up. The ignorance of this humble but indispensible art which the poorer classes show is a distinct obstacle to social progress.'[22] A series of minor famines intensified concern. Cookery instruction proved central to broader debates about theoretical and practical education as it offered a remarkably apt and illuminating example of a practical improving mechanism that might ameliorate the physical and social experience of the poor being inadequately addressed in the state-managed formal education system.

Analysis of the content of National School textbooks affirms contemporary judgement. Fannie M. Gallaher's *Short Lessons in Domestic Science,* distributed to students from 1894, offers a telling example. In this, Gallaher drily described cookery as 'the art by which the largest proportion of the nutritive elements is preserved for use, and where indigestible food substances are rendered digestible' and as a process that would rid food of injurious acrid properties and supplied tissues with fuel. Should too little food be consumed, Gallaher ominously warned, then bones, eyes and nervous systems suffered, loss of strength ensued, great prostration followed and, finally, death came, 'for the fire goes out when there is no more fuel to be burnt'.[23] Gallaher continued by elaborating on the properties of animal, vegetable and mineral foods, discussing in intimate detail how scientists believed that meat contained proteins, albumin, fibrin and gelatine which, in turn, provided bodies with nitrogen, carbon, oxygen and hydrogen. She conveyed this information in a language replete with references to molecules, atoms and internal combustion.[24] For Gallaher, to appreciate why some foods needed to be roasted depended upon an awareness that fibrin was insoluble in water, albumen soluble only in cold water and gelatine only in hot water.[25] Similarly, she discussed vegetables in relation to their organic acid, gluten and starch content. 'Not so long ago, when dietetic science was a thing unknown', Gallaher clarified, 'the ignorant idea prevailed that it was vulgar to introduce vegetables on the dinner table. As soon, however, as the constitution of the earth and its inhabitants began to arouse attention as a subject worthy of study, it was discovered that without plant life, animal life could have no existence, for without plants inorganic material could never become organic.'[26] Finally, Gallaher discussed tea in terms of its theine (caffeine), tannin and volatile oil content with an appended warning that 'if large quantities be consumed, [tea] causes insensibility, convulsions and death may be the result'.[27]

Evidently, Gallaher sought to promote a scientifically grounded understanding of food preparation. She presented food as more than simply nourishment. Instead, for Gallaher, purchasing decisions needed to be informed by a comprehensive appreciation of the chemical content of food and the molecular changes that occur while cooking. Otherwise, so she repeatedly stressed, ill-health and premature death would naturally result. As with nutritional advice dispensed during the Famine, Gallaher's model bypassed cultural preference, personal taste and the individuality of the human palate by offering a homogeneous model that provided one rule for all. In her model, cookery was rigidly defined, scientifically measured and appreciated solely in physiological terms. Ultimately, Gallaher's text proved to be impersonal and technical. It paid little recourse to personal experiences of cooking and consuming while her recurrent warnings of imminent death should her dietetic warnings remain unheeded were unconvincingly alarmist.

Gallaher's dry language and stern teaching methods contrasted sharply with the practical and seemingly more enjoyable training offered in convent schools. The convent school system had evolved in parallel with a dramatic rise in the numbers of nuns throughout late nineteenth-century Ireland.[28] The Commissioners routinely praised convent cookery instruction. When inspecting, they observed pupils preparing stirabout, bread, soups, potatoes and stews. Many convent schools had large, well-lit and well-ventilated kitchens, lavishly furnished with modern culinary utensils, scales and measures. As one inspector positively reported following a visit:

> The tables were beautifully covered, the range nicely polished, and the tins as bright as silver. The girls were dressed in cooking costumes – white pinafores and white sleeves. Their hands and nails were scrupulously clean, and their hair either cut short or nicely tied up. A more pleasing sight than this kitchen and these young girls I have never seen.[29]

Convent school instruction (mostly intended for wealthier students) offered an admirable, imitable vision of domestic harmony and cleanliness. The system also offered an idealised image of domestic education which the Commissioners hoped to apply to National School education to enrich the domestic life of the poor.[30]

Nonetheless, National School provision remained limited even despite the Commissioners arranging with the Royal Irish Association for the Technical Training and Employment of Women to dispatch qualified cookery teachers across Ireland from 1895.[31] Financial considerations partly explain this predicament. Ignoring decades of social commentary on Irish nutritional well-being, requests by Irish MPs to increase expenditure on cookery and laundry from £500 per year to £1,100 were refused in 1897 on the basis that the House of Commons was unaware of any 'great demand for instructors'.[32] In response, Irish MPs vociferously pointed to a 'national cry' for practical instruction and an urgent need for state bodies to invest appropriate financial resources.[33] They saw a dearth of adequate cookery education as deeply perturbing in an era marked by stark concern over nutritional well-being, excessive tea drinking and national psycho-physiological decline. This pervasive social backdrop provided a framework for considering the potential social utility of domestic instruction.

By 1900, the fact remained that educational approaches to two subjects that now seemed so critical to the future integrity of Irish society – agriculture and cookery – remained lacking. Reformers viewed both pedagogical forms as having resoundingly failed to improve agricultural productivity and food hygiene. Nor had they adequately tackled the pressing issue of national physical and socio-economic decline by sufficiently promoting nutritional health. Dispensing complex doctrines on the chemical composition and physiological functions of food tended not to produce individuals who could cook. Nor did theoretical agricultural instruction create efficient producers. In response, educational reformers strove to resolve the issue by rethinking the pathways between scientific knowledge and social practice. Education was still to be scientific in nature but teachers needed to convey scientific knowledge accessibly and practically.

Reforming education

Many turn-of-the-century educational reformers were acutely aware of the detrimental social ramifications of English industrialisation including endemic poverty and chronic public health concerns. Discussion of agricultural and domestic education took on distinctive forms in Ireland where many reformers envisaged a ruralised, agricultural pathway as most appropriate for the country. In light of this, they insisted that the sanctity of Irish society could be preserved by strengthening agricultural rather than industrial sectors. Thomas Carroll annually echoed this latter perspective in his annual reports on agricultural education. On one instance, he asked:

> Why do country folk not see that the future of those who leave the land for city life is fraught with much misery? Agriculture – that primeval occupation, and the cleanest of them all, means more than the growing and grain. It means, amongst other things, the engendering and achievement of patient even minds in sound enduring bodies, gifts of which after the first generation, the great towns rob those who dwell and labour in them.

Continuing his denunciation of urban life, Carroll declared that:

> There the hideous grinding competition of the age leaves little room for those whom the last possible ounce of brain or body work can be no longer pressed. They go to the wall, they sink to the slum and the dock-gate, and the house and the hospital ward. I say that from these great towns, with their aggregated masses of mankind, there rises an eternal wail of misery – the hopeless misery that, with all its drawbacks, the country does not know of those who, having fallen, are being trampled by those who stand. Such are the things of the cities, with their prizes for the few, their blanks – their despair – for the many.[34]

Evidently, Carroll equated rural life with health and vivacity and, accordingly, censured commercial, industrial and cosmopolitan living as something that sapped human vitality and created disadvantageous social conditions. His caveat can also be interpreted as a response to rising levels of emigration and internal migration from rural to urban areas.[35] Carroll believed that educating the young on the merits of country life might stem this worrying outward flow by incubating a sense that 'the knowledge of Nature's work, given in an attractive form, will induce young people to remain in rural districts, where they can revel in Nature and her works'.[36] Despite this elevation of rural life, it tended to be in Irish rural contexts where an absence of technical knowledge of modern forms of food production was most pronounced.

Small farmers were traditionally sceptical of agricultural science. Critics condemned the stubborn tendencies of less affluent farmers to view scientific education as a threat to their economic success.[37] In the 1890s – a decade clouded by anxieties over Ireland's economic future – concern about agricultural conservatism sharpened. Carroll explicitly referred to the threat of foreign competition to justify his opinion on the practical worth of agro-scientific knowledge. Referring to contrasting Danish experiences, he argued a case for state-supported training by insisting that:

> The time has come when we can no longer afford to ignore the higher scientific demands of farming. It is true that much harm has been done through ill-advised efforts to prove that 'scientific farming' was alone the remedy for agricultural losses and that book learning and science alone would enable a man to farm profitably. The enthusiasts who endeavoured to lead us on to believe that science should be placed above practice in the studies of the agriculturist injured the cause which they had hoped to serve. Science must be hand in hand with practice, and the farmer who will be the most successful in the future will be the man who combines in his person the largest knowledge of farming practice and the most extensive acquaintance with the sciences bearing upon agriculture.[38]

Carroll was more willing than some of his predecessors to concede that agro-scientific information needed to be presented in a way attuned to the practicalities of Irish farming life if children were to internalise and apply it. In his view, agriculture needed to be pragmatically taught while remaining scientifically informed.

Pressure for reform mounted in the 1890s as groups such as the Irish Industrial League, chaired by Lord Muskerry, campaigned for state-supported educational provision.[39] The Chemico-Agricultural Society of Ulster also raised awareness by regularly criticising the educational system.[40] Various witnesses at the 1897 Commission on Manual and Practical Instruction raised the issue. The Commission was established to determine how far, and in what form, manual and practical instruction should be incorporated in National School curriculums. The Commission concluded, as had many contemporaries, that imparting agricultural theory alone had few practical benefits.[41] All of these actors saw reform of the pre-existing agricultural educational system, rather than the development of further private initiatives, as the most appropriate focal point of improvement.

Educational reformers also sought to tackle national physical deterioration by improving the quality of domestic instruction. For some decades, physicians had denigrated customs of consuming large quantities of stewed tea and white bread as a perversion of normative nurturing familial care. Turn-of-the-century ideas on how to update Irish domestic education were underpinned by various gender-based considerations. In fact, the ability of female household members to cook was upheld in this period as an enabler of familial harmony, social well-being and national health. The economic advancement of middle-class England in the

Industrial Revolution was commonly understood as having been made possible by the gendered division of labour. Men had laboured and produced while the extra wealth accumulated through industrial profit had allowed middle-class women to retreat into the home to raise and nurture the young. This faith in the social worth of gendered divisions formed the basis of middle-class opinion on how familial stability could be achieved by strengthening the female presence in the home. Throughout the nineteenth century, ideas such as these gained currency and slowly filtered down to working-class society.[42]

This enforcement of separate spheres of activity for men and women was central to late century discussion of Irish educational reform. According to this perspective, ensuring the physical well-being of their children and family members should be a main duty of housewives. This perspective was prominent in a provocative lecture delivered by Dublin physician Nicholas Whyte to the Rathmines and Rathgar Sanitary and Health Association in 1886. In this, Whyte declared that 'every particle of food wasted is a direct loss to the community'. Careless, or unskilled, food preparation was responsible for most of the diseases of modern life, so he suggested. Importantly, Whyte asserted that it was a woman's *duty*, whatever her social position, 'to know how to secure for her husband, her brother, or her sons, wholesome food to fit them for the battle of life'. To strengthen this point, Whyte argued that many Irish working-class mothers failed to instruct their children on how to select food when shopping, one consequence being newly married couples depending entirely on advice from tradesmen. This was a problematic situation, he insisted, given the proliferation of adulteration. Irish women, he insisted, should also assume familial and social responsibility for reducing the amount of tea being consumed at home.[43] Whyte's stance was an expression of a pervasive cult of domesticity that privileged the home as a repository of moral sanctity and as a space where properly nurtured individuals attained physical strength.[44]

Late century ideas on domestic instruction drew upon the presumption that nutritional problems often resulted from errant female domestic behaviour. This mindset was particularly apparent in an 1884 pamphlet penned by agrarian reformer and Bishop of Meath Thomas Nulty in which he suggested that the Commissioners should incorporate practical cookery into National School syllabuses to cultivate a particular mental culture at risk of being lost in the adverse economic climate of that period that, he thought, had produced a distinct loss of 'the nerve, the energy and the self-denial that shed such a lustre and imparted such a high value to the character and service of Irish girls'.[45]

Good cookery was intended to raise housewives as social beings; to render them and their homes desirable to male family members. By maintaining a healthy, nurturing home, housewives would strengthen the moral and physical resolve of male labourers who, in turn, would be more inspired and physically able to generate economic prosperity. In that way, public health campaigners once again connected personal acts of consuming food to broader activity in social and economic domains. When inaugurating a new session of Dublin's cookery school in 1884, Cameron remarked that 'women can influence men in many ways, but one most patent method is through the medium of the stomach. This is one of the best ways a workman's wife can control her husband. Give him a warm, savoury dinner and a cheerful, cleanly tea table, and he will soon appreciate the comforts of his own fireside and pass his evenings with his family.'[46] Cameron firmly believed that domestic harmony could shield male labourers from social vices detrimental to economic capacity, most importantly alcohol. He shared this perspective with an array of contemporaries. Edward Thomas, the Bishop of Limerick, also supported the training of young girls into housewives. In 1900, Thomas suggested that if Irish women knew how to keep their homes bright and clean, and offered their husbands comfortable, savoury meals, then the inevitable outcomes would be greater domestic happiness, less drunkenness and a gradual increase in thrift, comfort and prosperity.[47] Similarly, on the subject of domestic economy, cleanliness and thrift, co-operatist newspaper the *Irish Homestead* argued in 1898 that:

> None of these things is the poor Irish girl taught at her school; and when a young artisan, when the time for mating comes, chooses her or her comely face and bright spirits, none of this knowledge or capacity does he find in his wife. The consequences are disastrous to them both. How often does the working man in an Irish city, when he gets up in the early morning, find that there is no appetising breakfast in a cheery and tidy room prepared for him to start him on his day's work. The ever hospitable 'pub' is open, however, and, as the man must have some nourishment, he turns in and takes 'eating and drinking' in the form of a pint of stout. A day so begun is not calculated to develop and close propitiously.[48]

This is not to imply that all agreed upon the domesticated status of Irish women. Debates about the domesticated Irish female led to an ongoing discussion in *Ireland's Own* during 1902 and 1903. In November 1902, *Ireland's Own* published a letter by Helen Hawthorn entitled 'The Ideal Girl' in which she insisted that:

> Our young men like sensible girls with that graceful personal charm which so adorns those who possess it, and which might be an attribute of even the most up-to-date and smart girl of the day. They like thrifty, neat and intelligent girls, well versed in domestic science and the gastronomic art ... Cookery should be regarded as a *sine qua non* of every wife. A nice well-served meal and a neatly laden table is always a help to good humour, contentment and happiness in a man; while an ill-cooked one and an ill-cared for table make him irritable and quarrelsome – and not unnaturally so.[49]

One respondent, named Billie Lynch, argued on the contrary that:

> Now this may be all fine in high class circles. But I doubt very much if it be of any use in nine cases out of ten. For taking the rural districts, for instance, the lot of a peasant girl, be she poor or rich, is work while she is in it ... there is not much time left for the study of science or the gastronomic arts, the race for existence being so keen amid the hurry and bustle of the present day.[50]

A further respondent sardonically commented that:

> I myself have many lady acquaintances who, I am sure, would scarcely know how to cook a herring properly, as the saying is, and, yet, strange to say, most of them have taken lessons on scientific and up-to-date cookery.[51]

Nonetheless, much of the evidence on domestic instruction presented to the Commission on Manual and Practical Instruction in Primary Schools in 1897 focused intently on instilling domesticity in young girls to curb further national physical decline. Miss M'Carthy, cookery instructress at Baggot Street Training College, asserted that cookery instruction 'cultivates in girls a taste for home work, and therefore improves the comfort of the home, teaches girls to be more domesticated, and inculcates thrift and cleanliness in household affairs'.[52] Mrs Power Lalor insisted that National School cookery instruction should be offered continually rather than in the form of short courses as it was only after a number of years that its social worth would be felt locally and nationally.[53] Some witnesses noted that domestic instruction had failed in Belfast as local females had vehemently rallied against efforts to train them into cooks and laundry-maids.[54] Despite these occasional protests, the Commission concurred on the desirability of expanding domestic instruction provision and making financial aid available for buildings and equipment.[55] It also concluded that cookery was of prime importance as 'the labouring and artisan classes are sadly ignorant of the art of cookery, their food in consequence being seldom prepared in as economical or nutritious a manner as it might be'.[56] This latter perspective confirms Joanna Bourke's view that economic motivations underpinned the late century domestication of the Irish female. The closing decades of the nineteenth century saw a dramatic decline in female employment, partly due to the expansion of the creamery industry that, Bourke suggests, produced a residuum of redundant labour previously engaged in dairy work. Domesticity came to be construed as an essential precondition of economic growth.[57] Many educational reformers embraced these perspectives and targeted female behaviour when determining new ways of regulating familial behaviour.

David Fitzpatrick argues that the increased respectability of housekeeping in this period was an expression of diminished female utility rather than raised status.[58] However, it is worth noting that middle-class contemporaries framed the home more positively. They privileged it as a site from which economic growth and national progression would stem. In this discourse, domestic work became elevated to a practice with nationally felt benefits rather than simply disregarded as an inferior adjunct to male labour. Housework, reformers recurrently suggested, enhanced socio-economic life by securing the physical and moral health of future generations. According to F. M. F. Lovibond, writing in the *New Ireland Review* in 1904, 'the same turn of mind, the same aptitudes that are required to manage a private household successfully, are needed, though on a vast scale, to conduct much of the business of a nation'. Lovibund also rallied against those who blamed childhood hunger and starvation on a lack of familial compassion common among working-class women. Instead, he asserted these scenarios were rooted in ignorance, not lack of moral fibre.[59] Casting women as ignorant but transformable (instead of morally deficient) implied the manipulability and mouldability of the young female mind, a stance which, in turn, validated demands for practical instruction. This allowed reformers to conceive the Irish school curriculum as a powerful means of shaping socio-economic life across gendered lines and fashioning a new social order based upon dominant middle-class social values.[60]

Restructuring education

Educational reforms were formally initiated in 1900. In that year, the state established the Department of Agriculture and Technical Instruction (DATI) in Ireland.[61] DATI ostensibly sought to aid, improve and develop agriculture to stimulate self reliance. It specifically tailored its instruction to meet Irish needs.[62] The Department's functions were manifold. In 1902, DATI established clearer definitions of what constituted adulterated and unadulterated dairy produce.[63] It also dispensed information on yield improvement and the varieties of potatoes least susceptible to blight through pamphlets, lectures and public instruction.[64] Importantly, DATI also excelled in devising practical educational techniques intended to cultivate a rethinking of how and why agro-biological material could be productively and hygienically harnessed.[65] DATI's ideological perspectives can be gleaned from the prolific writings of its co-operatist and Unionist Vice-President Horace Plunkett who, in his *Memorandum on Agricultural Education for Ireland* penned in 1901, announced that the Department was to serve as a 'graft on the educational tree rather than a separate growth' although its success would rest upon the support of farming communities who, he confidently asserted – even despite the failure of agricultural education earlier in that century – would 'sustain the historic reputation of the Irish people as lovers of education'.[66] In Plunkett's view, agricultural instruction would create 'a vast addition to the nation's wealth, would greatly enhance the comfort and well-being of the people and would tend in some manners to check the deplorable drain of emigration'.[67] Notably, Plunkett's ideas were overly influenced by his desire to dilute the spread of Irish nationalism by demonstrating the benefits of state activity to the Irish populace.

Plunkett's reforms saw the appearance of a new educational figure: the agricultural instructor. This individual was, in Plunkett's phraseology, to be 'the guide, philosopher and friend of the existing farmers'.[68] The formation of this interpersonal relationship was intended, perhaps deliberately, to counteract popular associations of agricultural science with the more distant, often detested, landlord and as being 'an English hobby'. Instead, the relationship between instructor and farmer would be anchored in mutual trust and respect. The nature of the instructor's work would be altruistic and compatible with the needs of smaller farming communities rather than landed interests. For Plunkett, the ideal instructor would be an individual familiar with the conditions of Irish farmers. He had a first-class training in science but was also born to farming, being steeped in it from boyhood. These assets would well position him to estimate the difficulties that Irish farmers contended and to make use of his expert knowledge of the geographical and economic circumstances that impacted uniquely on food production in Ireland.[69]

From 1900, the Department had a penetrative influence on Irish agriculture. In 1904 alone, seventeen instructors delivered 1,159 lectures attended by an average of sixty-four people. Its staff also undertook 8,500 inspections of holdings and 974 field demonstrations in that year.[70] Between 1905 and 1906, thirty-one out of the thirty-three County Committees of Agriculture established in 1900 adopted schemes in agriculture, twenty-seven in horticulture, twenty-five in butter-making and thirty-two in poultry keeping, figures that illuminate the rapid spread of educational techniques.[71] Furthermore, DATI's commitment to redressing economic concerns was more than just rhetorical. The Department provided for the appointment of qualified butter-making instructors in each county to deliver daily dairying lessons.[72] Each instructor led classes containing up to fifteen pupils on practical butter-making.[73] Although DATI offered butter-making classes in just one district between 1900 and 1901, this figure rose to eighteen between 1903 and 1904.

The educational reforms of this period were distinguishable from earlier initiatives in two respects. Firstly, reformers forged the content of the reforms with reference to a distinct and recently created set of medico-scientific food discourses less concerned with maximising productivity alone and more intent on creating conditions of hygiene and purity. By 1900, purity had mutated into a moral and economic concern that imparted new social responsibilities onto producers who were now expected to ensure the cleanliness, hygiene and safety of food supplies. Accordingly, they were to cleanse and purify the biological material of dairy produce at micro-level to render it safe for human consumption. Quantity was now subordinated to quality, a pragmatic response to the elevation of purity into a national problem. Secondly, shifting gendered constructs embedded in the format of agricultural instruction helped to transform key areas of production into male-dominated preserves. The absorption of scientific regimes of cleanliness seemed to demand a technical mind which, to some, confirmed the suitability of the male sex in public economic domains. Accordingly, male producers tended to be indoctrinated in modern principles of hygiene and sanitation. Notably, DATI did little to arrest the declining role of female work.[74] If anything, its reforms mapped onto a broader trend of reorganising labour across gendered lines, a development that saw the transfer of dairy farming from a female to male preserve. For instance, from 1900 DATI allocated limited attention and financial support to female training undertaken at the Munster Dairy School, Co. Cork than was previously the case. The Department made no major changes to the function of the school, although it did set a considerable sum aside to extend the school's domestic science provision.[75]

These conceptual and practical adjustments were resonant in an era that witnessed a rapid expansion of the dairy industry. As Mary Daly argues, the switch to creameries in the 1890s was national and extraordinarily rapid.[76] Nonetheless, DATI and its inspectors routinely rebuked the creameries and dairy farms that sprang up for being unhygienic. In response, in 1902, DATI recommended that managers equip their creameries with pasteurising plants to allow milk to be heated to a temperature that destroyed pathogenic, lactic and harmless bacteria. The Department set aside £5,000 per annum for grants and loans to defray part of the costs.[77] The following year, the Department altered the training structure for creamery managers after observing the unsatisfactory condition of many buildings and equipment first-hand. It extended facilities at Glasnevin for technical training. It also devised new initiatives including certification, inspection and registration, as well as annual surprise butter competitions. Between 1903 and 1904, 102 creameries applied for registration, all of which were inspected. The Department held forty-six butter competitions adjudicated by key butter purchasers in Britain, Cork, Limerick, Belfast and Dublin.[78] New examinations contained rigorous questions on dairy bacteriology, the microscopial study of milk and the sources and effects of bacterial contamination. Questions on dairy technology coalesced around the composition and properties of milk, causes of variation, changes produced by heat and bacteria, butter and milk testing, and packaging.[79] These new educational and inspectorial regimes were intended to encourage a rethinking of the relationship of man to the microcosmic realm of germs and microbes.

If educational reforms set the workplace apart as a male terrain of scientifically guided production then, by default, it also affirmed the domestic sphere as a suitable domain of female influence. As with agricultural training, reformers helped to reconfigure Irish cookery instruction in 1900. A revised National School programme allowed instruction to commence in the first standard and to continue throughout the entire educational programme.[80] Like DATI, the Commissioners of National Education sought to create and perpetuate gendered divisions by forging housewives. In 1900, they announced that they:

> Disapprove of the introduction now or at any future time of 'fancy' cookery or 'ornamental' laundry work into the National Schools. Their object in respect of these branches is similar to their object in respect of Manual Instruction generally – they do not wish to train cooks or laundresses, but to impart such information about these and cognate domestic sciences as shall enable the average primary school girl, when she assumes the position of a housewife, to perform the ordinary culinary and washing operations that may appertain to her.[81]

In 1900, DATI established twenty scholarships at the Kildare Street School of Cookery for teacher training.[82] Three years later, it acquired control over the institution which embarked on a career as the Irish Training School of Domestic Economy.[83] Curriculums were revised, student numbers increased, premises improved and conditions for obtaining a teaching diploma rethought.[84] The school was now prepared to produce a core of trained instructresses to be dispatched across Ireland upon qualifying. In 1905–6 alone, sixty-two students attended the school to train as instructresses.[85] Regional demand for these instructresses was also high. Between 1900 and 1901, DATI received ninety applications in an academic year in which just twenty scholarships were on offer. This nationally orientated system replaced a more restricted Dublin-orientated system of training National School teachers. Between 1893 and 1897, the numbers of teachers trained in practical cookery nationwide totalled just 566. The key training centres were the Commissioners' Training College, the Church of Ireland Training College and Our Lady of Mercy Training College. Just over half of this total was trained at the Commissioners' College while only five teachers trained at district centres.[86] In contrast, by July 1901, fifty-six teaching centres had been formed throughout the country.[87] Leinster and Munster boasted over twenty each of these, although Connaught established only six, and Ulster just five.[88] In 1904, sixty-three domestic instructresses delivered a total of 360 courses, with an average attendance of forty-two pupils, complemented by 300 house visits.[89] Courses of instruction lasted for seven weeks, five of which were devoted to cookery and two to laundry and which would often take place between five and eight in the evening.[90] In subsequent years, the Commissioners allocated money for travel expenses and lodging where necessary.[91] The training itself appeared to run smoothly, although in 1908, William Moore, MP for Armagh North, claimed that the Commissioners sometimes intimidated female teachers by withholding salary increments if they refused to attend cookery lectures, although the Commissioners swiftly denied this.[92]

According to one Commissioners' report, cookery was awarded such high priority because:

> It is found that the dietary of the people is to a large extent innutritious and uneconomical, and one of the purposes kept in view in this instruction is to enable the housekeeper to understand how to obtain more nourishing food in a more economical way and, in rural districts, to increase and vary the food supply by growing vegetables and learning how to cook them.[93]

In light of this, DATI announced that poultry keeping, horticulture, home industries and manual work were all to become subservient to domestic economy for women. DATI portrayed this step as an improving strategy that specifically targeted apprehension about nutritional decline.

However, the promptness and efficacy that had characterised the spread of agricultural instruction after 1900 was not equalled in provision for domestic training. Legislation had demanded the national extension of domestic instruction but most National Schools were small and lacked equipment. Upon returning from training, many teachers faced a dearth of funding that might have allowed them to buy utensils and materials.[94] Initially, many of them relied upon the resources of those convent schools willing to allow teachers and pupils to use their well-equipped kitchens.[95] This restrictive scenario was condemned throughout the echelons of educational administration. In 1901, one senior inspector insisted that 'the want of funds will, I fear, prevent the introduction of cookery and laundry work into the great majority of schools, unless the

Commissioners can see their way to make an equipment grant to each school'. To clarify his point, he observed that cookery instruction had commenced in only one school in his city despite fifteen teachers having received training in the previous year.[96] Even Miss Fitzgerald, organiser of the training scheme, conceded that 'the poverty of some districts will, I fear, render the teaching of cookery or laundry, without financial aid, practically impossible'. For Fitzgerald, it was possible, at best, to instruct on cleanliness, domestic economy and the theory of cooking, but little more could be expected.[97]

The Commissioners certainly strove to secure additional funding but their efforts proved fruitless. In 1901, they requested an allocation of three shillings per annum to each pupil from the Treasury in addition to contributions to building costs.[98] However, the Treasury decided not to provide money.[99] In the years that followed, the Commissioners repeatedly lamented the barriers encountered in implementing organised nationwide cookery instruction and the ongoing confinement of domestic education to convent schools and larger schools.[100] On one occasion, they suggested that responsibility could be transferred to DATI.[101] This proposition was also dismissed.[102]

This absence of financial support had practical implications. The staff at Newry Model School who, as detailed above, had struggled to secure funds to build a new schoolroom and were offered only a small scullery extension, were exasperated with the new legislative demands placed on them from 1900 and signed a petition stipulating that educational authorities had failed to take limited space and facilities into account. In 1901, the school's headmistress began afresh with her request to construct a new room, pointing out to the Commissioners that the proposed scullery 'was considered very small even when we only expected to teach cookery to a few of the pupils, but now that it is to be taught to the whole school, and laundry work in addition, I do not think we could manage without better accommodation than this would afford'.[103]

If space was unavailable in schools, then it had to be sought elsewhere. In Kilkenny, teachers delivered cookery classes in abandoned houses, rented rooms and cramped, poorly ventilated converted dwelling houses. Throughout Co. Wexford, they taught in an array of unsuitable sites including unoccupied dwelling homes, courthouses, a security room attached to a church, a stockroom, a spare room in a disused mill, a joiner's workshop and even in barns and coach-houses.[104] In 1903, the *Irish Technical Journal* asserted that 'the pupils who attend regularly under these conditions are heroes without knowing it. Neither the teachers nor the pupils, however, can do the best work when their work is done in a vitiated atmosphere'. The *Journal* concluded this article by stating: 'it is absurd to give courses of lectures on Hygiene in a "Black Hole"'.[105] Issues such as these caused consternation for years. However, it was only in 1907 that the Chief Secretary of Ireland agreed to receive a deputation on the matter. As Reverend Father Dowling vociferously asserted at this deputation, 'we have, therefore, the curious position that we have a scheme for technical instruction but no provision whatever for housing it'. Dowling proceeded by announcing:

> If you preach technical instruction as the cause of the economic salvation of the country and then point to an old jail or some such building as the centre from whence this panacea of the wants of Ireland were to come, it creates a bad impression. The moral effect of having these unpresentable buildings mentioned in this report as the centres from which Technical Instruction is to spread is considerable.[106]

In 1906, the Commissioners finally agreed to contribute five shillings per pupil enrolled on two-year cookery classes.[107] In the following year, they convinced the Treasury to sanction grants for schools with three or more teachers, or with at least 160 pupils.[108] However, the Lord Lieutenant refused requests to provide separate rooms for domestic training and cookery in schools containing at least eighty pupils on the basis that he was not prepared to sanction a standard of accommodation for Ireland exceeding that offered in England.[109] In response, the Commissioners angrily denigrated his decision as 'a retrograde step, and one that would seriously interfere with the teaching of these subjects in larger schools'.[110]Nonetheless, the number of schools offering cookery rose dramatically from 936 by December 1907 to 1,596 in 1908, 2,342 in 1909 and 2,672 in 1910.[111] The issue of facilities also persisted well into the following decade, as is evidenced by ongoing debates about the water supply of the School of Rural Domestic Economy in Clifden, Co. Galway. In September 1912, staff reported water from the school pump as dark in colour and of poor taste, declaring it as suitable only for flushing and washing. As an alternative, children used rain water to cook with. DATI only took a sample in May 1913 and, in the following month, made a grant of £90 available to cover the costs of piping, hydrants and valve bends. Yet the landlord who owned the lake proved difficult to reach and communicate with. Eventually, in 1915, he consented to allowing teachers to draw water from his lake, by which time the Department was forced to withdraw its grant due to a wartime reallocation of finances.[112]

And what of the teaching itself? The public often favourably received the optimistic aspirations that underpinned reformist tendencies. In 1903, District Inspector Headen reported positively that 'the children are very fond of cookery, which, through the habits of cleanliness and attention to details which it induces, is likely to have a permanent beneficial effect on the social condition of the country'.[113] In the same year, Fitzgerald confidently announced that parents were pleased with the instruction of their children in cookery, adding that they considered it to be 'the most useful thing that has ever been taught, and will bring comfort to our homes'. She went so far as to claim that many children now cooked 'comfortable dinners' at home each weekend and that they wished to remain at school longer to learn cookery.[114] Despite these confident assertions, cookery instruction for younger pupils was not as encompassing as originally hoped. Infants in the first class learnt only matters of personal cleanliness and hygiene. Similarly, the second class was marked by an emphasis on cleanliness, although students learnt how to prepare potatoes and cabbage for cooking, the purpose of salt and how to toast bread. It was only in the third class that teachers allowed pupils to actually cook their potatoes and cabbage and to make colcannon, tea, coffee and cocoa, boiled eggs and fried potatoes. Teachers devoted the remaining years to more advanced forms of cookery involving bacon, sausages, mutton and beef.[115]

In terms of pedagogical style, one notable change was the pragmatic manner in which teachers now instructed pupils. New textbooks such as Kathleen Ferguson's *Advanced Lessons in Cookery* refrained from meticulously outlining the scientific principles of cookery in the intricate detail that Gallaher had done. Instead, Ferguson systematically guided pupils through the practicalities of cookery, commencing with soups and fishes before proceeding to entrees, savouries and high-class puddings. For Ferguson, scientific theory alone had few edifying purposes in the classroom.[116] Josephine Redington's *Economic Cookery Book* adopted a similar tactic. Redington was head teacher at the Irish Training School of Domestic Economy.[117] Rather than instilling scientific principles, her text placed especial attention on obtaining value for money while purchasing as, according to Redington, domestic happiness depended on how housewives spent.[118] She also sought to dispel myths that skimmed milk was only fit for pigs and that Indian meal was a more suitable dish for animals than humans.[119] In addition, Redington insisted that both buttermilk and skim milk could be bought cheaply in rural regions. The loss of fat in these milks, she explained, could be compensated for by mixing dripping with potatoes or by preparing oatmeal puddings with chopped suet.[120]

National School examination questions demonstrate that some scientific theory was taught but that teachers encouraged pupils to consider how that science might be practically applied. Examination questions asked the months that herrings, cod and mackerel were in season; which joints of beef were most suitable for roasting and boiling; what different methods existed for trussing and stuffing fowls as well as what flesh-forming foods were supplied by the animal and vegetable kingdoms; why soups were both economical and nutritive; and what medicinal value vegetables had.[121] Cookery instruction had clearly evolved into a reactive mechanism that bore greater relevance to Irish day-to-day life and that sought to counter contemporary physical and social problems. Reformers initiated changes to end the practice of imparting theoretical scientific knowledge by focusing instead on practical aspects of female domestic work including budgeting and practical cooking. It was not the case that reformers sought to devalue scientific understandings of food. They did, however, agree upon it as an unsuitable starting point for social change. Nonetheless, the implementation of new forms of cookery instruction, although rooted in the same reformist foundations omnipresent in contemporary ideas on how to restructure agricultural instruction, failed to live up to its aspirations. Its advocates articulated preferred visions of domesticity and propagated the gendered division of society itself. Yet, in practice, the idea of the social worth of cookery instruction was not matched with a corresponding allocation of material resources.

Conclusion

In 1900, educational reformers reorganised Irish domestic and agricultural education to render it more practical. In line with dominant gendered ideologies, this step involved segmenting agricultural food production into a male terrain and domestic education into a female one. Although influenced by contemporary gendered constructs, these shifts were also intended to resolve many of the food-related concerns that had arisen since the Famine. Educational reformers sought to tackle deficient cookery knowledge in Ireland as well as economic problems relating to food purity, unhygienic practices and the need to form a response to foreign economic competition. Reformers sought to regulate aspects of life ranging from the nutritional health of citizens to the eradication of germs and microbes from foodstuffs. The simultaneous implementation of these schemes complemented one another by carving out and reinforcing new social roles for men and women who were now expected to socially perform in different ways but for the same elusive goal: national improvement.

Combined, the four chapters in Part II of this monograph demonstrate the pervasive sense of national decline that followed the Famine and the continuing identification of problems in post-Famine food consumption and production. The post-Famine institution was a site where anxieties arose about the consequences of subsisting on an innutritious diet and the potential impact of institutional dietary regimes on the future health of the rising generation. The regulation of food was more feasible in the institution than in the general community. As reliance on the potato as a dietary staple gradually diminished throughout much of Ireland, new anxieties arose about the poor purchasing decisions being made by the less affluent. In this context, working-class mothers found themselves exposed to blame for neglecting their family members. Concerns such as these contributed to a gloomy narrative of national decline and degeneration that was mirrored in contemporary discussion of a persistent lack of economic advancement. Food purity was a further arena in which Irish medical figures intervened during the late nineteenth century although food analysts faced considerable public and business opposition. Nonetheless, an apparent failure to adhere to new standards of food production continued to generate unease about the ever-declining health of the Irish economy. Combined, reformers targeted these problems by implementing structural changes in 1900. As the final part of this monograph demonstrates, a continuing lack of Irish socio-economic advancement was increasingly framed by opponents of British rule in relation to colonialism and Ireland's positioning in a broader Empire.

Notes

1 A. Gailey, *Ireland and the Death of Kindness: The Experience of Constructive Unionism, 1890–1905* (Cork: Cork University Press), p. 65.
2 *Report from Select Committee on Industries*, p. 10.
3 *Fifty-Sixth Report of the Commissioners of National Education in Ireland*, H. C. 1890 [C.6074] xxx.89, p. 69.
4 *Sixty-First Report of the Commissioners of National Education in Ireland*, H. C. 1895 [C.7796] xxix.1, p. 117.
5 *Sixty-Third Report of the Commissioners of National Education in Ireland*, H. C. 1897 [C.8600] xxviii.1, p. 115.
6 T. Baldwin, *An Introduction to Practical Farming* (Dublin: Alex. Thom and Co., 15th edn, 1877), p. 86.
7 T. Carroll, *Introduction to Practical Farming (new edition)* (Dublin: Alex. Thom and Co., 1898), pp. 265–6.
8 'Agricultural teaching in Irish schools', *House of Commons Debates* (21 July 1899), vol. 74, c. 1551.
9 *Sixty-Fifth Report of the Commissioners of National Education in Ireland*, H. C. 1899 [c.9446] xxiv.377, p. 228.
10 *Appendix to the Forty-Fifth Report of the Commissioners of National Education in Ireland*, H. C. 1878–9 [C.2312–I] xxiv.553, p. 24.
11 'Scientific Cookery', *Irish Times* (9 March 1881), p. 7.
12 *Fifty-First Report of the Commissioners of National Education in Ireland*, H. C. 1884–5 [C.4458] xxiv.75, pp. 410–11.
13 *Fifty-Seventh Report of the Commissioners of National Education in Ireland*, H. C. 1890–1 [C.6411] xxix.1, p. 14.
14 *Irish Times* (11 March 1876), p. 4.
15 Data collated from *Reports of the Commissioners of National Education in Ireland* (1875–95).
16 McElligott, *Secondary Education in Ireland*, p. 5.
17 PRONI, ED/8/1/145, Communication relating to the establishment of Belfast Model School, 1895.
18 PRONI, ED/8/1/214, Communication relating to the erection of Carrickfergus Model School, 1899.
19 PRONI, ED/8/1/212, Communication relating to the erection of a cookery room at Newry Model School, 1898–1900.
20 'Motion for leave', *House of Commons Debates* (22 February 1892), vol. 1, cc. 968–99.
21 *Sixty-Second Report of the Commissioners of National Education in Ireland*, H. C. 1896 [C. 8142] xxviii.1, p. 26.
22 *Fifty-Ninth Report of the Commissioners of National Education in Ireland*, H. C. 1893–4 [C.7124] xxvii.265, p. 160.
23 F. M. Gallaher, *Short Lessons in Domestic Science* (Dublin: Browne and Nolan, 2nd edn, 1894), pp. 85–6.
24 Ibid., pp. 112–14.
25 Ibid., p. 122.
26 Ibid., pp. 152–3.
27 Ibid., p. 172.
28 T. Fahey, 'Nuns in the Catholic church in Ireland in the nineteenth century', in M. Cullen (ed.), *Girls Don't Do Honours: Irish Women in Education in the Nineteenth and Twentieth Centuries* (Dublin: Women's Education Bureau, 1987).

29 *Fifty-First Report of Commissioners*, p. 250.
30 For discussion of the middle-class ideologies of convent schools, see C. Clear, *Nuns in Nineteenth-Century Ireland* (Dublin: Gill and Macmillan, 1987), pp. 114–16.
31 *Sixty-Second Report of Commissioners of National Education*, p. 407.
32 'Cookery and laundry teaching (Ireland)', *House of Commons Debates* (19 July 1897), vol. 51. c. 412.
33 'Class IV', *House of Commons Debates* (15 July 1898), vol. 61, cc. 1233–79 on 1278–9.
34 *Sixty-Sixth Report of the Commissioners of National Education in Ireland*, H. C. 1900 [Cd.285] xxiii.189, p. 158.
35 W. E. Vaughan and A. J. Fitzpatrick (eds), *Irish Historical Statistics, Population 1821–1971* (Dublin: Royal Irish Academy, 1978), pp. 261–3.
36 *Sixty-Sixth Report of Commissioners of National Education*, p. 159.
37 T. Carroll, 'Education in agriculture', *New Ireland Review*, 4 (February 1896), 336–40 on p. 337.
38 *Fifty-Sixth Report of Commissioners of National Education*, p. 868.
39 'Irish Industrial League', *Freeman's Journal* (5 February 1891), p. 6.
40 'Chemico-Agricultural Society of Ulster', *Belfast Newsletter* (28 January 1893), p. 6.
41 *Final Report of the Commission on Manual and Practical Instruction in Primary Schools under the Board of National Education in Ireland*, H. C. 1897 [C.8923] xliv.1, p. 3.
42 See, for instance, L. Davidoff and C. Hall, *Family Fortunes: Men and Women of the English Middle Class, 1750–1850* (Chicago: University of Chicago, 1987).
43 'Food: Its Preparation and Variety', *Irish Times* (1 April 1886), p. 8.
44 See J. Calder, *The Victorian Home* (London: Batsford, 1977).
45 T. Nulty, *The Relations Existing between Convent Schools and the Systems of Intermediate and Primary National Education* (Dublin: Browne and Nolan, 1884), p. 36.
46 'Practical Cookery', *Weekly Irish Times* (15 November 1884), p. 2.
47 E. Thomas, *Technical Instruction* (Dublin: Browne and Nolan, 1900), p. 14.
48 'The Feeding of the People', *Irish Homestead* (12 March 1898), pp. 237–8.
49 H. Hawthorn, 'The Ideal Girl', *Ireland's Own* (26 November 1902), p. 8.
50 B. Lynch, 'The Ideal Girl', *Ireland's Own* (3 December 1902), p. 8.
51 *Ireland's Own* (10 December 1902), p. 8.
52 *Third Report of the Commission on Manual and Practical Instruction in Primary Schools under the Board of National Education in Ireland*, H. C. 1897 [C.8618] xliii.401, p. 139.
53 Ibid., p. 26.
54 *First Report of Commission on Manual and Practical Instruction*, p. 29.
55 *Final Report of Commission on Manual and Practical Instruction*, p. 3.
56 Ibid., p. 42.
57 *Bourke, Husbandry to Housewifery*, pp. 26–7, p. 262.
58 D. Fitzpatrick, 'The modernisation of the Irish female', in P. O'Flanagan, P. Ferguson and K. Whelan (eds), *Rural Ireland 1600–1900: Modernisation and Change* (Cork: Cork University Press, 1987), p. 167.
59 F. M. F. Lovibond, 'Women and hygiene in modern life', *New Ireland Review*, 21 (April 1904), 74–82 on pp. 74–5.
60 J. Harford and D. Raftery, 'The education of girls within the national system', in D. Raftery and S. M. Parkes (eds), *Female Education in Ireland 1700–1900: Minerva or Madonna* (Dublin and Portland, OR: Irish Academic Press, 2007).
61 Agricultural and Technical Instruction (Ireland) Act, 1899 (62 & 63 Vict.), c. 50. See also M. Daly, *The First Department: A History of the Department of Agriculture* (Dublin: Institute of Public Administration, 2002).

62 *First Annual General Report of the Department of Agriculture and Technical Instruction*, H. C. 1902 [Cd.838] xx.522, p. 1, p. 14.
63 Ibid., p. 88.
64 Ibid., p. 150.
65 Ibid., p. 22.
66 H. Plunkett, *Memorandum on Agricultural Education for Ireland* (Dublin: DATI, 1901), p. 2.
67 Ibid., p. 4.
68 Ibid., p. 11.
69 Ibid., p. 12.
70 *Fourth Annual General Report of the Department of Agriculture and Technical Instruction*, H. C. 1905 [Cd.2509] xxi.261, pp. 1–3.
71 *Sixth Annual General Report of the Department of Agriculture of Technical Instruction*, 1907 [Cd.3543] xvii.241, p. 18.
72 *Second Annual General Report of the Department of Agricultural and Technical Instruction*, H. C. 1902 [Cd.1314] xx.817, pp. 183–4.
73 *Fourth Annual General Report of DATI*, p. 34.
74 Bourke, *Husbandry to Housewifery*.
75 *First Annual General Report of DATI*, p. 34.
76 M. E. Daly, *Social and Economic History of Ireland since 1800* (Dublin: Educational Company of Ireland, 1981), p. 59.
77 First Annual General Report of DATI, p. 46.
78 *Third Annual General Report of the Department of Agriculture and Technical Instruction, 1902–3*, H. C. 1904 [Cd.1919] xvi.435, p. 45.
79 *Third Annual General Report of DATI*, p. 188.
80 *Sixty-Eighth Report of the Commissioners of National Education in Ireland*, H. C. 1901 [Cd.1198] xxx.403, p. 77.
81 Ibid., p. 78.
82 *Second Annual General Report of DATI*, p. 24.
83 *Third Annual General Report of DATI*, pp. 85–6.
84 *Third Annual General Report of DATI*, p. 87.
85 *Sixth Annual General Report of DATI*, p. 91.
86 Data compiled from 'Index of Teachers Qualifying at Training Colleges', NAI, Department of Education, ED 8/2.
87 *Appendix to the Sixty-Seventh Report of the Commissioners of National Education in Ireland*, H. C. 1902 [Cd.954] xxx.1, pp. 89–91.
88 Ibid., p. 91.
89 *Fourth Annual General Report of DATI*, p. 6.
90 *Appendix to the Sixty-Ninth Report of the Commissioners of National Education in Ireland*, H. C. 1904 [Cd.1903] xx.195, p. 187.
91 National Library of Ireland (hereafter NLI), Minutes of the Proceedings of the Commissioners of National Education in Ireland, 1902, p. 104.
92 'Instruction in cookery in Irish Schools', *House of Commons Debates*, 4 March 1908, vol. 185, c. 696
93 *Fourth Annual General Report of DATI*, p. 6.
94 Ibid., p. 8.
95 *Appendix to Sixty-Seventh Report of Commissioners of National Education*, pp. 89–91.
96 Ibid., p. 9.
97 Ibid., p. 90.
98 NLI, Minutes of the Proceedings of the Commissioners of National Education in

Ireland, 1901, pp. 250–1.
99 Ibid., p. 317.
100 NLI, Minutes of the Proceedings of the Commissioners of National Education in Ireland, 1905, p. 30.
101 NLI, Minutes of the Proceedings of the Commissioners of National Education in Ireland, 1904, p. 154.
102 NLI, Minutes of the Proceedings of the Commissioners of National Education in Ireland, 1905, pp. 102–3.
103 PRONI, ED 8/1/212.
104 NAI, Department of Agriculture, 92/1/26, Building Grants for Technical Instruction.
105 'Funds for building Technical Schools', *Irish Technical Journal* 4 (July 1903), pp. 72–4.
106 NAI, 'Building Grants for Technical Instruction'.
107 *Seventy-Second Report of the Commissioners of the National Education in Ireland*, H. C. 1906 [Cd.3154] xxix.635, p. 18.
108 *Seventy-Fourth Report of the Commissioners of National Education in Ireland*, 1908 [Cd.4291] xxvii.841, p. 6.
109 NLI, Minutes of the Proceedings of the Commissioners of National Education in Ireland, 1907, p. 98.
110 Ibid., p. 101.
111 *Appendix to Seventy-Seventh Report of the Commissioners of National Education in Ireland*, H. C. 1912–3 [Cd.5935] xxi.409.
112 NAI, Department of Agriculture Files, 92/2/302.
113 *Appendix to the Seventieth Report of the Commissioners of National Education in Ireland*, H. C. 1905 [Cd.2373] xxvii.403, p. 104.
114 Ibid., p. 206.
115 *Sixty-Eighth Report of the Commissioners of National Education*, p. 92.
116 K. Ferguson, *Advanced Lessons in Cookery* (Athlone: Athlone Printing Works, 1903).
117 J. Redington, *The Economic Cookery Book* (Dublin: M. H. Gill and Son, 1906), p. ii.
118 Ibid., p. 1.
119 Ibid., p. 14.
120 Ibid., p. 3.
121 *Sixty-Eighth Report of Commissioners of National Education*, p. 93; *Appendix to Sixty-Ninth Report of Commissioners of National Education*, p. 35.

III

Food, imperialism and resistance, c.1900–22

7

Voluntarism, the state and the feeding of the young

Who ought to assume responsibility for feeding the young? Were mothers who failed to do so neglectful individuals or simply lacking in dietetic and nutritional knowledge? And what role should the state adopt in relation to infant and child welfare and, by extension, securing the future health of the citizen body? Questions such as these were pivotal to a prominent turn-of-the-century Irish food discourse that exerted a strong influence on contemporary conceptions of infanthood, childhood and motherhood. The problems highlighted by these questions were simultaneously personal, biological and socio-political. Furthermore, they formed the basis of a new array of improving strategies designed to improve the health of the young. In Ireland, childhood health was a concern that rested primarily in the hands of voluntary groups who sought to persuade the state to assume greater responsibility.[1] This chapter explores the ideas and work of two voluntary groups: the Women's National Health Association (WNHA) and the Ladies School Dinners Committee (LSDC). Although these groups held contrasting political agendas, they united around the precept that feeding the young was a matter of national importance and strove, in different ways, to increase state intervention.

Importantly, the very presence of these groups is indicative of the post-Famine spread of dietary knowledge. By the turn of the century, middle-class women had absorbed dietary and nutritional knowledge to such a degree that they were now able to confidently position themselves as authorities on food. Unlike in earlier decades, those dispensing knowledge no longer had to be medical or scientific experts, although philanthropic women certainly referred to medico-scientific knowledge to validate their perspectives on domesticity and good motherhood. Instead, these were figures – mostly female – that had grasped and appreciated the social utility of the science of food, developed a nutritional consciousness and started to present themselves as appropriate vectors of dietary knowledge. They sought to carve out new areas of social intervention and to forge new forms of bodily governance that exerted considerable influence over the vulnerable young. Nonetheless, the quest to enact nutritional improvement ultimately remained confined to voluntary schemes rather than state action. This scenario, as this chapter demonstrates, allowed nationalist opponents to British rule to ask whether imperial governance was in fact helping to determine the conditions that had caused Irish national decline rather than helping to remove them, a theme that forms the basis of Part III of this monograph.

Infant welfare

During the late nineteenth century, the individualistic *laissez-faire* principles that had once dominated British politics gradually began to fall out of fashion to be replaced by new forms of liberal social intervention.[2] Contemporaneously, ideas gained currency of childhood being a sacred period of health and maternal protection that the young had a right to enjoy.[3] These developments coincided with mounting concern over national deterioration and a related uptake of the idea that promoting the health of the young would guard against further national decline. Strengthening the physical and psychological stamina of the rising generation, it seemed, would ensure future national collective health. Although observations of the weak calibre of military recruits following the Boer War have traditionally been depicted as the driving force behind turn-of-the-century initiatives to counter degeneration in Britain, Vanessa Heggie presents a more nuanced picture, persuasively demonstrating that contemporary debates on national decline were equally, if not predominantly, concerned with long-standing, non-military social issues such as diet and health.[4] This argument is affirmed in early twentieth-century Irish contexts where, more often than not, discussion coalesced around now familiar issues such as excessive tea drinking and post-Famine nutritional decline rather than imminent conflict. In this context, pessimistic nineteenth-century accounts of national decay and decline gradually gave way to a new, more optimistic, neo-hygienist approach. At its heart, neo-hygienism espoused the value of scientifically educating parents on infant and childhood health to attack national decline at its physiological root.[5]

In the early twentieth century, the extent to which state bodies ought to intervene in personal matters such as child rearing remained undecided. French obstetrician Aldophe Pinard had recently and influentially posited that childhood health could be productively cultivated if mothers heeded the doctrines of nutritional and physiological science. Subsequently, the French state began to actively intervene in matters of motherhood and infanthood under the pretext of ameliorating national physical decline. Shortly afterwards, discussion was sparked in other European countries about the value of state intervention in those arenas, although sceptics retorted that state intrusion would result in mothers becoming reliant rather than independent.[6] Physicians and health reformers referred to, and productively contributed to, these narratives by sponsoring new regimes of infant and childhood health care intended to ensure a normal growth into adulthood. They also interacted with the state in complex ways.[7] Anna Davin convincingly demonstrates that British concerns over infant life and child health arose in this period as the value of a strong and numerous young population came to be gradually realised as a potential national resource that would provide citizens to populate an ever-expanding Empire and produce soldiers to fight against competing imperial powers.[8] Accordingly, a sequence of new policies was initiated in Britain including compulsory medical inspection, national insurance and school meals legislation. These legislative measures generated a lively discussion of the acceptable boundaries of state intervention in personal and familial health.[9] In addition, by 1900, the nature of public health had shifted away from a sole focus on regulating unhealthy environments to managing more personal aspects of daily life and social relations.[10]

In Ireland, mothers, children and infants emerged as new objects of close medical governance. Philanthropic groups formed to tackle nutritional problems among the less affluent and often raised awareness of problems left unaddressed in the formal education system. Although the reform of domestic instruction had been welcomed as a potentially important driver of social reform, it seemed inconceivable to some that, alone, it could successfully avert problems in post-Famine dietary customs. The Bishop of Ross, when giving evidence to the Inter-Departmental Committee on Physical Deterioration (1904), conceded that the Commissioners of National Education had striven admirably to remedy issues such as excessive tea drinking. However, according to the Bishop, 'the causes are like a torrent sweeping away the population and the remedies are only like a drop, and it will take a very considerable time before we have the current on the other side'.[11] Voluntarism was a further key resource for remedying deficient dietary customs through the targeting of mothers, infants and children.

The Women's National Health Association and infant welfare

The WNHA was founded in 1907 by the Countess of Aberdeen Ishbel Gordon – popularly known as Lady Aberdeen – who was the wife of Lord Lieutenant John Campbell Hamilton-Gordon.[12] The organisation's 19,000 members rapidly established 150 branches nationwide with the aim of stemming high infant mortality rates, promoting new regimes of child welfare and tackling tuberculosis.[13] At the turn of the century, Irish infant mortality rates were significantly higher than in many other countries. In fact, incidences of infant deaths were declining in Britain and America.[14] The ideological aspirations of the Association can be neatly situated within emerging neo-hygienist doctrines that often apportioned blame for poor infant health to maternal ignorance. To counter this perceived lack of knowledge, the Association exhorted education. Notably, the proposed reform of motherhood affirmed ideas that Irish society needed to be divided along gendered lines to maximise national socio-economic potential. As Greta Jones suggests, the WNHA adopted tactics of health management that upheld female domesticity as a means of 'civilising' working-class homes.[15] It was from the home that improvement would stem.

Middle-class interventions in working-class domestic life were buttressed by a strong scientific ethos. The WNHA's knowledge of nutrition helped the organisation to justify its philanthropic presence in working-class homes. For instance, a key strategy deployed by its members involved stressing the pivotal importance of milk to infant health. The status of milk had recently shifted from a hazardous – potentially adulterated or contaminated – drink to one that, if clean and uninfected, strengthened infant bodies and helped to prepare the young for a healthy adult existence. Research conducted in the 1890s by individuals such as Thomas Rotch, Professor of Childhood Diseases at Harvard University, demonstrated that milk contained valuable quantities of casein, fat, sugar and salt.[16] Through lectures and pamphlets, the Association stressed the importance of breast-feeding, bottle-feeding and securing pure milk and also outlined the dietary causes of diarrhoea, vomiting and constipation and the practical importance of good cookery.[17] In addition, the Association's members vociferously rallied against popular beliefs that porter increased milk quantity, insisting instead that breast milk ought to be of a high quality and that nursing mothers should avoid alcohol, tea, coffee, mustard and spices.[18]

Philanthropists also drew attention to issues of hygiene in public milk supplies. Public health officials such as Charles Cameron had recently forged concrete associations between milk and tuberculosis infection. In the late nineteenth century, connections between tuberculosis and milk had remained heavily disputed as the idea of intra-special disease transmission was novel, controversial and open to contestation. However, bacteriologists had more convincingly established these links by 1900.[19] One important outcome was the declining sway of understandings of tuberculosis as a hereditary condition. Instead, tuberculosis was understood as a bacterial problem.[20] Shifting medical emphases fostered new preventative strategies. The WNHA proclaimed the importance of eradicating bacteria and germs from domestic life and, in doing so, reinforced morally charged doctrines of cleanliness and order. As Nancy Tomes details in relation to America, middle class reformers exposed working-class housewives to a nascent 'gospel of germs'. They achieved this by transforming themselves into 'domestic scientists' whose self-proclaimed mission was to modernise, rationalise and cleanse domestic space under the aegis of stemming contagion.[21] Bacteriological eradication in the home, and in substances such as milk, was visibly enshrined in the WNHA's campaign. Promoting the consumption of (uninfected) milk worked on two interconnected and encompassing levels: milk stimulated healthy infant growth while the closer regulation of supplies helped to combat tuberculosis. Combined, these strategies offered a socially utilitarian strategy intended to lower infant mortality rates and avert further degeneration.

Pasteurising milk was a key initiative promoted by the WNHA. Directly inspired by developments in bacteriology, pasteurisation involved heating milk at a high temperature to purify the substance of germs. As the Association's publication *Sláinte* warned in 1909:

> The tender digestive organs of little babies, intended as they are by Nature to deal with 'mother's milk', which is sterile – that is, free from germs – are cruelly upset

> by the countless swarms of ordinary dirt germs which are present in milk as usually supplied. In every drop of such milk, when the weather is warm, over a million of dirt germs can be found![22]

Although alarmist, accounts such as these were calculated to instil an awareness of the invisible, but potentially harmful, content of milk. In 1908, the Association established a pasteurised milk depot near Phoenix Road, Dublin, an initiative influenced by similar schemes operating in France and British cities such as Glasgow.[23] The WNHA also established the depot in response to the ongoing difficulties faced by Dublin's urban poor in obtaining good quality, unadulterated milk. Milk supplies received at the depot were guaranteed to have come from healthy cows kept in humane conditions and who had been hygienically milked. To counteract the poor taste and palatability caused by intensive heating, the Association's members added cream, sugar and water to 'humanise' the milk. The concoction would then be made up in different strengths according to the different ages of infants.[24] In 1911, the Association extended this scheme by setting up a milk depot in Naas, Co. Kildare, after becoming aware of seasonal milk scarcities in that region. However, it was not enough to simply provide milk. Mothers, so the WNHA insisted, also needed educating if they were to be improved. Accordingly, managers dispensed detailed information on nutrition and infant feeding when providing milk and refused to sell milk to mothers who arrived brandishing a dirty jug.[25]

This blending of practical and conceptual considerations was also embodied in the WNHA's baby clubs, a scheme that served the dual purpose of improving the health of both mothers and children. The first of these opened in Belfast in 1908 and operated between three and five o'clock on Mondays and Fridays. The site reportedly received forty mothers in its first month of operation alone. Although the WNHA charged mothers ½ d. for their baby to be weighed, the Association offered tea and buns to mothers as well as educational material in return. Mothers could buy feeding bottles at the baby clubs on the condition that they listened to basic advice on simple methods of preparing and storing milk. On alternate Fridays, the Association provided cooking lessons where housewives learnt how to budget 12 s. 9 d. per week to feed an entire family nutritiously. The Association felt so assured of the cumulative benefits of their baby clubs that its members confidently asserted in 1909 that not one infant had succumbed to diarrhoea in Belfast in the autumn of that year – a direct upshot of the milk distribution scheme.[26]

Evidently, philanthropic women in Ireland amalgamated theories of nutrition and disease transmission to assemble an active social programme that aimed to foster improvement in personal, social and national domains. The social outlook of the WNHA captured the spirit of neo-hygienist agendas as it portrayed Irish mothers as morally sound individuals capable of forming strong emotional bonds with their children but whose lack of knowledge caused unintentional suffering for children and, indeed, for mothers themselves should their infants succumb to disease and ill-health. Accordingly, their strategies hinged on tackling ignorance, not negligence. Rejecting derogatory, but previously influential, perspectives on intentional neglect as responsible for infant mortality, the Association contradictorily insisted that improper feeding resulted from mistaken ideas about the digestive capacities of the young and a lack of awareness of infant nutritional needs. By insinuating that working-class mothers lacked knowledge, new social relations crystallised that empowered philanthropic middle-class ladies to offer scientific guidance to the uninformed. The notion of ignorance in itself justified the very presence of middle-class ladies in the working-class home.

Yet the Association reached an impasse when it attempted to draw upon its successful voluntary schemes to campaign for a systematic state-supported scheme. Its members intended voluntary milk depots to provide a model for an anticipated state-assisted system. This was evident in the proceedings of the Vice-Regal Commission on the Irish Milk Supply, appointed in May 1911 and presided over by Aberdeen's husband Hamilton-Gordon. The Commission referred to the achievements of the WNHA to reinforce its opinion that Irish municipalities and urban authorities should be awarded powers to contribute to depots from the rates. In turn, so the Commission insisted, children would reap the socio-physical benefits of healthier constitutions and enjoy protection from disease, thereby decreasing the future financial burdens of ratepayers.[27] Impressively, the Commission made a thorough national investigation of milk supplies to draw attention to dramatic regional variance. It identified many small towns as suffering from seasonal milk scarcities and demonstrated that milk was virtually unprocurable in remote rural regions in Co. Meath, Co. Donegal and Co. Galway. The Commission established that graziers fattened milch cows for retail as meat in those areas instead of rearing strong milk-producing cattle.[28] Some witnesses cited popular prejudices against the condensed milk returned from creameries as a secondary problem. One witness claimed that condensed milk had a 'vile, sour, venomous taste' as it had been heated at a high temperature.[29] However, despite having gathered persuasive evidence about the economic determinants of low milk consumption, the Commission ultimately rejected lack of availability as the root cause of milk's unpopularity. The poor, they asserted, did not enthusiastically buy milk even in regions with relatively high availability.[30] Instead, its members predictably blamed the ignorance of mothers in nutritional matters; a stance that further legitimised the perceived need for voluntary organisations and local authorities to encroach into working-class domestic space.[31]

This conclusion allowed the Commission to sponsor personal instead of social or economic reform. It sought to modify individual domestic behaviour rather than promote change in the conditions that created, encouraged and sustained poverty. Some witnesses went so far as to claim that poor purchasing choices made by mothers were partly to blame for Ireland's unfavourable economic climate. This perspective was palpable in the claims of William Henry Thompson, Professor of Physiology at Trinity College, Dublin. Linking personal matters of consumption to the economic vitality of the nation, he asserted that:

> I think the race really is affected by the ability or the inability of the mothers to nurse their children, and this is very largely at bottom a question of the nutrition of the mother. The mothers among the poor children are really not, I think, sufficiently fed to be able to nurse their children, and then I think the whole question of the nutrition of the working man has the greatest influence upon his willingness and capacity as a worker. In fact, I think the lack of interest in his work, what is called by some the laziness of the Irish workman, is largely a question of feeding him. So that the question has an intimate relation with the economic condition of the country.[32]

Thompson elaborated by depicting milk and tea consumption as interconnected contours of a vicious circle. Tea, he argued, was most popular during seasonal periods of milk scarcities. Local populations quickly became addicted to the substance and remained so even when milk supplies once again became available. Infants and young children were particular prone to becoming accustomed to the taste of tea, reported Thompson, in the way that adults might become addicted to alcohol. Intense tea cravings, coupled with the development of a life-long repugnance for milk, caused debilitation, anaemia, scurvy, abscesses and rickets, he claimed, while adult life, should a child get that far, passed with heightened susceptibility to epidemic disease.[33] Ignoring overriding factors such as poverty, as well as the influence of popular fears of adulteration and disease transmission, Thompson, like many other witnesses, firmly subscribed to the view that education was essential if purchasing habits were to be altered.

Despite the forcefulness of the Commission's evidence and conclusions, DATI failed to set its recommendations in place, a scenario that forced the WNHA to send a deputation to DATI three years later who reminded the Department of the outcomes of the Commission. At this meeting, Aberdeen suggested that DATI's domestic economy instructresses could help to distribute information on the nutritious value of milk to local communities and even offered to distribute pamphlets on the subject on behalf of DATI. Aberdeen also offered the services of the Association in managing milk depots and clubs.[34] The fact that a scheme never came to fruition might be attributable to a subsequent restructuring of financial outlay as the First World War commenced. What is significant, however, is that the WNHA operated within, and strove to assist, pre-existing political administrative structures in managing infant mortality. Their close allegiance with the state and official bodies shaped, if not dictated, their approaches to tackling infant feeding. However, the Association was ultimately unable to go beyond the bounds of voluntarism to encourage state bodies and local authorities to intervene.

'School-day starvation'

Questions of who should assume responsibility for childhood feeding became remarkably tense in the immediate pre-Independence period as female nationalists seized opportunities to challenge the state's ostensible preoccupation with childhood welfare. They sought to expose transparency in official interest in motherhood and child-rearing by querying why the state had not initiated appropriate welfare policies in Ireland. Debates on this matter coalesced around school meals. School-day feeding had emerged as a topical subject after the implementation of the Irish Education Act in 1892. This made school attendance compulsory for pupils aged between six and fourteen on at least seventy-five days of each half year. However, the measure aroused opposition as it was seen to remove young family members from the economic unit of the family. Critics also raised questions about formal provision not having been put in place for school-day feeding.[35] Organised opposition emerged slowly. Although a group of teachers formed the Midday Meal Hour Movement in 1901, their campaign was short-lived.[36] The minute books of the Commissioners of National Education reveal that in 1901, Anthony Traill, provost of Trinity College, Dublin proposed the fixing of a thirty-minute midday interval to allow National School pupils to return home to eat. The Commissioners disproved of this plan and the issue remained notably absent in subsequent meetings.[37]

Interest resurfaced in 1906 when the Home Office implemented the Education (Provision of Meals) Act across the rest of the British Isles.[38] John Burnett emphasises the significance of this measure in that it was implemented in the face of strong concern about the spread of socialist ideas and the potential of school meal provision to diminish self-help.[39] According to James Vernon, school meals provision signalled the state finally assuming responsibility for hunger – a step that he portrays as having constituted a profound shift in state approaches to feeding the poor.[40] Notably, however, John Welshman warns of the dangers of focusing on the symbolic meanings of legislation alone as school meals were in reality adopted unevenly and gradually.[41] Official explanations for Ireland's exclusion from the Act often dwelled upon the fact that National Schools were not under the control of a Local Education Authority. The English act allowed schools to defray expenses out of local rates. According to one English MP, the work of philanthropic ladies and nuns was enough for Ireland.[42] But were other factors in play? Burnett notes, in relation to Britain, that religious opposition to school meals coalesced around the idea that school day feeding dissipated parental responsibility for feeding and nurturing.[43] It is certainly plausible to hypothesise that the architects of the School Meals Act were wary of antagonising a Catholic Church that held an ingrained hostility to the principle of non-denominational education. In 1913, the Archbishop of Dublin adopted a cautious approach when he warned of the dangers of indiscriminate assistance and undeserving children being given food.[44]

This strict ideological perspective failed to convince many of those working in the school system who came face-to-face with hungry children on a daily basis. Disheartened by an absence of formal provision, some Irish schools opted to voluntarily serve meals. This was the case at Oblates National School, Inchicore, Co. Dublin, where in 1905 headmaster T. P. O'Brien, also Vice-President of the South Dublin National Teachers' Association, established facilities to allow pupils to buy a midday meal of bread and butter, jam and cocoa. O'Brien's scheme was financed through local subscriptions and supported by prominent local ladies who provided food.[45] The WNHA also distributed penny dinners at Celbridge, Co. Kildare. The Association distributed up to a hundred dinners in the opening four weeks of the scheme at a charge of 1 d. for older children, and ½ d. for younger children. The school was fortunate enough to hold a cooking range meaning that the Association had only to supply bowls, spoons, pots and a kettle at a total cost of £2 18 s.[46] The success of these schemes was contingent on schools having a pre-existing cooking facility which, as concurrent debates about domestic education demonstrated, was often not the case.

Debates on school meals were divided around ideological questions on the desirability of parental or state responsibility. Some female nationalist groups such as the United Irishwomen resolutely opposed the principle of school meals provision. When Mary Lawless delivered an address at the organisation's annual general meeting in 1911 entitled 'Feeding Schoolchildren in Rural Districts', she insisted that feeding children from local rates would demoralise parents by freeing them from their natural parental responsibilities. As an alternative, Lawless promoted a system where parents contributed to the cost of ingredients.[47] Later that year, United Irishwomen president Anita Lett asserted in the *Irish Times*:

> Why cry to the British government to help us to feed our children? . . . There is, no doubt, something very wrong in a system which causes the deterioration of the race, and our best efforts should be put forward to alter that system, and until we have altered it to one more suitable to the tender years and delicate constitutions of our children, let us at least feed them ourselves.

The United Irishwomen held little confidence in a state-organised scheme, as exemplified in Lett's appended announcement: 'Let us do something and do it quickly; something to meet this obvious and terrible evil which is undermining the health of the race, and causing unknown suffering to our children, and let us do it without pauperising our people or wasting our money on State-aid and State officials.' Lett proposed instead that a committee of women be formed in each parish to prepare dinners.[48]

Nonetheless, those with contrasting perspectives stressed that school feeding was too large an undertaking to be organised by private initiative alone. According to this viewpoint, state intervention was the only feasible solution. In this context, the absence of state provision in Ireland evolved into an important and emotive issue that captured the attention of leading intellectual figures such as Reverend Thomas A. Finlay. Finlay was a Professor of Classics, Philosophy and Political Economy at University College Dublin and was also renowned for his active role in the Irish Renaissance, having edited its leading publications *New Ireland Review* and *Irish Homestead*.[49] The issue of school meals provision blended Finlay's interests in education and social improvement and it is unsurprising to find him, while serving as President of the Child Study and Food Hygiene section of the Public Health Congress in 1906, offering a provocative indictment of a system that, in his view, enforced a cruel act of forcing half-starved children to undertake intense mental work. For Finlay, a lack of school feeding provision was acutely problematic in impoverished western regions where children were already under-nourished.[50] Concern also surfaced in the 1907 Royal Commission on Congestion when witness W. J. D. Walker insisted that food was a necessity for education. Children reared on bread and tea, Walker warned, were not fit subjects for a National School education.[51] By connecting scanty feeding with decreased intellectual capacity, advocates of school meals were able to argue that the young required food to operate efficiently, both physically and mentally, in educational environments.

Female nationalists were often the most vocal figures who trenchantly objected to an absence of school meals policy for Ireland. Nationalists attached themselves to the cause because what they dubbed 'school-day starvation' offered an evocative platform upon which they could attack the legitimacy of imperial influence in Ireland and the authenticity of state interest in childhood health. In their view, the state had effectively forced children out of the home without pausing to consider how they were to be fed. Assertions that state legislation (or an absence of it) damaged the health of children held deep resonance. If British interest was bound up with the needs of Empire and creating a generation to oversee it, as Davin suggests, then Ireland's legislative exclusion from a key welfare policy implied, for some, a subservient, rather than active, colonial function. This allowed female nationalist groups to portray Ireland as a space where the state was weakening bodies rather than strengthening the young to perform an important imperial role. Campaigners queried colonial logic by insinuating that state policies in Ireland were in fact sustaining poor childhood health conditions and contributing to ongoing national physical and psychological deterioration. Turning on their head notions that ignorant, tea-addicted mothers were to blame for precarious Irish childhood health, they insinuated that deficient state policies were fertilising poor Irish well-being.

The trope of starvation served useful rhetorical purposes. Women's republican newspaper *Bean nÉireann* emotively presented Ireland's legislative exclusion as constituting a deliberate policy of schoolroom starvation. It also adversarially situated an absence of provision in a much longer lineage of imperial agendas of starving the Irish populace, a narrative that provocatively conjured images of the Famine. 'England cannot prevent the long families in Ireland', so one editorial claimed, 'but she can arrange to weaken in dietary the health of the Irish citizen. It suits her policy even better than emigration, for the Irish in America are sometimes troublesome.'[52]

In the midst of these heated debates, the Ladies School Dinners Committee formed in 1910, marking the commencement of a sustained campaign for state provision. In contrast to the WNHA, the Committee adopted a strikingly confrontational ethos that, although frequently emotive, makes it difficult to disentangle the extent to which their activities and public outcries arose from a genuine, deep concern over the fate of children or whether Irish exclusion from legislation offered yet another trope for challenging British governance. The Committee's leader was the revolutionary, feminist and actress Maud Gonne, best remembered for her turbulent relationship with poet W. B. Yeats but also as a central female nationalist figure.[53] Gonne's reflections on school meals can be gleaned from an article published in the *Irish Review* in 1911, in which she asserted:

> A great wrong is being done in our midst. Hundreds of child lives are being sacrificed; thousands of Irish boys and girls are being condemned to life-long physical suffering and mental inefficiency by school-day starvation. Under pain of imprisonment Irish parents are by English law obliged to send their children to school, and from nine thirty to three o'clock the children are obliged to remain in school. No provision is made for feeding the children thus taken into custody. Growing children need more frequent food than adults, they have tissues to make, and they expend more nervous energy; and in all free countries where education is compulsory, for the sake of the future of the race, arrangements are made to ensure school children are fed.[54]

Gonne's poignant rendering of 'school-day starvation' not only reveals how she chose to subsume her critique within a broader condemnation of British influence in Ireland, but also how she evocatively invoked a sense that future Irish physiological decline was being propagated under British rule rather than resolved. She inverted the logic of policies ostensibly committed to reversing degeneration by asserting that the educational system supported by the state itself was perpetuating the physical and psychological weakening of Irish subjects. Notably, her statements were also intended to challenge the Irish Parliamentary Party whose brand of constitutional nationalism was proving unpopular in Ireland.

The colonial-orientated content of Gonne's public assertions proved persistent in her later critiques. In October 1912, she proclaimed that 'it is no unusual thing for a child to faint from hunger in an Irish National School' and declared that 'some of our Irish National Schools appear terrible and tragic factories for the destruction of the race'.[55] Her writing, although hyperbolic, depicted images of injustice and forced legal obligations to an unwanted and alien legislative presence. In this account, the schoolroom itself was portrayed as allegoric of all that seemed wrong in the fraught relationship between Britain and Ireland. It presented the bodies of Irish citizens as being deliberately weakened from childhood as the bodies of the young failed to grow if their surpluses of nervous energy were expended when unfed at school. For Gonne, Irish schoolrooms served as metaphoric spaces where imposed power relations and systems of governance were played out and where policies of subjugation were being physically inscribed upon the fragile bodies of the Irish young.

Explicit in her claims were broader questions of whether Ireland was a benefactor of policies associated with imperial motherhood or, rather, a subject country whose vitality was being sapped to benefit the expansion and maintenance of the British colonial system.

Although Gonne adopted an overtly propagandist and anti-imperialist tone, her arguments did point to pertinent social issues. After all, many children in poverty-stricken districts were indeed underfed and might have benefited from school-day feeding. On one occasion, she argued that over half of the children from Dublin's poorest districts failed to bring lunches into school with them and, in consequence, were being educated on empty stomachs. Furthermore, Gonne suggested, many families had finished their dinners by the time their children returned home, by which time the male breadwinner had consumed most of the food. In Gonne's words, 'little is left for the children after their long cruel school fast but bread and tea again'.[56] Yet Gonne strove to direct blame away from the mother herself by presenting her as a caring, compassionate individual whose disadvantageous circumstances dictated hunger, rather than a lack of emotional feeling towards her children. 'No mothers are tenderer than the Irish mothers', so Gonne later claimed in *Bean hÉireann*, 'and it is absurd to suppose a mother would let her children go hungry if she saw any way of preventing it, and there is a side of this children's tragedy of which I dare hardly think, and that is the agony of the mothers who watch their little ones fading and know the cause and cannot remedy it.'[57]

Gonne also implicitly attacked the nature of the medico-scientific ideologies underpinning influential perspectives on the desired reform of motherhood. These had coalesced around facilitating normal physical, mental and moral growth through improved nutrition. Offering a counter-argument, Gonne insisted that high mortality rates, widespread tuberculosis and rising insanity levels were all ascribable to policies of 'school-day starvation'. To fortify this powerful claim, she drew attention to an address given earlier that year by nationalist physician and writer Oliver St John Gogarty of Meath Hospital in Dublin who had claimed that of the 3,000 children whom he had examined in the previous four years, a high proportion of physical and psychological complaints had developed in consequence of the strain of long hours of study without nourishment. Gonne also validated her assertions with evidence given by John O'Conor Donelan, assistant medical officer of Richmond Asylum, Dublin, who attributed numerous incidences of mental breakdown among the young to the excessive strain and long hours of schooling, coupled with insufficient physical nourishment. Having endorsed her arguments with expert medical authority, Gonne pondered whether 'the responsibility for this child murder will not rest on the community who allows it to go on without a protest'.[58] Gonne's use of medical evidence allowed her to complicate images of medicalised interest in mothers and children by positing that even if infant health was secured, degenerative impulses still existed in other areas of life that could be, and should be, regulated.

Gonne's statement clearly aimed to generate public feeling on the subject by conveying apocalyptic warnings about Irish national vitality and future decline. Simultaneously, she also formed a response to very real concerns about the fragility of Irish childhood. By 1912, her Committee was distributing 450 meals per day at St Audoen's and St John's Lane National Schools, two of the poorest schools in Dublin. Its members served Irish stew four times per week and rice and jam on Fridays at a cost of 1 d. to older children and ½ d. to younger children.[59] However, the Dublin Corporation refused to provide a grant to aid this work.[60] Gonne was later forced to manage the school meals campaign remotely after fleeing to France to care for her son, under fear that Irish authorities would take him out of her care if she stayed. Yet she never lost touch with the Committee, corresponding weekly and visiting at least three times a year. Like the WNHA, Gonne hoped that her school meals schemes at St Audoen's and St John's Lane in Dublin would reveal, through practical demonstration, the benefits of school meals provision. The value of her work rested not in the provision of food to an admittedly limited group of schoolchildren, but instead in its symbolic worth. She intended her efforts to demonstrate what could be achieved even with relatively limited resources in order to imply that much more could be achieved with extensive legislation and secure financial resources. To deflect arguments about the potential decline of parental responsibility, those pupils who could afford to pay did so.[61] Nonetheless, the scheme faced problems. In 1913, the Committee raised £278 15 s. However, the amount spent on dinners at the two Dublin schools had amounted to £328 7 s. 9 d.[62]

In 1912, Stephen B. Walsh elaborated upon the lack of financial support awarded to the Committee in an emotive article published in the *Irish Review* in which he suggested that provisions made for schools to appoint medical officers were worthless because the state had 'instituted a vast, elaborate, and costly scheme for discovering and tabulating defects in school children, but made not the slightest extra provision for treatment'.[63] In the same year, Gogarty drew further attention to Gonne's cause by arguing in the *Irish Review* that:

> The hours are far too long – 9.30am to 3.30pm at the earliest. The poorer children are left with a little piece of bread for lunch, even if they have as much as that. Some come breakfastless to school. Adults could not stand this treatment, much less could they assimilate learning, or fix their attention for half the time that is required for the children. We must not forget that the amount of disease in the world is daily and hourly rapidly increasing, because ethics and science are encouraging and increasing the duration of life. Lunacy is increasing in this country. The unfit are being propagated and preserved. There is neither law to protect the children nor law to save the future generation from unfit parents. Soon there will be no one healthy. But we must not deliberately hasten this morbid millennium. It may be in some way delayed, and the most important way of delaying it is to protect the rising generation. Feed the school children. The school children must be fed.[64]

Although witnesses to the Vice-Regal Committee of Inquiry into Primary Education (Ireland) of 1913 mostly skirted the issue, Alfred Purser, Chief

Inspector of the Board of National Education in Ireland, insisted in his evidence that food was important for the mind. However, he faced concerted opposition by Committee members who proceeded by pondering over the irrelevant question of whether the minds of schoolchildren could become overloaded and packed with food if fed at school, the inevitable outcome being 'mental indigestion'. Purser, although not a medical man, staunchly denied the existence of this so-called 'mental indigestion', asserting instead that if the mind of the child was overloaded then the mind would naturally reject excess food. Nonetheless, this furnished Committee members with further evidence that it was inadvisable to place food in the mind in the first place.[65] Gonne's efforts to convince the Dublin Corporation to provide school meals received a fresh impetus from the Dublin Lockout, a nine-month period of industrial tension that raised concern about the underfeeding and potential starvation of the children of working-class employees who were temporarily out of work.[66] The situation was eventually resolved through the introduction of the Education (Provision of Meals) (Ireland) Act of 1914 that allowed, but did not compel, local authorities to provide school meals via a central School Meals Committee. The Act also allowed Committees to distribute money for the purchasing of cooking equipment. Significantly, the structure of the Act went some way towards reaching a compromise between those who argued that responsibility for feeding rested with the family and those who favoured state intervention. It allowed some parents to be charged while stipulating that children who 'are unable by reason of lack of food to take full advantage of the education provided for them, could apply to the Local Government Board to spend money out of the rates'.[67]

Nonetheless, the execution of the Act raised further issues. The school meals organising committee consisted primarily of men – a situation that alarmed Helen Chenevix of the suffragist Irishwomen's Reform League who angrily pointed out in 1914 that the Committee lacked the skills and expertise that female philanthropic groups had developed.[68] The underlying reasons for this development were not quite as gendered as they appear on the surface. Gonne and her colleagues, after all, represented a highly reactionary element of Irish society, openly supporting revolutionary nationalist causes. Little surprise, then, that local bodies operating in Ireland failed to establish cordial relations with them, even despite their experience. The Committee was certainly in a less enviable position than the WNHA, a group more able to exert influence in official commissions. Further problems emerged when revelations surfaced of the School Meals Committee forcing teachers to supervise and assist in meals provision even though the Act had declared that this should not fall under the duties of the teacher. As trade unionist Ronald J. P. Mortished argued in a letter published in the *Irish Independent*, 'surely there are numbers of women, and perhaps, not a few men, who would be quite willing to do the work for nothing'. He also observed that doctors did not form part of the Committee, despite the obvious medical dimensions of school feeding. Nor had representatives of workers been appointed, the consequence being that children might be overcharged as the Committee lacked an understanding of average working-class family budgeting circumstances.[69] Nonetheless, the issue of school meals was one that captured the attention of various nationalist critics of British rule who saw the issue as emblematic of broader problems in Anglo-Irish relations. It offered a provocative trope that, for some, further validated the need for Ireland to govern itself. Indeed, in this instance, resistance to British rule coalesced around the Irish body and the need for schemes to be set in place to strengthen it and shield it against further national deterioration.

Conclusion

At the turn of the century, public and official interest in infant and childhood nutritional health increased, as did the public role adopted by philanthropists. The WNHA sought to address matters relating to infant feeding. Yet placing blame on the ignorance of mothers was a strategy that ignored other causative factors of infant mortality such as poverty. Importantly, the Association sought to resolve the issue of childhood health constitutionally. In sharp contrast, groups such as the LSDC picked up on the inherent weaknesses of ideologies that targeted mothers and inverted them by questioning the legitimacy of state approaches to improving the health of the Irish young or, conversely, asking if, as an imperial subject, Ireland was exempt from the broader agenda of strengthening the young. Individuals such as Gonne implicated state bodies in deliberate policies of weakening imperial subjects to cater for the needs of British expansionism and strove to expose the illogical behaviour of a government purportedly set on tackling infant mortality. Exploration of these debates further renders visible the intricate connections between food, the Irish population and the British state, as well as demonstrating the multiplicity of actors who now involved themselves in food matters for a variety of reasons.

Notes

1 For an overview of pre-independence child welfare strategies, see L. Earner-Byrne, *Mother and Child: Maternity and Child Welfare in Dublin, 1922–60* (Manchester: Manchester University Press, 2007), pp. 8–23.

2 G. Finlayson, *Citizen, State and Social Welfare in Britain, 1830–1990* (London: Clarendon Press, 1994).

3 H. Cunningham, *Children and Childhood in Western Society since 1500* (Harlow: Pearson Longman, 1995), pp. 171–8; For Irish contexts see A. Mauger and A. Mac Lellan, 'Introduction' in Mac Lellan and Mauger (eds), *Growing Pains*.

4 V. Heggie, 'Lies, damn lies, and Manchester's recruiting statistics: degeneration as an "urban legend" in Victorian and Edwardian Britain', *Journal of the History of Medicine and Allied Sciences*, 63:2 (April 2008), 178–216.

5 N. S. Rose, *The Psychological Complex: Psychology, Politics and Society in England, 1869–1935* (London: Routledge and Kegan Paul, 1985).

6 W. H. Schneider, 'Puericulture and the style of French eugenics', *History and Philosophy of the Life Sciences*, 8 (1986), 265–77.
7 L. Featherstone, 'Infant ideologies: doctors, mothers and the feeding of children in Australia, 1890–1910', in C. K. Warsh and V. Strong-Boag (eds), *Children's Health Issues in Historical Perspective* (Waterloo, ON: Wilfred Laurier University Press, 2005), p. 131.
8 A. Davin, 'Imperialism and motherhood', *History Workshop*, 5 (Spring 1978), 9–65 on pp. 9–13. See also J. Lewis, *The Politics of Motherhood: Child and Maternal Welfare in England, 1900–1939* (London: Croom Helm, 1980).
9 D. Dwork, *War is Good for Babies and other Young Children: A History of the Infant and Child Welfare Movement in England, 1898–1918* (London: Tavistock, 1987); Finlayson, *Citizen, State and Social Welfare*; B. Harris, *The Health of the School Child: A History of the School Medical Service in England and Wales* (Buckingham: Open University Press, 1995).
10 D. Armstrong, *The Political Anatomy of the Body: Medical Knowledge in Britain in the Twentieth Century* (Cambridge: Cambridge University Press, 1983), pp. 10–13.
11 Minutes of Evidence taken before the Inter-Departmental Committee on Physical Deterioration Volume II, p. 412.
12 See A. Evans, 'The Countess of Aberdeen's health promotion caravans', Journal of the Irish Colleges of Physicians and Surgeons, 24:3 (July 1995), 211–18.
13 Jones, '*Captain of All these Men of Death*', p. 101.
14 M. Daly, 'Death and disease in independent Ireland: a research agenda', in C. Cox and M. Luddy (eds), *Cultures of Care in Irish Medical History, 1750–1970* (London: Palgrave Macmillan, 2010), p. 230.
15 Jones, '*Captain of All these Men of Death*', p. 118.
16 R. Apple, *Mothers and Medicine: A Social History of Infant Feeding, 1890–1950* (Madison, WI: University of Wisconsin Press, 1987), pp. 24–5.
17 M. McNeill, 'A campaign for the babies', *Sláinte*, 1:8 (August 1909), 169–72.
18 Women's National Health Association, *Lecture on the Health of the Child* (Dublin: Waller & Co., 1909), pp. 31–2.
19 Hardy, 'Animals, disease and man', p. 205
20 Jones, '*Captain of All these Men of Death*', p. 102.
21 N. Tomes, *The Gospel of Germs: Men, Women and the Microbe in American Life* (Cambridge, MA: Harvard University Press, 1998), pp. 135–6.
22 E. J. McWeeney, 'Why children's milk should be pasteurised', Sláinte, 1:1 (January 1909), 39–40.
23 For international perspectives, see Dwork, *War is Good For Babies*, pp. 93–123, and A. H. Ferguson, L. T. Weaver and M. Nicolson, 'The Glasgow Corporation milk depot 1904–10 and its role in infant welfare', Social History of Medicine, 19:3 (December 2006), 443–60.
24 J. Lumsden, 'The result of six months' experience of Dublin Pasteurised Milk Depot', *Sláinte*, 1:3 (March 1909), 41–8.
25 *Vice-Regal Commission on the Irish Milk Supply: The Final Report of the Irish Milk Commission*, H. C. 1914 [Cd.7129] xxxvi.601, p. 8.
26 'The "Babies Clubs" of Belfast', *Sláinte*, 1:1 (January 1909), 13–14.
27 *Vice-Regal Commission*, p. 8.
28 Ibid., p. 11.
29 Ibid., p. 4.
30 Ibid., p. 2.
31 Ibid., p. 3.
32 Ibid., p. 13.

33 Ibid.
34 NAI, Department of Agriculture, 92/1/686, Women's National Health Association: Deputation to Vice President Concerning Recommendations of the Commission on the Irish Milk Supply, 1912.
35 J. Burnett, 'The rise and decline of school meals in Britain, 1860–1990', in J. Burnett and D. J. Oddy (eds), *The Origins and Development of Food Policies in Europe* (London and New York: Leicester University Press, 1994), p. 57.
36 Parent, 'Midday Meal Hour for National School Children', *Irish Times* (20 February 1901), p. 7.
37 NLI, Minutes of the Proceedings of the Commissioners of National Education, 1901, pp. 228–9.
38 Education (Provision of Meals) Act, 1906 (6 Edw. 7.), ch. 57.
39 Burnett, 'The rise and decline of school meals'.
40 Vernon, *Hunger*, p. 161.
41 J. Welshman, 'School meals and milk in England and Wales, 1906–45', *Medical History*, 41 (1997), 6–29.
42 'Feeding of Children in Schools Bill', *House of Commons Debates* (16 February 1911), vol. 21, c. 1406W.
43 Burnett, 'The rise and decline of school meals', p. 59.
44 S. C. Harrison, 'Question of School Dinners', *Irish Independent* (30 October 1913), p. 9.
45 'Meals for School Children', *Irish Independent* (19 February 1906), p. 6.
46 A. O'Brien, 'Penny school dinners at Celbridge', *Sláinte*, 1:6 (June 1909), 1.
47 'United Irishwomen: Annual General Meeting', *Irish Times* (16 November 1911), p. 10.
48 A. Lett, 'State-Aid or Irish Self-Help', *Irish Times* (9 December 1911), p. 7.
49 T. J. Morrissey, *Thomas A. Finlay S. J., 1848–1940: Educationalist, Editor, Social Reformer* (Dublin: Four Courts Press, 2004).
50 *Irish Independent* (3 July 1906), p. 4.
51 Fourth Report of the Royal Commission on Congestion in Ireland, Reports of Commissioners, Commons, 1907 [Cd.3508], vol. xxxvi.1, p. 35.
52 'Feeding the School Children', *Bean nÉireann*, 8 (January 1910), p. 5.
53 For Gonne and feminine nationalism, see K. Steele, *Women, Press and Politics during the Irish Revival* (Syracuse, NY: Syracuse University Press, 2007), esp. pp. 66–105.
54 M. Gonne, 'Responsibility', *Irish Review*, 1:10 (December 1911), 483–5 on p. 483.
55 M. Gonne, 'Meals for School Children', *Irish Times* (16 October 1912), p. 9.
56 Gonne, 'Responsibility', p. 483.
57 M. Gonne, 'The Children Must be Fed', *Bean na hÉireann*, 20 (January 1911), p. 6.
58 Gonne, 'Responsibility', p. 484.
59 Gonne, 'Meals for School Children'.
60 Lett, 'State-Aid or Irish Self-Help'.
61 Military Archives, Cathal Brugha Barracks, Dublin, Bureau of Military History 1913–21 files, 'Statement of Miss Helena Molony', pp. 13–15.
62 'Dinners to School Children: What the Ladies Committee are Doing. Seven Hundred Children Fed Daily', *Irish Times* (28 February 1914), p. 8.
63 S. B. Walsh, 'Food and the hungry school children', *Irish Review*, 2:21 (November 1912), 494–501 on p. 500.
64 O. St J. Gogarty, 'The need of medical inspection of school children in Ireland', *Irish Review*, 2:13 (March 1912), 12–19 on p. 18.
65 *Appendix to the Second Report of the Vice-Regal Committee of Inquiry into Primary Education (Ireland)*, Reports of Commissioners, Commons, 1914 [Cd.7229], vol. xxviii.5, p. 26.

66 P. Yeates, *Lockout: Dublin 1913* (Dublin: Gill and MacMillan, 2000), p. 366.
67 Education (Provision of Meals) (Ireland) Act, 1914 (4 & 5 Geo. 5.) ch. 35.
68 H. S. Chenevix, 'Meals for School Children' *Irish Independent* (21 November 1914), p. 6.
69 R. J. P. Mortished, 'The Position of Teachers', *Irish Independent* (15 December 1914), p. 4.

8

Anticipating a second Famine: consumption, production and resistance during the First World War

> We ought to have a well understood national policy in regard to our food supplies at time of war, a policy which our public men and the Press ought never to let us forget, consideration of which would influence legislation, the work of the Department, and the Farmer's Association. If we don't formulate such a policy we may starve sometime, and the sometime may be no distant date.[1]

This gloomy foreboding, published in the *Irish Homestead* in 1911, expressed rising apprehension about Ireland's food surplus as Europe mobilised for conflict. As war loomed, the question of whether Ireland was at risk of starving evolved into a topic of lively debate. Ultimately, this concern created a set of food-related controversies of a profundity and character not witnessed in Ireland since the Famine. In the years leading up to the First World War, the *Homestead* strove relentlessly to establish a sense of Irish physical and economic vulnerability. One editorial poignantly warned that 'our bodies are like lost sheep wandering about without anybody to look after them or give them proper meals and as a result Irish bodies contain a higher percentage to the square inch of the microbes of insanity, tuberculosis, typhoid, and such like diseases than bodies born in other countries which are properly looked after'. True to its co-operative spirit, the *Homestead* placed little faith in state bodies to satisfactorily oversee food distribution should war erupt. Instead, if Ireland were to be shielded from the domestic ramifications of conflict, then local societies needed to form whose members could feed the populace using the country's national resources. Citizens could cure their own bacon and corn their own beef. These steps, the *Homestead* insisted, would forestall food reserves being 'instantly bought up by the great wholesalers to feed the teeming population in English cities'. Importantly, the *Homestead* claimed that these actions would guarantee that Ireland did not find itself in 'the same position as in the years of the Great Famine when we grew enough food for our wants, exported it, and starved'.[2] During the First World War, the threat of famine was more than just an allegoric trope. Mass starvation was something that, to some, seemed tangible, realistic and immediate.

The imminency of conflict provided an occasion to re-evaluate the trajectory of post-Famine food reform. Prior to the war, questions resurfaced about the Irish poor's precarious dependency on consuming imported tea and cheap meat while Irish food producers exported goods of higher nutritional value – particularly beef – to Britain and beyond. Recurrent trade union disruption rendered the volatility of Anglo-Irish economic arrangements further apparent. When English railway workers went on strike in 1911, Irish bacon and pork provisions rapidly diminished, granting the *Homestead* an opportunity to reinforce its remonstrations about over-depending on imported goods for consumption.[3] Later that year, supplies were once again disturbed when the Dublin Operative Bakers and Confectioners' Trade Union went on strike, encouraging the *Homestead* to declare the existence of a 'bread famine' across the city.[4] It seems surprising, with the benefit of hindsight, to find the newspaper virtually alone in its dogged determination to present these localised disruptions as microcosmic examples of what might happen in Ireland should sustained war interrupt trade. 'It is no use for a country at the last moment to think of adjusting its national domestic economy to a state of war', warned a 1912 editorial, for 'when the house is on fire is not the time to think of fire insurance.'[5]

This chapter explores the centrality of food in debates about national existence during the First World War. More specifically, it argues that conflict forced a rethinking of Irish food networks and how these had evolved since the Famine. For critics, the post-Famine economy had primarily benefited imperial needs while weakening the Irish physical condition, an argument brought out by Maud Gonne in her school dinners campaign and that became articulated in further new ways during wartime. This chapter also posits that the exigencies of conflict encouraged closer governance of Irish food production as state bodies attempted to mobilise national resources. However, the state's primary interest was in boosting agricultural productivity. State bodies put relatively few measures in place to ensure that the Irish populace retained access to a nutritionally adequate diet, fortifying claims being made by those who sought to demonstrate that Ireland's positioning within a broader imperial system had impacted adversely on national physical well-being. However, wartime Irish discussion of food is best conceived as a forum of discussion where pre-existing debates on nutritional health and food production were revisited and lent urgency. Questions about female domesticity, milk supplies, infant welfare, education, agricultural modernisation, national physical health and the Famine all flowed into wartime anxieties about national vitality, a confluence that sparked fresh perspectives on why and how Ireland could be, and should be, politically and economically independent.

Historians have tended not to fully explore food when assessing the domestic impact of the First World War in Ireland. This period of war witnessed a strengthening of militant Irish nationalism which encouraged the formation of powerful critiques of British rule. Ben Novick demonstrates that from 1917 republican political party Sinn Féin exploited the emotive threat of a second

Famine to amass support.[6] Nonetheless, Novick's approach obscures a wider genealogy of food anxieties that intersected with and fuelled new forms of political critique during the war. From 1914, food prices rose, imports decreased and fears of starvation escalated. Old concerns resurfaced as nationalists resuscitated long-standing debates on Anglo-Irish encounters. This was particularly the case when critics invoked the cultural memory of the Famine to negatively appraise wartime policies that, according to some, implicitly supported the exportation of food to Britain while leaving Ireland hungry. This chapter suggests that concern over the consequences of this scenario in many ways unified diverse sections of Irish society irrespective of politics or religion. Responses to the handling of food supplies were more than just knee-jerk reactions to wartime exigencies. On the contrary, according to those opposed to British rule, they rendered visible a far longer lineage of adverse British influence in Ireland. In turn, wartime experiences created a firm conviction that Irish food systems needed to be permanently reconfigured in a way that truly benefited Ireland.

Conserving and producing food

Wartime techniques of preserving Irish food supplies and nutritional health typically sought to regulate food purchasing behaviour through propaganda and persuasion. The limitations of this strategy ultimately added to a sense that the state was unwilling to take realistic steps to ensure that Ireland would not starve. Fears about limited food availability surfaced at the onset of conflict. When war erupted in July 1914, customers panic bought. Some shopkeepers responded by raising prices. The *Irish Times*, continuing its long tradition of championing working-class food causes, daily rebuked opportunistic grocers who artificially raised prices, on one occasion declaring that their names should be publicly announced and their shops boycotted.[7] In return, the Dublin Retail Purveyors' and Family Grocers' Association publicly protested against the indiscriminate use of terms such as 'miserable parasites' being habitually attached to their profession in the newspaper's furious editorials. Grocers, they insisted, were compelled to raise prices.[8] Allegedly objectionable trade practices, coupled with fears of dwindling provisions, implied an urgent need for an organised food distribution system. But who was best equipped to oversee this? The Irish co-operative movement certainly believed that it was. During summer 1914, Lionel Smith-Gordon, one of its leading members, co-published a pamphlet with Home Rule journalist Francis Cruise O'Brien entitled *Ireland's Food in War Time*. In this, the authors depicted a 'consuming public' ignorant of the nature and extent of food supplies and a 'producing public' uninformed about which foods needed to be produced to alleviate shortages. The authors urged both 'publics' to make themselves more aware of how much food was being grown, imported and exported and also recommended the establishment of food distribution organisations to shield consumers from the insecurities of the market economy.[9] Nonetheless, the ideal of co-operatism was far from universally agreed upon and, in any case, remained relatively inconsequential throughout the war.

Official efforts were severely hampered by a financial and practical inability to implement collective solutions, meaning that state bodies resorted to extolling individual responsibility and self-regulation. In 1914, DATI, newly entrusted with the task of managing food supplies, initiated a campaign predicated on what it termed 'productive thrift'. A key component of 'productive thrift' was a war on waste, denounced by Thomas Patrick Gill, DATI's president, as 'at all times reprehensible' and during wartime 'doubly so'. Dissociating thrift from meanness, Gill sought to infuse 'a habit of order, method and avoidance of waste' in household management. He portrayed thrift via waste reduction as a 'supreme and patriotic virtue' and one that 'must become a national habit', ominously adding that the whole nation was suffering in consequence of wastefulness, a claim that underlined interconnections between personal and national activity. In the Department's 1916 pamphlet *Productive Thrift*, he declared that:

> It is not possible to enumerate even the commoner forms of wastefulness, but an examination of the majority of town dust bins would provide a damaging epitome – the rejection of cinders which, mixed with coal, form an excellent fuel; bones which, by boiling, would make excellent stock; potato parings unnecessarily thick; scraps of fat, which should have been melted down and utilised; crusts of bread, every crumb of which could have been used for puddings of various kinds, or dried in the oven and crushed to make bread crumbs. These evils call for vigorous amendment.[10]

Gill presented waste avoidance as an important step towards protecting food resources that could be taken through simple household actions and individual responsibility.

'Productive thrift' was a multi-layered concept that simultaneously sought to preserve nutritional health in the face of food shortages. Concern over nutritional well-being resonated in wartime as the dietary well-being of the Irish poor, even in pre-war times, seemed to be at a remarkably low ebb. Since the Famine, state bodies had intervened in communal consumption habits only infrequently, an important exception being the poorly financed network of National School cookery instruction initiated in 1900. Wartime contingencies deepened public unease about the extent of under-nourishment across vulnerable populations who, more so than ever, needed to be strong and healthy if Ireland's war effort was to succeed. Predictably, Gill lambasted over-reliance on tea and white bread as uneconomical and unhealthy. Instead, he insisted, if the Irish public consumed vegetables, oatmeal, wholemeal flour, cheese and milk, national health would improve and financial savings be made.[11] These ideas were hardly new, but war lent them extra urgency.

Given the shared commonalities between the ethos of 'productive thrift' and the agendas of contemporary voluntary groups, it is unsurprising that the Department successfully enlisted the support of both the WNHA and William

H. Thompson.[12] In their pamphlets and public lectures, all three agents – a group encompassing official, philanthropic and scientific perspectives – strove to popularise ideas that food offered more than just nourishment; that it strengthened bodies and supplied the physical energy needed to labour efficiently. Gill, for instance, drew attention to meat's usefulness as a flesh-forming, muscle-building food. In contrast, he presented the potato – a crop often turned to when meat supplies dwindled – as replete with starch and sugar but no muscle-building material. Accordingly, he instructed his readers that cheap but healthy nourishment could be instead obtained from cheese, oatmeal, milk, peas, beans and lentils. There was just as much nutrition, Gill affirmed, in 4¾ d. of oatmeal or 1 s. 9 d. worth of cheese as there was in 5 s. 10 d. of beef.[13] Similarly, Gill upheld oatmeal as an economical foodstuff, partly because of its cheapness but also on the basis of its nutritional value.[14]

Thompson's pamphlet *War and the Food of the Dublin Labourer* (1915), published by the WNHA, elucidated how war had detrimentally impacted on nutritional health. Expanding on his investigations undertaken earlier that year, Thompson calculated that Dublin labourers, prior to conflict, had subsisted on pig's heads, bacon, fish, butter, milk, beef, sugar, bread, potatoes, vegetables and tea. Their diet, according to Thompson's calculations, allowed an average of 2,600 units of energy to be assimilated per day. However, he continued by warning that wartime prices had raised the cost of a pig's head from 11 d. to 3 s 6 d. Thompson cautioned that this problem threatened nutritional well-being as labouring families now bought less nutritious shoulders, ribs and picnic hams. The least affluent now bought sausage, tripe and trotters. Thompson presented these purchasing choices, coupled with a limited intake of wholemeal, oatmeal, pulse foods and cheese, as damaging to work capacity.[15] Like Gill, he encouraged the consumption of dairy and grain products, in part to end over-reliance on tea, white bread and potatoes among the poor. Although Thompson concerned himself with wartime problems, his pamphlet can also be situated in a far broader lineage of concern over, and investigations into, the diet of the Irish poor. In many ways, war added new contours to ongoing debates about Irish dietary customs rather than generating entirely new concerns.

Notably, war affirmed contemporary conceptions of the centrality of female domestic work to national endurance. When the Ministry of Food dispatched actress, suffragist and wartime relief worker Elizabeth Robins to encourage Irish female participation in the war effort in 1917, she reiterated the importance of economising. 'The day might easily come', warned Robins on the subject of inflation in one public lecture, 'when even with £100 in one's pockets, one could not buy a pound of flour.' Robins suggested that if women failed to voluntarily ration, compulsory rationing would be enforced. She continued by stressing how saving one teaspoonful of crumbs per person per day could preserve 100,000 tons of flour per year. Robins also provocatively asserted that a remarkably efficient voluntary system had evolved in Germany and, in view of that, she 'was more afraid of the German housewife than she was of anything else Germany could produce'. Concluding, Robins castigated

Ireland, England and America for being the three most wasteful countries. 'Facing this crisis', she preached, 'she [the housewife] had to put into housekeeping more brains and conscience than ever before; she must defend her section of the trench, and this war would be won by the housekeeper and the woman at the kitchen range.'[16] Robins's approach offered an illustrative example of how state propaganda sought to inculcate a sense that positive domestic actions bolstered national success. Instilled with guilt at their relative lack of patriotism, it was hoped that Irish housewives would eagerly maximise domestic resources by conserving food.

For sceptics, however, the gloss of state interest in Irish hunger concealed significant structural and financial difficulties and a lack of real solutions. Disquiet over infant welfare intensified during the war. In 1916, Lady Aberdeen lamented:

> Fancy what an America city would say if it were told that it had no power either to maintain a municipal Pasteurised milk depot for the benefit of weakly babies, nor to give a grant to such a milk depot already running under voluntary workers and proved to have done excellent work in saving scores of babies' lives! Yet that is what the Dublin municipality was informed by the Law Officer and the Local Government Board. And accordingly, the said milk depot had to be closed after the first few weeks of war owing to the diversion of voluntary subscriptions to war purposes; and the doctors agree that an increase of infant mortality in the city of Dublin is the result.[17]

Similarly, cookery institutions such as Marlborough Street Training College suffered as rising prices began to impinge upon the ability to deliver classes.[18] Local teachers' associations passed resolutions to urge the Commissioners of National Education to increase fees in line with rising costs of food and utensils.[19] Nonetheless, state activity remained clearly dependent on persuasion. Importantly, the public rhetoric of productive thrift also subtly skirted contentious questions about the continuing exportation of Irish-produced food.

DATI's intercession in consumption was scarcely comparable to its vigour in boosting agricultural production. Its interjection in that arena was ostensibly framed in a rubric of long-term agricultural improvement. In many ways, the promise of permanent, enduring development helped to legitimise state encroachment into Irish production. In 1916, Gill reassured farmers that by producing more food they would not only:

> be doing a good public service both in health and in pocket, but will be encouraging the Irish farmer in his transition to sounder methods. It all works together towards protecting the country against economic danger and advancing her upon a line of policy which is not merely called for by the present emergency, but which has long been advised by the Department as the true road of her agricultural and industrial welfare.[20]

Statements such as these preyed upon perpetually distant hopes of national progress to ensure public consensus.[21] Improvement itself served as a key bargaining mechanism that might placate objections to a dramatic increase in state intervention and regulation.

State bodies sought to boost production of grain and winter crops as they believed that consuming bread and vegetables would help to resolve wartime nutritional problems.[22] This was a problematic tactic as the post-Famine economy had been increasingly characterised by cattle production and, later, dairying. According to Cormac Ó Gráda, the value of wheat, oat and barley dropped dramatically between 1876 and 1908.[23] Persuading farmers to return to tillage therefore presented a momentous obstacle. Regardless, in August 1914, DATI summoned its instructors to a national conference to advise them to arrange for the planting of winter crops and cereals, make certain that seed merchants purchased extra supplies, dispense relevant information in leaflets and local newspapers, request that clergymen make agricultural announcements in parishes and deliver regular lectures.[24] DATI dispersed leaflets nationwide in September that urged farmers to increase wheat acreage, sow oats, barley and rye, produce more cabbage and feed animals frugally.[25]

This proposed shift towards tillage hardened attitudes to the already unpopular grazier community.[26] Speaking to the Statistical and Social Inquiry Society of Ireland in 1914, landowner and prominent lawyer Charles A. Stanuell warned that Irish farmers had long forgotten how to farm, having instead become content with cattle-watching and ranching. Stanuell also conjectured that in spite of decades of protests against graziers and landlordism, few farmers, upon securing land, had truly departed from pasture. He was particularly anxious about farmers who refused to till on the basis that it did not pay as well as grazing. On this, Staunell provocatively asserted:

> Are the farmers of Ireland prepared to do nothing but wait and see starvation prevailing over the land, as it did in 'forty-eight'? Starvation brings with it disease, ruin, suffering, hopeless misery and death to men, women, and children. It will be too late if preparations are not made now, and if the provisions be not required to save life they will still be of the usual value in the market.[27]

In Stanuell's view, the state needed to set strict persuasive measures in place to foment a rapid shift from grazing to tillage and avoid a second Famine. His statement also points to the class-based tensions in play in wartime discussion of food production and the manner by which the alleged greed and selfishness of the wealthy grazing community could be presented as having detrimental consequences for the Irish poor. Predictably, graziers objected. One grazier asserted in the *Irish Times* in 1915 that 'the man in the city, who goes for a picnic in the fields on a fine day, does not consider when he sits down to abuse the farmers for not doing what he would not do himself if he were in their place'. Crucially, however, the author stated that 'it takes a very self-sacrificing man to work hard all the year round at tillage farming when can make quite as much profit in walking about looking at his cattle doing the trick'.[28]

In the face of grazier objections, state intervention further increased the following year when the Departmental Committee on Food Production met to consider how to raise a good harvest.[29] Its members pondered over how to boost tillage output, furnish farmers with modern machinery and conserve artificial manure.[30] A majority concurred that the state needed to closely regulate agricultural output and promote permanent improvement.[31] Yet incongruity punctuated the proceedings of the Committee. State intervention, a minority insisted, was 'open to abuse' whereas co-operatism offered collective security and collective responsibility. Horace Plunkett was the key espouser of such views. Tensions between DATI and Plunkett's co-operative movement were long running. In 1914, Gill had publicly accused creameries of artificially raising the price of butter and bacon although Plunkett had quickly debunked this suggestion, pointing out, somewhat convincingly, that Irish creameries did not even manufacture bacon.[32] What infuriated Plunkett most about the Committee was its implicit rejection of co-operatism even though that movement, in Plunkett's view, had radically reformed Irish dairying practices in preceding decades.[33] Plunkett angrily reminded the Committee that he was a spokesman for 'tens of thousands of farmers whose opinions and wishes I am in a position to know'. For these reasons, he refused to append his signature to the Majority Report.[34]

For Plunkett, the feeling lingered that state-led agendas of long-term agricultural improvement were inauthentic. Accordingly, he queried the necessity and usefulness of increased state influence in production. The co-operative movement had sought to incubate progress for some decades and felt naturally threatened and unconvinced by the spectre of state control of agriculture. Plunkett also asserted that the state would cease propping up Irish labour markets once war stopped and predicted, perhaps insightfully, that the Irish economy was bound for depression once soldiers returned home – a period to be woefully characterised by acute economic decline and plagued by high food costs and mass unemployment. Frustrated, Plunkett also accused the Committee, and by default the state, of contemplating policies that were anchored in an insensitive, naive and uninformed approach to Irish agriculture.[35] He concluded that 'the Irish Agricultural Organisation Society, in the days of governmental neglect of agriculture and before central or local institutions administered state aid, successfully initiated a far more complicated and difficult reform in dairying than that which has now to be undertaken in general agriculture', a stance that unabashedly articulated his annoyance at the rejection of his vast agricultural experience.[36] The *Irish Times* concurred with Plunkett by commenting that 'it is quite clear that the main object of a majority of the Committee was not the increase of tillage, but the prevention of the co-operative principle from winning any sort of official footing in Ireland'.[37]

Nonetheless, state intervention in agriculture continued to expand. The Maintenance of Live Stock Act of 1915 granted DATI powers to stop farmers slaughtering breeding stock.[38] DATI allocated financial resources to Glasnevin to support experiments in milk and potato production and also to determine the most efficient means of animal feeding, although ideas that pigs could be fed on cod liver oil rather than potatoes prompted terse responses from butchers who protested that their pork would become tainted with a fishy flavour.[39] However, it was crop production, above all other considerations, that persistently formed the primary basis of state interest. Anticipating ongoing reluctance among graziers to turn to tillage, DATI expended considerable energy attempting to instil a psychological mindset in that community that gravitated towards patriotic responsibility, not profit. Public speeches delivered by the Department's Vice-President Thomas Russell were undeniably propagandist in nature. In 1915, he presented the following message to farmers:

> You as a class are being charged – I do not say the charge is well founded – you are being charged, you and your sons, with avoiding all the responsibilities of this war. It is held by some people that, while you are allowing the full weight of the struggle to fall upon others, you are reaping whatever benefits have arisen out of the war in the shape of good markets and high prices.[40]

This statement was characteristic of Russell's efforts to promulgate an ethos of national agricultural responsibility. And it was not without basis, as many graziers were indeed accumulating profit from a high demand for meat in wartime England.[41] In response, at one public lecture delivered in 1915 in Dundalk, Co. Louth, Russell expounded that although Ireland was one of the most fertile lands in Europe, she tilled only 16 per cent of her arable land, adding that 'if the enemy countries tilled only this percentage the war would certainly have been over by now'. He fortified his stance by claiming that Russia had ploughed 78 per cent of her land, Germany 65 per cent and France 55 per cent. Russell also carefully reminded his audiences that tillage campaigns were not calculated to depreciate the cattle trade. On the contrary, increased tillage allowed for increased cattle feeding, claimed Russell, or 'more food for man and beast'. He concluded by announcing that:

> The farmer was simply asked to perform a duty which he owed to the Empire of which he was a citizen; he was asked to minister to his own well-being and that of his family; he was asked to look beyond the present crisis; to lend a hand in lifting Ireland out of the evil rut into which she had fallen and to set in motion a life that was vital to the economic salvation of his country.[42]

Evidently, the opening years of war witnessed a palpable state encroachment upon Irish life. A range of strategies of governance emerged that targeted different social groups in differing ways. An array of actors promoted, or became the subjects of, activities that aimed to harness Ireland's physical and agricultural resources. These included nutritional scientists alarmed at the bodily ramifications of food shortages; co-operative societies reluctant to concede to increased state intervention; mothers and housewives being pressurised to economise; tradesmen fearful of the changes to their business practices implied by wartime demands; and state bodies forced to re-orientate their improving strategies to suit an adjusting socio-economic climate. Apprehension about poor nutrition that had long lingered now seemed more menacing. At stake, for the first time since the Famine, was national survival.

Food and Anglo-Irish relations

State bodies took considerable steps to optimise agricultural output throughout the conflict. However, some wondered if these actions primarily benefited British consumers given that little was being done to curb Ireland's lively food export trade to Britain. Of course, the *Irish Homestead* had striven to draw attention to inherent problems in that import/export scenario for some years. But it was only when war commenced that the disconcerting instability of Anglo-Irish economic interactions truly mutated into a more controversial topic. Smith-Gordon and O'Brien's aforementioned pamphlet penned in 1914 ascertained that only around 18.5 per cent of Irish-bred cattle was being consumed in the country. The authors also demonstrated that less than half of butter being produced in Ireland was being domestically consumed.[43] Although the authors conceded that Irish production was important to Britain, they also cautioned that Ireland itself needed to be protected from depleting food supplies. Ireland needed a food surplus for its own consumption.[44]

Newspaper editorials held diverse opinions on the matter. Adopting a moderate tone, the Unionist-minded *Irish Times* reported that 'we do not suggest for a moment that Ireland should adopt a selfish attitude, or neglect the needs of the English consumer, but we do suggest strongly that Irish supplies adequate, at least, to the minimum need of the Irish people should be retained in this country'. The editorial reveals conflicting priorities: whether to aid the British war effort or ensure Irish survival.[45] That same month, nationalist outlet the *Irish Independent* adopted a more adversarial stance when it declared:

> We remember that in the years of the Great Famine food enough to feed the Irish people was produced here and was being exported while our people starved. We do not want anything of the kind to occur again. So long as the mob in London, Liverpool, Manchester, Birmingham and other big cities can get fed and can be kept from rioting, the troubles of little Irish country towns will not be heeded.[46]

This account invoked the Famine as a highly evocative trope. Although directly referring to immediate food supply problems, this discussion of the wartime import/export system served as a prism through which recollections of past British unjustness could be reconsidered to demonstrate a continuing, perhaps concealed, long-term pattern of Irish needs being subsumed to imperial interests. Intermittent outbreaks of potato blight did little to abate fears of mass starvation. In 1915, blight re-appeared in remote islands in Co. Galway and later in Clifden, Cork and Kerry. Enlisting the help of the Royal Irish Constabulary, DATI took steps to ensure that farmers sprayed potatoes by circulating 20,000 leaflets on the matter.[47] When blight struck again in the following year, the Department privately discussed the complete failure of the potato crop and asked for the Chief Secretary's consent to immediately halt potato exportation.[48] Publicly, however, DATI stressed that the potato crop had not failed.[49] Owing to the partial failure of the 1916 potato crop, DATI prohibited potato exports, although only temporarily, except under special licence.[50]

There was one useful aspect of Ireland's role as food exporter, at least from the Irish standpoint: its utility in arguments against national conscription under the National Registration Act (1915), a measure successfully defended in Ireland until 1918.[51] Although the volatile Irish political situation of the period resulted in a disinclination to enforce conscription, advocates of Ireland's exclusion also recognised the importance of Irish food production to the war effort. In 1915, Jonathan Samuel, British MP for Stockton-on-Tees, insisted in the House of Commons that Ireland performed a vital role: feeding England. Anticipating a probable 'meat famine' in England should Irish labourers be forced into fighting rather than producing, Samuel conjectured that 'it would be a very serious matter if we were to create any disturbance in Ireland'.[52] Clearly, British political opinion was not always averse to siding with an agenda of preserving Ireland as a fruitful food source for England.

The idea that Ireland should serve as Britain's allotment antagonised those who asked: what was Ireland to eat? Thompson was exceptionally active in drawing attention to the problematic import/export situation. On one occasion, he blamed the failed implementation of an effective domestic education system in National Schools for having inadequately prepared the Irish populace for wartime conditions. In his *War and the Food of the Dublin Labourer* (1915), Thompson lambasted educational reformers for having failed to cultivate an ample awareness of nutrition and its importance to bodily strength and work efficiency. In Thompson's words:

> We are content with teaching a modicum of domestic science to a small number of our women, chiefly trained cooks, forgetful of the fact that the health and vigour of the nation as a whole, depend more intimately than on anything else, on a right knowledge of the nourishing qualities and uses of foods. No greater or more lasting good could be done to the country than would accrue from preaching this doctrine; and from inducing those who are in a position to do so, to take measures to spread accurate knowledge far and wide on questions relating to food, till this knowledge becomes part and parcel of the everyday life of the least educated member of the population.[53]

Thompson presented education as a key to overcoming prejudices against oatmeal that was traceable back to the Famine and countering a 'supreme contempt for soups'.[54] In his later pamphlets, he more explicitly conflated the issue of food exports with wartime health concerns. In *Food Problems: Supplies and Demand in Ireland* (1916), he lamented that 94 per cent of Irish-produced wheat was being exported, that only a quarter of Irish-produced potatoes was being consumed as human food and that two-thirds of Irish-produced oat supplies was being fed to animals. His further calculations established that the Irish consumed only 30 per cent of pigs and 20 per cent of cattle produced in Ireland. The physiological consequence of this, according to Thompson, was a dangerously low level of fat intake among manual workers who then derived their energy instead from potatoes, bread and tea. This, declared Thompson, was both economically unsound and physiologically unhealthy.[55]

Others went further than Thompson by invoking 'starvation' as an emotive rallying call – a less precise rendering than Thompson's scientifically informed vocabulary of fats, proteins and carbohydrates but a far more emotive one. This rhetoric proved all the more effective as Anglo-Irish relations deteriorated. The precariousness of food supplies became remarkably visible in the 1916 Easter Rising. Prior to the Rising, militant nationalist groups made preparations for potential food shortages should they engage in hostile activity. The Irish Volunteers arranged regular lectures for its members to instruct them on what to eat, and why, in the event of sustained militancy against the state.[56] When the Easter Rising erupted in 1916, communication was immediately cut between Dublin city centre and the suburban districts. Bakers, grocers, milkmen and butchers struggled to deliver to customers. Butter prices trebled, flour and meal sold out, bread supplies diminished as Messrs Boland bakery was taken over, and gangs broke into the suburban properties of large market gardeners to steal cabbages and cauliflowers.[57] Local committees formed to secure food. Churches donated money to labourers who were unable to collect their wages. The Parish Priest of Fairview even transported 1,000 loaves of bread from Belfast to Dublin.[58] Likewise, Father Patrick O'Doyle of Naas, Co. Kildare – a figure intimate with leading Republican individuals such as Michael Collins and George Gavan Duffy – departed to Dublin in a car loaded with food upon hearing word of food shortages.[59] Small farmers also prided themselves on their active involvement in the Rising. One of them recalled that:

> While the dwellers of Dublin city were being bombarded in Easter week, the cows from which is drawn the milk for those babies who are fortunate enough to escape Sir Charles Cameron's microbes, nearly went mad one morning (Wednesday morning, to be precise) because the dairy boys were unable to find their way out of the town to perform their task of 'stripping them'. We small farmers came to the rescue and organised gangs of milkers morning and evening, and for several days did our neighbours' work as well as our own.[60]

For some, the search for food was exceptionally fraught. Mary Flannery Woods, member of republican women's volunteer group Cumann na nBan, later recalled that her husband secured a military pass to allow him to help distribute food. One day, he noticed that the stables of a local butter merchant on Westland Row were ablaze. Although Woods set the horses, frantic with fright, free, he injured himself while doing so. Some days later, a group of local nuns asked Woods to secure margarine from the city centre. While returning, the weight of his box of margarine caused Woods to topple off his bike, permanently straining his back. Despite his injuries, according to his wife, 'all that week of terror he never rested, leaving home early in the morning after a breakfast of stale bread and tea and maybe an egg exchanged for something, for there was great scarcity of food, his next meal [being] at or after midnight on his return home'.[61]

Shortly after the Rising, the *Homestead* reported that thousands of citizens had faced famine during the brief period of conflict, not only in Dublin but also in the countryside where it now seemed apparent that food supplies quickly expended if imports failed to arrive in, and be distributed from, the capital. On this matter, the newspaper optimistically reported that:

> People had never before been brought face to face with the fact that they had only a few weeks' supply of food stuffs in this country and that they were so dependent on foreign countries. They had often been told it, but they never fully realised it until now and are having it brought home to them in reality. I think there will be no difficulty in getting those who were slow in the past to exert themselves in the future and set about making themselves independent of foreign food stuffs.[62]

Agitation to curb food exports mounted during the year. The Belfast House Tenants' Defence Association organised a large conference in Belfast in November to consider how to persuade the state to halt food exportation. This event was attended by representatives of trade unions, labour unions, co-operatives, friendly societies and women's workers' organisations who planned a mass demonstration and arranged to write to Irish MPs about the solemn menace of starvation in Belfast. According to the Association's president Thomas Kennedy, 'we believe that the present high prices are uncalled for, and would not have obtained had the Government used ordinary business foresight at the outbreak of war by re-organising the available food, compelling tillage, and regulating prices'.[63]

Debates about the import/export system offered nationalists a rich resource for casting aspersions on the long-term impact of British influence in Ireland. They routinely deployed the memory of the Famine as a provocative rhetorical device that would, it was hoped, disclose the true nature of British policy in both the past and present. In December, Andrew E. Malone argued in nationalist outlet *New Ireland* that 'in 1848 the rural economy of this country was perhaps less of a money economy than it is today. In 1848 this country produced more of what it consumed and consumed more of what it produced than it does today'. Malone elaborated by asserting that Ireland had gradually *been made* dependent on consuming food imports, observing that 'for the potatoes and oatmeal of seventy years ago we have substituted American white flour and Indian tea' and adding that 'under any reasonable agricultural regime it might so easily have been otherwise'. He concluded by denouncing the free trade policies that had long infiltrated Irish economics and produced a country that now sold its most nutritious products to Britain. 'We are surely in a sorry plight', asserted Malone, as 'a self-governing Ireland might have made a stand against the tremendous economic pressure of the nineteenth century. An Ireland without any control, either economic or political, was bound to succumb.'[64] Here, Malone blamed one-sided interactions between central and peripheral powers for the country's current predicament; a stance predicated to affirm a need for political independence.

Maud Gonne went further by proclaiming that the wartime state had initiated a deliberate policy of starving Ireland. In a personal letter written in December 1916 to New York lawyer and art collector John Quinn, she predicted that all of Europe would be in a condition bordering upon famine by summer. Gonne claimed: 'I go further, in the case of Ireland, I think England is wilfully preparing another '46–7.' To justify this contentious viewpoint, she wrote that the state was maintaining the pre-existing export system in the face of visible food shortages and condemned military authorities for requisitioning meat and vegetables, one consequence being further price increases. 'The military are like locusts', she wrote, 'eating up everything in Ireland. And in spite of the urgent need of men in France, 40,000 English men are encamped in Phoenix Park and some 100,000 in other parts of Ireland, eating up the food of the people!' Gonne added her regret at being unable to leave France to oversee her school dinners scheme which, in her absence, had 'been let to drop' because of a shortage of potatoes, the price of which had risen from £3 to £10 per tonne.[65] Although Gonne over-estimated the genocidal nature of British intent in Ireland, she was certainly correct in asserting that the state seemed complacent about, even disinterested in, an apparent need to curb exports. And her views reflected a growing consensus that the state was neglecting Irish dietary needs in a period of crisis, an opinion shared by individuals and groups with diverse, often opposing, political views. At worst, this allowed critics to construe current state neglect as a problematic replaying of the past, a rerun of events that had caused Ireland to starve some seventy years earlier.

Increasing state intervention

In 1916, the wartime government established a Food Department which exercised compulsory powers under the Defence of the Realm Act (DORA), headed by the Food Controller Lord Davenport.[66] Its prime purpose was to increase productivity across the British Isles. DATI was entrusted with enforcing this measure in Ireland, instituting compulsory tillage in late 1916.[67] This meant that occupiers of ten or more acres of arable land were now legally obliged to cultivate an additional tenth of their land that was already being cultivated.[68] Publicly displayed posters offered visual reminders of the Department's newly granted powers to enter land and forcefully arrange cultivation. DATI imposed high penalties for misconduct involving either a fine of £100, six months' imprisonment or even both.[69] Evidently, an important shift had occurred in that state bodies now had to rely on compulsion to bolster agricultural production. Although cloaked in promises of permanent improvement, the scheme was in reality primarily concerned with short-term wartime agendas. In 1917, DATI appointed eleven temporary inspectors[70] and appointed an Advisory Committee familiar with Irish agriculture, although Plunkett's absence from this was notable. The Department also suspended most of the ordinary activities of the County Committees and concentrated energies instead on co-ordinating compulsory tillage.[71] In the first year of compulsory tillage, DATI exercised its powers of entry in 242 cases.[72] Its inspectors distributed seed supplies[73] and it made loans for agricultural machinery available.[74] DATI also purchased several thousand hand sprayers to combat blight.[75] The Irish Agricultural Organisation Society (IAOS), although critical of DATI's general tactics, assisted by distributing war posters and circulars and impressing a sense of national duty upon its members. It also formed societies that allowed farmers to buy expensive machinery and to loan them to fellow members.[76] Notably, the Commissioners of National Education remained adamant that children would be spared from the war effort. Teachers' associations gave short shrift to ideas that schools could be closed to allow children to harvest and gather potatoes,[77] and when DATI suggested that National Schools could set their pupils to work on urban allotments, the Commissioners refused, expressing their opinion that this was undesirable.[78]

Although the extent of regulation in food production was relatively pervasive given the persistent sway of *laissez-faire* economic approaches, problems in implementation proliferated. Labour availability was a significant obstacle: DATI was inundated with requests for leave from military service to provide additional labour. The Department tended to support the release of soldiers from service and wrote numerous letters to the War Office in favour as, in DATI's view, production was of greater national value than military service. Yet the War Office responded leisurely to such appeals. At worst, the Department felt that the Office was ignoring their opinions. When fish merchant Hugo Flinn sought military leave after his senior partner became ill, a tribunal was held after which members of both the Congested Districts Board and DATI complained about their views having been disregarded.[79] Delays in acquiring equipment further hindered the implementation of tillage schemes. County Committees of Agriculture remained adamant that potato-spraying machines should be bought by farmers, rather than hired or shared, a firm nod against co-operatism.[80] However, the Department struggled to acquire equipment and the Four Oaks Spraying Machine Company faced recurrent difficulties making machines due to copper shortages. The issue took months to resolve and was compounded by slow responses from the Ministry of War.[81]

The success of compulsory tillage also hinged on enthusiasm. At worst, the idea was met with apathy, even hostility. As David Fitzpatrick notes, many farmers were indignant about state efforts to control Irish agriculture, especially when they saw this step as primarily benefiting Britain.[82] Some contemporaries identified a lack of awareness of Irish farming practicalities as a serious hindrance to implementing compulsory tillage. According to Richard Ball, writing in *Studies*, DATI announced food production schemes too late in the year meaning that farmers in the west only become aware of them in January and resented the lack of time permitted to buy machinery, hire labour and conserve manure supplies. 'Do half these people who cry out for the tilling of Meath and Westmeath know what they are talking about? I think not', asserted Ball.[83] Graziers also proved persistently unwilling to turn their land to tillage, a scenario that, as Fitzpatrick also notes, led to rising incidences of cattle-driving (driving a herd from the land) in 1917.[84] In that year, MP Martin Flavin revealed in the House of Commons that fifteen landowners and graziers in North Galway had failed to commence tilling, despite only one having applied for exemption. At Ardfert, Co. Tralee, landlord Mr Crosbie reportedly owned

275 acres of land on which he had grown no food since war had begun. Local residents appealed to Flavin after Crosbie advertised his land for sale for grazing purposes. Flavin announced that 'he [Crosbie] has no right to stand between the people and the safety of the Empire or between them and their avoidance of starvation'. He then wrote to Crosbie reminding him that 214 families lived around the ranch, 120 of which did not have holdings over five acres and over 100 of which did not have land to grow even a stalk of potatoes. Even despite this, Crosbie still refused to till his land.[85] In the special edition of *Studies*, Edward Lysaght insisted that the destruction of graziers or ranchers must be accomplished as cattle producers were motivated by economic intentions instead of patriotism. 'Ireland will remain predominantly a grazing country no matter what legislation be passed to subdivide the grazing land, so long as pre-war conditions prevail', he explained. 'Why should any man', asked Lysaght, 'unless his farm be too small to support him by grazing alone, undertake the arduous and anxious task of raising crops in a treacherous climate, when with less risk and less hard work he could command a better income by not doing so?'[86]

In light of considerations such as these, opinion formed on the centralised food control system as being unsuitable for Ireland. On one occasion, a call was made in the House of Commons for Ireland to have its own independent Food Controller.[87] Even Chief Secretary Henry Duke wrote privately to the Cabinet arguing that a localised method of food control was preferable. Duke warned that 'in Ireland one of the effects of every blunder of a Government department is to aggravate the prevailing discontent, and a blunder which affects the prices of cattle, cereals or potatoes, has its effect in every parish'.[88] Nationalist MP for Sligo North, Thomas Scanlan, was remarkably outspoken on this matter and insisted in the House of Commons that the Chief Secretary had simply consulted a few officials and then 'decided on a scheme without taking any account of the needs of the country, the possibilities of the country, and the help which he could have got from the people of Ireland if he had taken the best means of consulting the views of practical agriculturists and those responsible for county government'.[89] Scanlan thought that many British MPs had insensitive perspectives on Irish realities and resolutely rallied against this in the House of Commons. In June 1917, Major Newman, MP for Enfield, claimed to have heard that forty wagon-loads of potatoes had been left to rot at Great Northern Railway, Dublin. He unsympathetically suggested that Irish producers were hoarding potatoes so that they could later sell these to Britain at a high price upon having created an artificial scarcity. The Chief Secretary and Flavin strongly refuted these suggestions, insisting that Irish labourers now depended on those potatoes in consequence of the high cost of Indian meal and flour, and reiterated that exports should cease.[90]

From 1916, an array of concerned actors continued to emphasise the relative lack of concern over access to food in Ireland. In this context, the vulnerable Irish body, threatened by poor nutrition and physiological decline even in normal times, evolved into a powerful tool of political and social critique.

Nonetheless, it proved persistently difficult to disentangle wartime nutritional problems from pre-war concerns. MPs made impassioned pleas in the House of Commons, including Patrick Meehan of Queen's Co. who warned that wartime scarcity was depriving Irish children of milk.[91] During 1917, DATI distributed questionnaires to secure information on the milk supply. An overwhelming majority of responses confirmed that milk was indeed scarce in regions across Ireland. However, they also observed that milk was no scarcer than usual, as it had been difficult to procure for some decades.[92] By disregarding milk shortages as a relatively normal state of affairs in Ireland, justification was provided for minimal state action. The Department did make some efforts to instigate compulsory winter dairying under DORA, yet it concluded that uniform improvement in the milk supply could probably not be secured until 1918 or even 1919.[93] The publication of co-operatist and scientist David Houston's *The Milk Supply of Dublin* also raised concern about adulterated milk and its contamination with cow-dung particles and swarms of germs. In its foreword, Oliver St John Gogarty, in characteristically hyperbolic fashion, announced that 'thousands of little children are yearly sacrificed and slowly, painfully and unobtrusively put to death'.[94] Again, the issue of milk purity was hardly unique to war.

Connections between food, poverty and war also became conflated. Father MacSweeney's *Poverty in Cork*, a product of Catholic social doctrine, did much to draw attention to Irish urban poverty and starvation upon its publication in autumn 1917. His study inquired into the living conditions of 1,010 families (a total of 5,058 people) whom he deemed representative of all skilled and unskilled workers. Borrowing from influential British sociologist Seebohm Rowntree's classification of poverty, MacSweeney divided his subjects into different classes of poverty. He categorised the worst of these – Class A – as living in a conditions of chronic want and suffering from bad housing and bad food. Class B had a slightly higher income – between 19 and 21 shillings per week – but still remained poverty-stricken, MacSweeney suggested, as these families were forced to curtail food purchasing to pay high rents. MacSweeney calculated that the bare minimum amount of food necessary for families cost a weekly minimum of fifteen shillings. However, most of Class A had incomes ranging between fifteen and eighteen shillings per week, an issue that impacted significantly on the amount and quality of food that could be procured. MacSweeney foresaw the destruction of home life and rampant immorality potentially arising from this situation.[95] The content of MacSweeney's work was undeniably provocative. But, again, stories of deep Irish poverty were far from novel. MacSweeney's timing simply coincided with escalating interest in the condition of the Irish poor in consequence of rising food prices and socio-political tension.

There was one exception, Smith-Gordon and O'Brien's emotively titled *Starvation in Dublin* (1917) – a pamphlet penned to call attention to the social conditions of Dublin's working classes. It tackled the issue of wartime starvation more directly and, uniquely, strove to separate normal conditions from wartime ones. The authors warned that the children of the urban poor were dying daily in Ireland from a want of food and that families were admitting them to hospitals in half-starved conditions in consequence of wartime food shortages. Smith-Gordon and O'Brien depicted hard-working men being driven out of their homes nightly by the sounds of their children crying for food. Worse still, the authors presented these dietary arrangements as an almost incomprehensible, unspeakable step down from an already insufficient diet of tea and bread that, the authors reminded, was not conducive to the rearing of healthy children.[96] They once again advocated better control and distribution of food supplies and the dissemination of appropriate information and advice.[97] The authors also ominously warned that if administrators in Britain did nothing, then a certain mood would envelop the people just as it had done in France in 1789, when grain scarcity had preceded the French Revolution, and in Russia in 1917. This claim was emotive given that hostility to British rule had intensified since the Easter Rising and become increasingly militaristic throughout the war. 'We hear distant murmurings from the people which make us fear that the matter is urgent', warned Smith-Gordon and O'Brien.[98] *New Ireland* commended the authors for having produced a 'coldly scientific' rather than 'warmly partisan' piece, one that was careful not to appear supportive of political causes or movements and which had 'no axes to grind, either social or political'.[99] The *Irish Homestead*, too, commented on the authors' findings by sceptically suggesting that state intervention in urban food problems would probably only occur if the government perceived a serious political threat in Ireland.[100]

And political threats certainly did exist. The potential of starvation, whether real or imagined, offered a remarkably effective trope for nationalists who played upon concern over the vulnerable Irish body to legitimate their anti-Union position. The harrowing theme of hunger surfaced recurrently in the rallying calls of Sinn Féin leader Éamonn de Valera who informed his supporters on one occasion that 'it was better to die with arms in their hands than from starvation'.[101] From late 1917, the Sinn Féin Food Committee, presided over by de Valera, campaigned vigorously to halt exports of oats, milk, butter, bacon and potatoes. At a meeting held in December, revolutionary nationalist, suffragist and socialist Countess Markievicz declared that England had adopted a deliberate policy of diverting Irish food supplies to feed her own people. The chairman concluded that if Ireland had a government of its own, the crisis would be resolved in twenty-four hours.[102]

In 1917, *New Ireland* also adopted a hostile approach to state food management and warned:

> Let us remember '47. To our farmers, our merchants, our shippers, to the British Government and to all whom it may concern, we must make it very clear that we do not contemplate with equanimity a repetition of the misery, destitution and death of 1847. Commerce may demand that supply follows the greatest price, but famine is too great a price to pay for a rigid adherence to the theory of economics. We have before set the 'laws' of economics at defiance and nothing very terrible happened, we obeyed them once and we starved our people to death.[103]

In January 1918, the publication claimed that:

> The poor are living on the very edge of starvation. A woman was found dead in her room recently who had evidently died of starvation, her limbs were wasted, and her hands were covered with ashes, as if she had been searching the dustbins of the city for food – a custom very widespread in this city of hunger.[104]

These accounts were undeniably hyperbolic in nature. Yet they served as responses to a very real diminution of food supplies and an absence of state-organised distribution. This is not to suggest that the government took no action whatsoever. The Butter (Ireland) Order, 1918 went some way to halt the shipping of butter out of Ireland.[105] Nonetheless, steps such as these had a minimal impact on problems of hunger and allowed nationalists to play upon fears of an imminent second Famine and to insinuate that Ireland had been part of a colonial economy since at least the Famine. Sinn Féin members insisted that Ireland could only be saved from starvation if producers sold food internally for Irish consumption only. The party's members also provocatively warned that they would treat anyone discovered making money by creating an artificial famine in Ireland as a common enemy of the country, a threat aimed principally at the unpopular grazier community.[106] Sinn Féin groups throughout Ireland attempted to wrestle control of the food situation by urging urban citizens and rural farmers to work together to reduce exports. In 1918, the East Mayo Executive of Sinn Féin formed Vigilance Committees to see that food did not leave the country and that surplus supplies remained available in towns and cities.[107]

Reflecting unionist perspectives, the *Irish Times* responded unsympathetically by insisting that Sinn Féin 'raises the cry that nothing must be exported to Great Britain, and seeks, by fomenting a panic about national starvation, to stampede the country into this idiotic and fatal policy'. The newspaper feared that prohibitions would tarnish English attitudes to Ireland and create perceptions of the country as disloyal and selfish. 'If we extend these prohibitions beyond the point of absolute necessity', warned the newspaper, 'we shall invite retaliation; and, if England begins to retaliate, we shall be starving in less than a month'.[108] The *Kildare Observer* also cautioned against hard-line approaches to the import/export issue and dismissed claims of an impending famine as grossly exaggerated.[109] The mixed opinion in existence on the matter did little to deter Diarmuid Lynch, the Sinn Féin Food Controller, who was arrested in Dublin in March 1918 on the charge of partaking in a conspiracy to seize pigs and other animals from their owners to prevent their exportation. Between twenty and thirty Sinn Féiners had lynched Michael Bowe, a farmer residing in Glasnevin, and took possession of seventeen of his pigs. Having secured them, Lynch and his colleagues proceeded to slaughter them, cut them up and prepare them for sale in Ireland. This act ultimately resulted in Lynch's deportation.[110]

Evidently, food evolved into a remarkably contentious issue during the First World War. Increased state intervention in agricultural practice demanded important shifts in food production. Contemporaneously, food shortages among an already under-nourished population rendered the implications of the post-Famine evolution of the Irish diet further visible. For critics of the import/export system, the apparent tentative approach of state bodies to improving or safeguarding Irish dietary health implied that Britain itself was indifferent to, if not responsible for, acute conditions of Irish physical and economic weakness. Although propagandist literature routinely invoked the Famine, it also pointed to the post-Famine development of a damaging economic relationship that seemed to have left the population physiologically vulnerable.

Conclusion

The First World War saw a clear intensification of strategies designed to harness human and agricultural resources in Ireland under the aegis of improvement. The state ostensibly promised dramatic reforms in both physical and economic life on the condition that bodily and agricultural productivity was maximised for the war effort. This stance formed part of a broader lineage of promoting national reform through attempting to adjust bodily and economic behaviour. Yet antagonism to state efforts had an equally long genealogy. By the end of the war few were persuaded by an increasingly unconvincing rhetoric of improvement. In fact, many critics saw increased state intrusion in Irish food matters as primarily serving British, imperial and military needs to the detriment of Irish needs. This idea appeared to have been confirmed by the rigorous approach to maximising food production adopted at the very same time that state agencies ignored Irish hunger and starvation. By the close of the war, it seemed apparent that Ireland could never return to its long-standing import/export system given the clear national precariousness of that arrangement. In 1917, Gill posited that 'it has required the super-submarine and the world's crop shortage to bring us to Compulsory Tillage and to shake our agriculture suddenly forward along a road it would take it twenty years to travel otherwise. We may be thankful that, when the need for the great effort which is now called for has come, we have at our command the groundwork of teaching and organisation which has been laid during some recent years.'[111] Official perspectives such as this could however be interpreted as propagandist in nature, with promises of future development being critically perceived as a bribe to increase short-term productivity but which carried false hopes for the future. Ball asserted that 'though we may dream and plan, we have no indication of what the morrow will bring; and may not the Irish farmer find that the Government, peace having been declared, will embark upon an open-handed policy of free trade? What then?'[112] The *Irish Homestead* also continued to warn of the dangers of further state intervention, frequently reiterating that a worldwide food shortage was likely to follow the war. On one occasion, the newspaper depicted Irish farmers as no longer having the right to plant what they liked as the state had now become an overlord who had taken away rights to the private ownership of land.[113]

Nonetheless, for many it had become apparent that Ireland needed to be self-supporting; a goal that could never be achieved without new forms of food reform. Regardless of political persuasion, critics unified around the idea that post-war Ireland needed to abandon a system of exporting its most nutritious foodstuffs while relying on the consumption of imported goods. For Russell, 'Ireland's economic machinery was just as dangerous a threat to the country as German submarines'.[114] War had confirmed his point. Lysaght, meanwhile, ruefully looked back to a period seventy years ago when Irish farmers had been self-supporting and hoped that the experiences of war would drive farmers back to consuming their own wheat and oats.[115] Agricultural instructor A. O'Sullivan believed that war had demonstrated the importance of the agriculturist, a figure previously neglected by statesmen and governments catering for industrial needs. He suggested that formal education should be remoulded to offer continuous courses in tillage until the age of fifteen.[116] Finally, for nationalist-minded groups, the experience of war had fortified their understandings of the need to gain independence from the imperial state which had, they believed, until now dictated Irish economic policy to its detriment. According to one *New Ireland* editorial, 'food was the great requirement of English industrialism and Ireland was simply converted into a ranch for the production of the roast beef of old England'.[117]

Notes

1 'The Commissariat', *Irish Homestead* (7 January 1911), pp. 1–2 on p. 2.
2 Ibid., p. 1.
3 'The Lessons of the Strike', *Irish Homestead* (26 August 1911), pp. 665–6 on p. 666.
4 'Rotunda Hospital without Bread', *Irish Times* (7 October 1911), p. 5; 'A Strike Policy for Farmers', *Irish Homestead* (7 October 1911), pp. 784–5.
5 'Food in War Time', *Irish Homestead* (9 November 1912), pp. 901–3.
6 B. Novick, *Conceiving Revolution: Irish Nationalist Propaganda in the First World War* (Dublin: Four Courts Press, 2001), pp. 181–7.
7 'Food Prices and the War', *Irish Times* (7 August 1914), p. 6.
8 'Food Prices: Position of Dublin Grocers', *Irish Times* (10 August 1914), p. 6.
9 L. Smith-Gordon and F. C. O'Brien, *Ireland's Food in War Time* (Dublin: Plunkett House, 1914), pp. 31–2. For international perspectives, see M. C. Dentoni, 'Black bread and social peace: Italy's dietary politics during the First World War', in J. Burnett and D. J. Oddy (eds), *The Origins and Development of Food Policies in Europe* (London and New York: Leicester University Press, 1994), p. 8.
10 *Productive Thrift* (Dublin: Department of Agriculture, 1916), p. 7.
11 T. P. Gill, 'Productive thrift', *Journal of the Department of Agriculture and Technical Instruction*, 16:2 (January 1916), 349–52.
12 W. H. Thompson, *Food Values, with a note on the Conservation of Irish Food Supplies* (Dublin, 1916); W. H. Thompson, *War and the Food of the Dublin Labourer* (Dublin: Women's National Health Association of Ireland, 1915).
13 Gill, 'Productive thrift', p. 350.
14 *Productive Thrift*, p. 7.
15 Thompson, *War and the Food of the Dublin Labourer*, p. 13.

16 'Food Economy in Ireland: What Women can Do', *Weekly Irish Times* (19 May 1917), p. 4.
17 Lady Aberdeen, *The Sorrows of Ireland* (1916), p. 70.
18 NLI, Department of Agriculture Minute Books, 1914, pp. 278–9.
19 NLI, Commissioners of National Education Minute Books, 1916, p. 182.
20 Gill, 'Productive thrift', p. 351.
21 As noted in relation to Italy in Dentoni, 'Black bread', p. 8.
22 NLI, Department of Agriculture Minute Books, 1914, p. 38.
23 Ó Gráda, *Ireland Before and After the Famine*, p. 154.
24 *Fourteenth Annual General Report of the Department of Agriculture and Technical Instruction*, H. C. 1913–14 [Cd.7839] vi.1, p. 24.
25 D. Kelly, *The War and Ireland's Food Supply, an Appeal to the Irish Farmer* (Dublin: Department of Agriculture and Technical Instruction, 1914).
26 Jones, *Graziers*, p. 206.
27 C. A. Stanuell, 'The effect of the war on Irish agriculture', *Journal of the Statistical and Social Inquiry Society of Ireland*, 95 (1914), 223–30 on p. 226.
28 Southern Farmer, 'Irish Food Production', *Irish Times* (9 September 1915), p. 6.
29 *Fifteenth Annual General Report of the Department of Agriculture and Technical Instruction*, H. C. 1916, [Cd.8299] iv.413, p. 15.
30 *Report of the Departmental Committee on Food Production in Ireland*, H. C. 1914–16 [Cd.8016] v.799, p. 2.
31 *Report of Departmental Committee on Food Production*, pp. 4–5.
32 'Food Prices in Dublin', *Weekly Irish Times* (15 August 1914), p. 4.
33 *Report of Departmental Committee on Food Production*, p. 11.
34 Ibid., p. 12.
35 Ibid., p. 14.
36 Ibid., p. 16.
37 'Irish Food Production', *Irish Times* (31 August 1915), p. 4.
38 Maintenance of Live Stock Act, 1915 (5 & 6 Geo. 5) 65.
39 NAI, Department of Agriculture, 92/1/1151, Conference of Instructors in Agriculture: Reports of Proceedings, 1915.
40 'Food Production in Ireland: Meeting in Dublin', *Irish Times* (27 August 1915), p. 5.
41 *C. Wills, That Neutral Island: A Cultural History of Ireland during the Second World War* (London: Faber and Faber, 2007), p. 237.
42 'Food Production in Ireland', *Irish Times* (14 September 1915), p. 9.
43 Smith-Gordon and O'Brien, *Ireland's Food in War Time*, p. 5.
44 Ibid., pp. 31–2.
45 'War, Finance and Food', *Irish Times* (1 August 1914), p. 6.
46 'Ireland in Time of War', *Irish Independent* (8 August 1914), pp. 633–4 on p. 634.
47 'Report on the prevalence of potato blight in Ireland up to the 17th July 1915', *Journal of the Department of Agriculture and Technical Instruction*, 15:4 (1915), 755–6.
48 NLI, Department of Agriculture Minute Books, 1916, p. 6.
49 'The Department of Food Production: Its Powers and Programme', *Weekly Irish Times* (30 December 1916), p. 4.
50 *Seventeenth Annual General Report of the Department of Agriculture and Technical Instruction*, H. C. 1918 [Cd.9016] v.383, p. 85.
51 A. Gregory, '"You might as well conscript Germans": British public opinion and the decision to conscript the Irish in 1918', in A. Gregory and S. Pašeta (eds), *Ireland and the Great War: 'A War to Unite Us All'?* (Manchester: Manchester University Press, 2002).

52 'Clause 14 (application to Ireland)', *House of Commons Debates*, 8 July 1915, vol. 73, cc. 572–601, 593–5.
53 Thompson, *War and the Food of the Dublin Labourer*, p. 14.
54 Ibid., p. 17.
55 W. H. Thompson, *Food Problems: Supplies and Demand in Ireland* (1916).
56 Bureau of Military History, WS1043, Statement of Colonel Joseph V. Lawless, pp. 36–7.
57 'The Food Supply', *Irish Times* (2 May 1916), p. 3.
58 Ibid.
59 Bureau of Military History, WS0807, 1.
60 Bergamot, 'The Milk Supply of Dublin', *Irish Homestead* (27 May 1916), pp. 325–6.
61 Bureau of Military History, WS0807, p. 43.
62 'Making Ready for the Future', *Irish Homestead* (20 May 1916), pp. 304–5 on p. 304.
63 'Belfast Workers and Food Prices', *Irish Times* (13 November 1916), p. 5.
64 A. E. Malone, 'Peace and potatoes', *New Ireland* (23 December 1916), 110–11.
65 NLI, Maude Gonne correspondence.
66 See Burnett, *Plenty and Want*, pp. 274–6.
67 *Seventeenth Annual General Report of DATI*, p. 13.
68 Ibid., p. 74.
69 NAI, Department of Agriculture files 92/1/1703, Parliamentary Questions and Correspondence: Cost of Food Production in Ireland, 1916.
70 NAI, Department of Agriculture, 92/1/1426, Food Production Scheme, 1917; Appointment of Inspectors, 1917.
71 *Seventeenth Annual General Report of DATI*, p. 14.
72 Ibid., pp. 76–7.
73 NAI, Department of Agriculture, 92/1/1703, Parliamentary Questions and Correspondence relating to the Cost of Food in Ireland, 1917.
74 Ibid.
75 *Seventeenth Annual General Report of DATI*, p. 14.
76 R. A. Anderson, 'The IAOS and the food problem', *Studies: An Irish Quarterly Review*, 6:21 (March 1917), 8–14 on pp. 10–12.
77 NLI, Commissioners of National Education Minute Book, 1917, p. 308.
78 Ibid., p. 53.
79 NAI, Department of Agriculture, 92/1/1462, Leave from Military Service for Men Needed for Farming and Fishing in Ireland, 1917.
80 NAI, Department of Agriculture, 92/1/1547, Conference of Chairmen and Secretaries of County Committees of Agriculture to Consider Compulsory Spraying of Potatoes, etc . . .', 1917.
81 NAI, Department of Agriculture, 92/1/1594, 'Potato Spraying: General Papers', 1917.
82 D. Fitzpatrick, *Politics and Irish Life, 1913–21: Provincial Experience of War and Revolution* (Cork: Cork University Press, 1998), p. 69.
83 E. E. Lysaght, T. W. Westropp Bennett and R. Ball, 'The farmers and the food problem', *Studies: An Irish Quarterly Review*, 6:21 (March 1917), 21–34 on p. 31.
84 Fitzpatrick, *Politics and Irish Life*, pp. 72–3.
85 'Food production', *House of Commons Debates*, 8 February 1917, vol. 90, cc. 109–233 on 221–3.
86 Lysaght, Bennett and Ball, 'The farmers and the food problem', p. 24.
87 'Food control (Ireland)', *House of Commons Debates*, 2 July 1917, vol. 95, c. 740.
88 National Archives, Kew, CAB/24/23, p. 4.

89 'New clause: (extent of Act)', *House of Commons Debates*, 12 March 1917, vol. 91, cc. 813–65.
90 'Potatoes', *House of Commons Debates*, 18 June 1917, vol. 94, cc. 1404–5
91 'Milk (Ireland)', *House of Commons Debates*, 15 February 1917, vol. 90, cc. 780–1.
92 'Milk Production in Ireland', NAI, Department of Agriculture, 92/1/1500.
93 NAI, 92/1/1526; 'Winter dairying and creameries', *Journal of the Department of Agricultural and Technical Instruction*, 7:2 (January 1912), 281–303.
94 D. Houston, *The Milk Supply of Dublin* (Dublin: Co-operative Reference Library, 1918).
95 A. M. MacSweeney, *Poverty in Cork* (Cork: Purcell and Company, 1917).
96 L. Smith-Gordon and C. O'Brien, *Starvation in Dublin* (Dublin: The Wood Printing Works, 1917), p. 21.
97 Ibid., pp. 25–6.
98 Ibid., p. 6.
99 'The way to anarchy', *New Ireland* (19 May 1917), 21–2 on p. 21.
100 'Preparedness', *Irish Homestead* (26 May 1917), pp. 385–6 on p. 386.
101 National Archives, Kew, CAB 24/29.
102 'Food Shortage in Ireland', *Irish Times* (7 December 1917), p. 4.
103 'Remember '47', *New Ireland* (8 December 1917), 70–2 on p. 72.
104 'The ghouls of famine', *New Ireland* (19 January 1918), 173.
105 'Difficulties of Food Control in Ireland', *Weekly Irish Times* (12 January 1918), p. 1.
106 'Famine and the Ard-Chomhairle', *New Ireland* (5 January 1918), 139–40.
107 'Growing Necessity for Food Economy', *Weekly Irish Times* (5 January 1918), p. 1.
108 'The Public and Food Control', *Weekly Irish Times* (16 February 1918), p. 4.
109 'Is the Tillage Order a Farce?', *Kildare Observer* (9 February 1918), p. 5.
110 'The Commandeered Pigs', *Irish Times* (9 March 1918), p. 4.
111 T. P. Gill, 'The Department of Agriculture and the food problem', *Studies: An Irish Quarterly Journal*, 6:21 (March 1917), 1–8 on p. 3.
112 Lysaght, Bennett and Ball, 'The farmers and the food problem', p. 34.
113 'State Control of Agriculture', *Irish Homestead* (21 April 1917), pp. 285–6.
114 G. and A. E. Russell, 'The self-supporting community', *Studies: An Irish Quarterly Review*, 7:26 (June 1918), 301–6 on p. 301.
115 E. E. Lysaght, 'Irish agriculture', *Studies: An Irish Quarterly Review*, 7:26 (June 1918), 314–19 on p. 318.
116 A. O'Sullivan, 'Agriculture in the future', *Journal of Agricultural and Technical Education*, 4:39 (August 1918), 73–4.
117 'Irish economy after the war', *New Ireland* (8 June 1918), 70–1 on p. 70.

Conclusion

Between the Famine and independence, Irish food customs underwent profound adjustment. New ways of knowing food, and of consuming and producing it, infiltrated post-Famine food discourse. Conceptions of food gained influence that were anchored in empirical regimes of knowledge derived principally from medicine and science, disciplines that became increasingly professionalised as well as authoritative across the period in question. In many ways, the health of the nation – physical, economic and social – came to be prescribed as dependent on the uptake of biological and physiological definitions of food consumption and production. In addition, food continued to serve as a highly politicised issue far beyond the Famine. It remained an unremittingly controversial object, as did the forms of knowledge surrounding it that gradually penetrated physical, social and economic behaviour. In this period, state approaches to food matters wavered continuously. Prior to the Famine, direct state intervention in consumption, nutrition and diet had been relatively limited, even despite the centrality of the potato diet to the critiques of Irish culture made by political economists. Political economists foresaw the dislodgment of the ubiquitously popular potato as a key to effecting national transformation. Unusually, the Famine prompted state bodies to attempt to intervene. Members of the Scientific Commission and the Central Board of Health held deep faith in their medico-scientific – specifically nutritional – understandings of what modes of production and consumption ought to replace a monotonous mono-crop culture. However, between 1845 and 1847, nutritional knowledge became entangled with broader political controversies about relief policy; a scenario that damaged public perceptions of nutritional science.

In the years that followed, food, and the manner by which it was ingested and processed in the body, became scientifically known. Scientists and medical investigators delineated and defined new standards of dietary and nutritional health, producing new ways of appreciating food and diet that perpetually evolved to gradually incorporate new concerns such as the role played by the ingestion of germs in creating illness. Late nineteenth-century food discourses also formed part of broader cultural anxieties about degeneration and imperfect motherhood. Paradoxically, although a deep-rooted faith existed in the idea that reduced reliance on the potato would ultimately improve Irish socio-economic life, physicians and social commentators continued to problematise Irish consumption patterns long after the Famine. This was particularly the case from around the 1880s when physicians blamed and faulted bleak, insufficient diets consisting of tea and white bread for helping to perpetuate national socio-economic and physical backwardness. Various actors attempted to take centre stage by claiming expertise in dietary matters. Experts from medical and scientific communities provide an obvious example. Educational reformers also intervened from around 1900. Domestic and agricultural education was considered too technical in the late nineteenth century and, arguably, not scientific enough in the twentieth century. The educational reforms of 1900 offered a potentially major state initiative although practical difficulties surfaced when implementing a nationwide domestic instruction scheme through the National School system.

Other key players held varied, sometimes competing, views on the efficacy of state schemes and the validity of expert knowledge. After the Famine, critics often interpreted institutional feeding as unnecessarily weakening young Irish bodies, forming individuals who were socially useless upon release. In the late nineteenth century, traders and business groups routinely objected to the imposition of new standards of purity, the definition of which remained scientifically and legislatively loose. Philanthropic groups emerged who were intent on improving the nutritional and dietary health of the less affluent, although some of these – most notably Maud Gonne's Ladies School Dinners Committee – adopted a remarkably adversarial stance to the state's ostensible interest in improving the health of the Irish young. In the 1910s, Sinn Féin, too, presented wartime food policies as constituting a gross assault on the Irish body. Common to all these debates was a sense that British governance and imperial rule, by now characterised by attempts to biologically govern, had in fact created scenarios that compromised Irish health – a predicament worsened by the complex Irish system of social and political relations.

These viewpoints, sometimes self-consciously, inverted the promises of improvement that had underpinned the extension of state, medical and scientific intervention into various spheres of day-to-day activity. When urging peasants to abandon the potato, state bodies, as well as physicians and scientists, had guaranteed that physical, socio-economic and national improvement would come to all. Agriculturists saw attentiveness to new biological ways of understanding animal life and how to convert it into food – enshrined in the ethos of mid-century agricultural schools – as a crucial precursor of economic advancement. Public health officials framed food purity – increasingly defined by an absence of germs and set standards of water and salt content – as a potential improver of Irish economic life. Yet these improvements never really came. Ultimately, the upheaval of the First World War forced a rethinking of the pathways traversed in consumption and production since the Famine. Claims of British mismanagement were, of course, propagandist in nature. However, they brought food to the fore of discussion of post-Famine development (or a relative lack of it). In the 1910s, a broad consensus insisted that post-war Ireland needed to adopt independent, self-sustaining food policies and become less reliant on importing innutritious foodstuffs while exporting their more nutritious equivalents. For some, implicit in these hopes was a feeling that once Ireland freed itself from a London-based government that was unsympathetic, uninformed or, at worst, apathetic, to Ireland, improvement would finally ensue.

How far post-independence Irish state bodies met these aspirations is a debatable issue, and one that requires fuller investigation than can be offered here. An initial reading suggests that relatively little was initially achieved. Wartime critics had avowed that the imperial state displayed visible tendencies to intervene more pervasively in food production than in diet, consumption and feeding. The First World War made clear to some that state efforts to maximise agricultural output primarily benefited British consumers. Surprisingly, given the prevalence of these issues in wartime political critique, relatively little was initially achieved in curbing the problematic import/export system after 1922.

The immediate post-independence period was certainly marked by optimism about the potential to transform Irish agricultural practice. In 1921, the Commission of Inquiry into the Resources and Industries of Ireland, headed by Sinn Féin politician Darrell Figgis under the then legally unrecognised revolutionary government in the Dáil Éireann (Irish parliament), was primarily interested in making Ireland self-sufficient.[1] Further investigations into areas such as cattle breeding ascertained that Ireland lagged behind many other countries with regard to the breeds that it developed and the amount of milk yielded from each cow.[2] However, the state ultimately revitalised compulsory tillage in 1922, a step presented as an important means of providing employment to landless agricultural labourers in a period of international economic downturn. This stance was intended to counter a perceived decrease in enthusiasm for tillage evident since 1918 – viewed as an impediment to Irish improvement. Based on the Corn Production Act of 1917 that had made wartime tillage compulsory, individuals such as Irish Labour Party politician Thomas Nagle presumed that 'if they could do that for British ruling classes, then they ought to be equally willing to till to keep landless labourers from starvation'. However, the nature of such legislation smacked of an authoritarianism that struck right at the heart of the ideologies of what it meant to live in a free country. According to Denis J. Gorey, leader of the Farmer's Party, farmers ought to have free choice over what they grew rather than being coerced into further slavery by men who had 'never soiled their hands'.[3] Nonetheless, exactly how to motivate them to produce without an authoritarian approach remained uncertain. In fact, the new rhetoric of agricultural improvement differed little from that espoused by the Imperial state some sixty years earlier. Take, for instance, trade unionist Thomas Johnson's announcement in the Dáil in 1925: 'these farmers, if they would combine, if they would use scientific methods, unified methods of marketing, could improve their standard of living very greatly indeed'. Or: 'I have no hesitation in saying that the farming community, if they would organise and use scientific methods, could produce from the soil foodstuffs and all the requirements of life that would lead them to a standard of civilisation higher than we claim for our workmen.'[4]

Some argued that it was the state's responsibility to properly educate farmers and equip them with the technical expertise needed to increase output. In the 1920s, TDs (members of the Irish parliament) even suggested the construction of model farms and agricultural schools, mirroring the idyllic pedagogical ideas of the 1850s.[5] The Commission on Agriculture of 1924 proposed that a nation-wide model farm system should be initiated to encourage the uptake of agro-scientific ideals.[6] The Commission's proposals were far less radical in nature than expected and mostly echoed the tactics of the mid-nineteenth-century state whose efforts had been challenged by many agricultural communities. The Commission also openly appreciated DATI's network of agricultural education instigated in 1900 and merely recommended that male pupils remain in school up until the age of eighteen to receive intensive training on small-scale husbandry and agricultural accountancy.[7]

It might be expected that discussion of production became directed inwardly following independence to focus on ensuring high standards for a home market, especially given that Ireland was expected to produce her own foods following the Great War. However, as Cormac Ó Gráda and others demonstrate, the Cummann na nGaedheal government that came into power in 1922 perpetuated an outward-looking commercial policy that sought to maintain free-trade export links with Britain.[8] This led one outraged politician to assert in 1927 that 'our agricultural economy ... is rooted in the conditions of the country. Of course it is, but who made them the conditions of the country? Who stereotyped those conditions? The British. Is Britain still ruling us? Is our fiscal policy still dictated from Westminster or from Downing Street? If it is, let us know the worst.'[9] According to Roy Foster, Cummann na nGaedheal emphasised making Irish produce marketable for a British rather than domestic market.[10] When proposing plans for the improved marketing of Irish dairy produce in 1923, the Department of Agriculture dispatched inspectors to Liverpool and Manchester to determine why Irish produce had gained such a bad reputation. Inspectors later discovered that Irish butter melted quickly on shop counters due to problems with its fat content.[11] The Agricultural Produce (Eggs) Act of 1924 was intended to tackle quality issues with Irish eggs by ensuring that producers tested and graded produce before it left the country to ensure its suitability for human consumption and to stop retailers marketing poor quality eggs as Irish in origin.[12] In 1931, one politician suggested in the Dáil that recent legislation ensured that the best foodstuffs were being exported from Ireland, meaning that only second-rate food was left available for home consumption.[13] For sceptics, the visions of a self-supporting, healthy nation that preserved its most nutritious, healthiest foodstuffs for domestic consumption was yet to be realised.

Post-independence responses to ongoing nutritional and dietary needs among the poor were also relatively lacking. In 1922, the Cost of Living Committee enquired into the prices of commodities in Ireland and asked why Irish produce could be purchased much cheaper in England than in Ireland, although little seems to have arisen from this in the form of policy.[14] During the economic depression of the 1920s and 1930s, the state continued to channel relief principally through the pre-existing Poor Law system which remained subject to stigma. The first Dáil government denigrated workhouses as odious, degrading and foreign. The Democratic programme of 1919 even pledged that they would be replaced with a more sympathetic system. The Local Government Act of 1925 formally abolished Boards of Guardians across Ireland (with the exception of Dublin) replacing them with Boards of Health and Public Assistance although, as both Virginia Crossman and Diarmaid Ferriter observe, newer approaches to poverty continued to supply relief rather than grapple with the causes of poverty. In fact, standards of health care in the 1920s and 1930s left much to be desired.[15] Ferriter argues that the Cumann na nGaedheal government was so intent on asserting its political authority and ensuring the survival of the state that it remained removed and detached from adverse social conditions, failing resoundingly to tackle issues of poverty and destitution.[16] Similarly, Foster asserts that dreams of a social welfare utopia were shattered in the face of the realities of fiscal autonomy.[17] The practical implications of post-war economic downturn no doubt accentuated these conditions, yet new measures to replace the Poor Law were considered equally degrading. When relief providers gave food tickets to the poor in 1926, critics invoked the word 'workhouse' and asserted that relief seekers mostly shunned such schemes.[18]

Predictably, the diet of the poor continued to be problematised. Witnesses at the Commission into the Resources and Industries of Ireland of 1922 asserted that Ireland had once been renowned for its physical vigour due to the population's high levels of milk intake. The opposite was the case in the 1920s, so they concluded. The Commission blamed high infant mortality incidences on widespread reliance on margarine rather than butter, limited consumption of oatmeal on the lack of availability of milk and an enduring 'tea and shop bread culture'.[19] These claims resonated with anxieties routinely expressed in earlier decades, in many ways serving as an indicator of limited social progress in that area. Leading medical figure Thomas Hennessy, Irish medical secretary for the British Medical Association, was acutely aware of such issues. When interviewed by the *Freeman's Journal* in 1924, he declared that 'we are dealing in Ireland at present with a third rate population from the health point of view'.[20]

Although it was not uncommon in the 1920s for the Famine to be invoked in discussion of starvation and under-nutrition, what differentiated the situation now was that political figures in Ireland had no-one but themselves to blame for the failings of a new Irish state, being no longer able to persuasively implicate ineffectual British policy. Politician Timothy Joseph O'Donovan eagerly invoked the memory of 'Black '47' when detailing an account of a family in his West Cork constituency discovered in 1927 by a neighbour with the mother dead, and the father and five children in 'a hopelessly weak condition, with no beds except hay, no bed-clothes and no food. The only food in the house was a few pounds of yellow meal and a half loaf of bread.' O'Donovan continued by claiming that 'I do not think we have had such a calamitous state of affairs since

'47' and announced that all of the family members had died just three days later.[21] The reporting of incidents such as these, as well as a chronic lack of progress in areas such as school dinners provision, fitted uneasily with the doctrines of Dáil Éireann's democratic programme drawn up in 1919 which had stipulated that:

> It shall be the first duty of the Government of the Republic to make provision for the physical, mental and spiritual well-being of the children, to secure that no child shall suffer hunger or cold from lack of food, clothing, or shelter, but that all shall be provided with the means and facilities requisite for their proper education and training as Citizens of a Free and Gaelic Ireland.[22]

The formal education of poorly nourished children also persisted as a problematic issue, despite earlier decades of agitation by prominent female figures such as Maud Gonne. Irish provision contrasted sharply with the situation north of the border where the Education Act (Northern Ireland) 1923 stipulated that it was the duty of the Education Authority to offer food to children who struggled to learn due to their under-nourished physical condition.[23] In 1925, Labour Party spokesmen Tomas J. O'Connell recited the Democratic Programme in the Dáil. 'Children are attending school cold and hungry', O'Connell explained, adding that 'there is no provision for their relief either from cold or hunger', a statement that mirrored criticisms made much earlier in the century.[24] It was not until 1930 that the School Meals (Gaeltacht) Act was implemented outside of Dublin.[25]

Likewise, milk provision continued to create contention.[26] Despite improvements in quality, the price of delivered milk in Dublin rose from 3 d. per quart in 1914 to 7 ½ d. per quart in 1924, a significantly higher cost than customers in smaller cities such as Cork could expect to pay. Looking north of the border, official investigations revealed that milk in Belfast that had been cleansed, tested and delivered in sealed bottles cost just 5 d. per quart, thereby demonstrating that it was possible to produce clean milk cheaply. In Dublin, matters were not helped by sustained disputes between the Dublin Dairymen's Association and railway operators.[27] Eventually, in 1933, the State put aside £100,000 to provide needy children with milk, in part due to recognition that an absence of adequate supplies was a potent cause of childhood diseases, most notably rickets.[28]

It is perhaps ironic, given the extensive criticism of the potato diet prior to and during the Famine that almost a century later the official line on national diet reminisced about the simplicity and austerity of Irish food prior to the introduction of modern ways of eating. Speakers at the Celtic Congress held in Dublin in July 1934 reflected that if Celtic races were to flourish, they needed to be well fed on home-produced foods as they had been in the past. Speakers at the event depicted cosmopolitan foodstuffs as having undermined the health of the Celtic races with salvation being offered only by a return to home-produced national dietary systems that were admittedly simple but nonetheless essential for the rearing of healthy people. 'Our lands', one speaker claimed, 'are starving for want of proper fertilisation, because the farmers are impoverished by the importation of preserved foreign foods.'[29] Views such as these flourished after the rise of Fianna Fáil. Led by de Valera, this party formed in 1926 and came to power in 1932. It promised forms of economic radicalism entailing advances in welfare reform and a firm move away from the *laissez-faire* approaches that had dominated Cumann na nGaedheal policies.[30] Politicians in the Dáil began to look back to when Ireland had been a predominantly wheat-producing country prior to the Famine and to ask why Irish land could not be turned to wheat once again.[31] However, Fianna Fáil's approach left the party open to accusations of having primitive economic perspectives. 'Anybody who thinks that this State can exist merely by producing food and consuming it', explained politician and philosopher Desmond Fitzgerald in 1932, 'is living in a fool's paradise. I do not mind the odd politician living in a fool's paradise. What I do object to is the consistent attempt to mislead the people and to mislead them into paths which will mean their economic and moral ruin.'[32]

Notes

1 *Commission of Inquiry into the Resources and Industries of Ireland* (Dublin: The Commission, 1919–22).
2 *Report on Stock-Breeding Farms for Pure-Bred Dairy Cattle* (Dublin: Stationery Office, 1921), pp. 8–10.
3 'Compulsory tillage', *Dáil Éireann Debate* (19 September 1922), vol. 1, no. 7.
4 'Shannon electrification scheme: motion by Deputy Johnson', *Dáil Éireann Debate* (3 November 1925), vol. 13 no. 1.
5 'Committee on Finance: Office of the Minister for Lands and Agriculture – Vote 48', *Dáil Éireann Debate* (4 June 1925), vol. 12, no. 3.
6 *Report on Stock-Breeding Farms for Pure-Bred Dairy Cattle*, pp. 24–6.
7 *Reports of the Commission on Agriculture* (Dublin: Stationery Office, 1924).
8 C. Ó Gráda, *Ireland: A New Economic History, 1780–1939* (Oxford: Oxford University Press, 1994), pp. 385–403.
9 'Adjournment debates: distress in Cork', *Dáil Éireann Debate* (31 March 1927), vol. 19, no. 7.
10 R. F. Foster, *Modern Ireland, 1600–1972* (London: Penguin, 1989), p. 522.
11 NAI, Department of Agriculture files, 92/3/129.
12 NAI, Department of Agriculture files, 92/3/299; 92/3/453.
13 'In Committee on Finance: Vote 52 – agriculture', *Dáil Éireann Debate* (27 May 1931), vol. 38, no. 16.
14 *Report on the Cost of Living in Ireland* (Dublin: Ministry of Economic Affairs, 1922).
15 Crossman, *Poor Law in Ireland*, pp. 53–5; D. Ferriter, 'Local government, public health and welfare in twentieth-century Ireland', in M. E. Daly (ed.), *County and Town: One Hundred Years of Local Government in Ireland* (Dublin: Institute of Public Administration, 2001).
16 D. Ferriter, *The Transformation of Ireland, 1900–2000* (London: Profile Books, 2004), p. 299.
17 Foster, *Modern Ireland*, p. 519.
18 'Question on adjournment: relief of distress', *Dáil Éireann Debate* (10 March 1926), vol. 14, no. 14.

19 NAI, DE4/8/13.
20 'Third Rate Race: Need for Drastic Reform in Irish Public Health', *Freeman's Journal* (31 May 1924), p. 7.
21 'Adjournment debate: distress in West Cork', *Dáil Éireann Debate* (31 March 1927), vol. 19, no. 7.
22 'Democratic programme', *Dáil Éireann Debate* (21 January 1919), vol F, no. 1.
23 PRONI, LA/7/29BA/79.
24 'Policy of the Minister for Education: motion by the President', *Dáil Éireann Debate* (11 November 1925), vol. 13, no. 2.
25 School Meals (Gaeltacht) Act, 1930.
26 See, for instance, J. W. Bigger, 'Milk and the public health', *Dublin Journal of Medical Science*, 2:5 (April 1922), 87–9.
27 NAI, Department of Agriculture files, 92/3/68.
28 'In Committee on Finance: supplementary estimate. Vote 41: local government and public health', *Dáil Éireann Debate* (14 June 1932), vol. 42, no. 9.
29 'Food Problems of the Celts: The Plain Diet of Old Days', *Irish Times* (12 July 1934), p. 8.
30 See R. Dunphy, *The Making of Fianna Fáil Power in Ireland, 1923–48* (Oxford: Oxford University Press, 2005).
31 'Committee on Finance: office of the Minister for Lands and Agriculture – Vote 48', *Dáil Éireann Debate* (4 June 1925), vol. 12, no. 3.
32 'Supplementary and additional estimates: Vote no 73 – Emergency Fund grant-in-aid', *Dáil Éireann* (4 August 1932), vol. 43, no. 11.

Select bibliography

Archives

Military Archives, Cathal Brugha Barracks, Dublin
WS0807.

National Archives of Ireland (NAI)
92/1/1426, 92/1/1462, 92/1/1500, 92/1/1526, 92/1/1547, 92/1/1591, 92/1/1594, 92/1/1597, 92/1/1686, 92/1/1703, 92/1/26, 92/1/686, 92/2/302, 92/3/129, 92/3/299, 92/3/305, 92/3/453, 92/3/68, DE4/8/13.ED8/2, RLFC2/Z14434, RLFC2/Z14466, RLFC2/Z14518, RLFC2/Z15316, RLFC2/Z15556, RLFC/15866, RLFC2/Z16624, RLFC3/1/3417.

National Archives, Kew
CAB/24/23, CAB/24/28, CAB/24/29.

National Folklore Commission
lml.l.8344.

National Library of Ireland (NLI)
Department of Agriculture Minute Books (1914, 1916).
Minutes of the Proceedings of the Commissioners of National Education in Ireland (1901, 1902, 1904, 1905, 1907, 1916, 1917).
Maude Gonne correspondence.

Public Records Office of Northern Ireland (PRONI)
D2682/1/1, ED/8/1/145, ED/8/1/212, ED/8/1/214, LA/7/29BA/79, LA/7/3/JA/25.

UCD Archives
Albert Agricultural College Admission Registers, Records of the Albert Agricultural College, University College Dublin Archives, IE UCDA AAC1/14.

Royal College of Physicians in Ireland (RCPI)
Reports on the State of Public Health in Dublin (1864–94).

Debates

House of Commons Debates
Dáil Éireann Debates

Official reports and documents

Alleged Increasing Prevalence of Insanity in Ireland: Special Report from the Inspectors of Lunatics to the Chief Secretary, Reports of Commissioners, Commons, 1894 [C.7331], vol. xliii.647.

Annual Reports of the Commissioners of National Education in Ireland, Reports of Commissioners, Commons, 1847–48 [981], vol. xxix.219; 1849 [1066], vol. xxiii.91; 1850 [1582], vol. xlii.1; 1852–3 [1582], vol. xlii.1; 1860 [2593], vol. xxv.1; 1860 [2706], vol. xxvi.1; 1861 [2873], vol. xx.91; 1862 [3026], vol. xx.249; 1864 [3351], vol. xix Pt.II.1; 1871 [C.360], vol. xxiii.7; 1878–9 [C.2312–I], vol. xxiv.553; 1884–5 [C.4458], vol. xxiv.75; 1890 [C.6074], vol. xxx.89; 1890–1 [C.6411], vol. xxix.1; 1893–4 [C.7124], vol. xxvii.265; 1894 [C.7457], vol. xxx Pt.II.1; 1895 [C.7796], vol. xxix.1; 1896 [C.8142], vol. xxviii.1; 1897 [C.8600], vol. xxviii.1; 1899 [C.9446], xxiv.377; 1900 [Cd.285], vol. xxiii.189; 1901 [Cd.1198], vol. xxx.403; 1902 [Cd.954], vol. xxx.1; 1904 [Cd.1903], vol. xx.195; 1905 [Cd.2373], vol. xxvii.403; 1906 [Cd.3154], vol. xxix.635; 1908 [Cd.4291], vol. xxvii.841; 1912–3 [Cd.5935], vol. xxi.409.

Annual Reports of the Congested Districts Board for Ireland, Reports of Commissioners, Commons, 1893–4 [C.6908], vol. lxxi.525.

Annual Reports of the Department of Agriculture and Technical Instruction, Reports of Commissioners, Commons, 1902 [Cd.838], vol. xx.522; 1902 [Cd.1314], vol. xx.817; 1904 [Cd.1919], vol. xvi.435; 1905 [Cd.2509], vol. xxi.261; 1906 [Cd.2929], vol. xxiii.295; 1907 [Cd.3543], vol. xvii.241, 1913–14 [Cd.7839], vol. vi.1, 1916, [Cd.8299], vol. iv.413; 1918 [Cd.9016], vol. v.383.

Annual Reports of the Inspector appointed to visit the Reformatory Schools of Ireland, Command Papers, Reports of Commissioners, 1863 [3194], vol. xxiv.623.

Annual Reports of the Inspector appointed to visit the Reformatory and Industrial Schools of Ireland, Command Papers, Reports of Commissioners, 1872 [C.671], vol. xxx.661; 1873 [C.858], vol. xxxi.739; 1876 [C.1494], vol. xxxiv.777; 1880 [C.2692], vol. xxxvii.373.

Annual Reports of the Inspectors-General on the General State of the Prisons of Ireland, Reports of Commissioners, Commons, 1850 [1229], vol. xxix; 1851 [1364], xxviii.357; 1852–3 [1657], vol. liii.1; 1857 [2236], vol. xxii.173; 1866 [3690], vol. xxxiv.235.

Annual Reports of the Poor Law Commissioners, Reports of Commissioners, Commons, 1840 [253], vol. xvii.447; 1842 [399], vol. xix.1192; 1846 [704], vol. xix.1; 1851 [1381], vol. xxvi.547.

Appendix to the Second Report of the Vice-Regal Committee of Inquiry into Primary Education (Ireland), Reports of Commissioners, Commons, 1914 [Cd.7229], vol. xxviii.5.

Changes in the Food Chain since the Time of the Great Irish Famine (National Nutrition Surveillance Centre, University College Galway, 1995).

Commission of Inquiry into the Resources and Industries of Ireland (Dublin: The Commission, 1919–22).

Commission to Inquire into Child Abuse Volume 1 (Dublin: Stationery Office, 2009).

Committee of Butter Regulations: Minutes of Evidence, Reports of Commissioners, Commons, 1902 [Cd.944], vol. xx.123.

Fourth Report of the Royal Commission on Congestion in Ireland, Reports of Commissioners, Commons, 1907 [Cd.3508], vol. xxxvi.1.

Judicial Statistics Ireland, Commons, Command Papers, Accounts and Papers, 1865 [3563], lii.657; 1875 [c.1295], lxxxi.259; 1884–5 [c.4554], lxxxvi.243; 1895 [c.7799], cviii.323.

Minutes of Evidence taken before the Inter-Departmental Committee on Physical Deterioration Volume II, Reports of Commissioners, Commons, 1904 [Cd.2201], vol. xxxii.45.

Prison Dietaries (Ireland). Copy of a circular addressed by Inspectors General of Prisons to the Board of Superintendence of Irish county Prisons in reference to the Proposed Alteration in the Prison Dietaries, Accounts and Papers, Commons, 1867–8 [131], vol. lvii.533.

Report from the Select Committee on Adulteration of Food, Commons, Reports of Committees, 1856 [379], vol. viii.1.

Report from the Select Committee on Industries (Ireland), Reports of Committees, Commons, 1884–5 [Cmd.288], vol. IX.1.

Report of the Commissioners of Health, on the Epidemics of 1846 to 1850, Reports of Commissioners, Commons, 1852 [1562], vol. xli.

Report of the Committee appointed by His Excellency the Lord Lieutenant to inquire into the Dietaries of County and Borough Gaols in Ireland (1867–8), Reports of Commissioners, Commons, 1868 [3981], vol. xxxv.665.

Report of the Departmental Committee on Food Production in Ireland, Reports of Commissioners, Commons, 1914–16 [Cd.8016], vol. v.799.

Report of the Departmental Committee on the Irish Pig-Breeding Industry, Reports of Commissioners, Commons, 1914–16, Cd.7890, vol. v.855.

Report on the Cost of Living in Ireland (Dublin: Ministry of Economic Affairs, 1922).

Reports of the Commission on Agriculture (Dublin: Stationery Office, 1924).

Reports of the Commission on Manual and Practical Instruction in Primary Schools under the Board of National Education in Ireland, Reports of Commissioners, Commons, 1897 [C.8383], vol. xliii.1; 1897 [C.8618], vol. xliii.401; 1897 [C.8923], vol. xliv.1.

Reports on the State of Public Health (Dublin) (Royal College of Physicians in Ireland).

Report on Stock-Breeding Farms for Pure-Bred Dairy Cattle (Dublin: Stationery Office, 1921).

Returns from County Gaols and Workhouses in Ireland of Daily Diet allowed to Able-Bodied Men, Accounts and Papers, Commons, 1847–8 [486], vol. liii.

Returns of All Counties in Ireland in which Public Analysts have been Appointed, with Names, Dates of Appointment, and Salaries, Accounts and Papers, Commons [1874], C.410, vol. lvi.861.

Royal Commission on Congestion in Ireland: Appendix to the Sixth Report, Reports of Commissioners, Commons, 1908 [Cd.3748], vol. xxxix.701.

Royal Commission on Labour. The Agricultural Labourer. Vol. IV. Ireland. Part III, Reports of Commissioners, Commons, 1893–4 [C.6894–xx], vol. xxxvii Pt.1.265; *Part IV,* 1893–4 [C.6894–xxi], vol. xxxvii Pt.1.341.

Sixth Report of the Medical Officer of the Privy Council, Reports of Commissioners, Commons, 1863 [3416], vol. xxviii.

Vice-Regal Commission on the Irish Milk Supply: The Final Report of the Irish Milk Commission, Reports of Commissioners, Commons, 1914 [Cd.7129], vol. xxxvi.601.

ort of the Irish Milk Commission.

Newspapers

Bean nÉireann.
Belfast Evening News.
Belfast Newsletter.
Cork Examiner.
Farmer's Magazine.
Freeman's Journal.
Irish Independent.
Irish Times.
Kildare Observer.
Nation.
Nenagh Vindicator.
Sláinte.
Tuam Herald.
Weekly Irish Times.

Primary sources

Annual Report of the Chemico-Agricultural Society of Ulster (Belfast: Francis D. Finlay, 1847).
'Discussion of Dr Cameron's paper, "On an epidemic of fever caused by infected milk"', *Dublin Journal of Medical Science*, 91 (1 July 1879), 66–85.
'Dr. Letheby's third lecture on food', *Medical Press and Circular*, 5 (25 March 1868), 257–260.
'Famine and the Ard-Chomhairle', *New Ireland* (5 January 1918), 139–40.
First General Meeting and Council Dinner of the Chemico-Agricultural Society of Ulster (Belfast: Francis D. Finlay, 1846).
'Funds for building Technical Schools', *Irish Technical Journal*, 4 (July 1903), 72–4.
'Insanity and tea-drinking', *Lancet*, 138 (1891), 302.
Lancet, 49 (27 February 1847), 232.
'Letters from Dr W. N. Cote: diet of laborers in Ireland', *Medical and Surgical Reporter*, 11:2 (9 January 1864), 40.
'Meat inspection in Belfast', *Belfast Health Journal*, 3:4 (21 March 1905), 69.
'Ministers of the devil', *Dublin University Magazine*, 57 (June 1861), 696–709.
Productive Thrift (Dublin: Department of Agriculture, 1916).
'Remember '47', *New Ireland* (8 December 1917), 70–2.
'Report of L'Abbé J. O. Godin on his mission to Europe', *Statement of the Public Accounts of the Province of Quebec for the Fiscal Year Ended 30th June 1869* (Quebec: Augustin Cote, 1869).
'Report on the prevalence of potato blight in Ireland up to the 17th *July 1915', Journal of the Department of Agriculture and Technical Instruction*, 15:4 (1915), 755–6.
'Royal Agricultural Improvement Society of Ireland', *Irish Farmer's Gazette*, 10 (March 1851), 157–8.
'Symptoms produced by eating diseased potatoes', *Dublin Hospital Gazette*, 23 (1846), 166.
'Tea-drinking', *British Medical Journal*, i (1888), 812.
'The adulteration question', *Dublin Medical Press* (9 April 1856), 235.
'The Albert Model Farm, Glasnevin', *Farmer's Magazine*, 36 (July 1869), 20–2.

'The famine in the land: what has been done and what is to be done', *Dublin University Magazine*, 29 (April 1847), 501–40.
'The food of the Irish', *Dublin University Magazine*, 43 (February 1854), 127–46.
'The ghouls of famine', *New Ireland* (19 January 1918), 173.
'The sugar contract for the North Dublin Union', *Dublin Medical Press* (8 July 1863).
'The way to anarchy', *New Ireland* (19 May 1917), 21–2.
Transactions of the Central Relief Committee of the Society of Friends during the Famine in Ireland in 1846 and 1847 (Dublin: Hodges and Smith, 1852).
'Wholemeal bread', *Boston Journal of Chemistry*, 3:2 (1 August 1868), 27.
'Winter dairying and creameries', *Journal of the Department of Agricultural and Technical Instruction*, 7:2 (January 1912), 281–303.
A Catholic Layman, *Mixed Education: The Catholic Case Stated, or Principles, Working and Results of the System of National Education* (Dublin: John Mullany, 1859).
Abernethy, J., *Surgical Observations on the Constitutional Origin and Treatment of Local Diseases* (London: Longman, Hurst, Reese and Orme, 1809).
Aldridge, J., *On the Comparative Nutritive and Pecuniary Value of Various Kinds of Cooked Food* (Dublin, 1847).
Anderson, R. A., 'The IAOS and the food problem', *Studies: An Irish Quarterly Review*, 6:21 (March 1917), 8–14.
Arnott, J., *The Investigation into the Condition of the Children in the Cork Workhouse* (Cork: Guy Brothers 1859).
Association of Victuallers, *A Defence of the Dublin Victuallers* (Dublin: R. D. Webb and Son, 1882).
Baldwin, T., 'On the application of artificial manures part one', *Journal of the Royal Dublin Society*, 2 (October 1859), 309–21.
——, *An Introduction to Practical Farming* (Dublin: Alex. Thom and Co., 15th edn, 1877).
Bastable, C. F., 'The Irish export trade in butter, with special reference to the regulations of the Cork Market', *Journal of the Statistical and Social Inquiry Society of Ireland*, 8:60 (August 1882), 331–9.
——, *The Commerce of Nations* (London: Methuen and Co., 1892).
Beard, G. M., *A Practical Treatise on Nervous Exhaustion (Neurasthenia): Its Symptoms, Nature, Sequences, Treatment* (New York: William Wood, 1880).
Beaumont, W., *Experiments and Observations on the Gastric Juice and the Physiology of Digestion* (Plattsburgh: F. P. Allen, 1833).
Bellingham, O'B., 'Observations upon the potato disease as it prevailed in Ireland this year', *Dublin Medical Press*, 13 (1845), 359–64.
Bigger, J. W., 'Milk and the public health', *Dublin Journal of Medical Science*, 2:5 (April 1922), 87–9.
Burnett, J. T., *The Chemico-Agricultural Society of Ulster on Rotations of Cropping* (Belfast: Francis D. Finlay, 1846).
Cahill, M., *Remarks on the Present State of Dublin with Suggestions for the Improvement of Smithfield and the Erection of a General Abattoir and Carcase Market* (Dublin: Hodges, Smith & Co., 1861).
Cameron, C. A., *The Stock-Feeders Manual: The Chemistry of Food in relation to the Breeding and Feeding of Livestock* (London and New York: Cassell, Petter and Galpin, 1868).
——, 'Half-yearly report on public health', *Dublin Journal of Medical Science*, 3 (1 May 1872), 394–425.

——, 'On an epidemic of fever caused by infected milk', *Dublin Journal of Medical Science*, 91 (1 July 1879), 1–23.

——, 'Report on public health', *Dublin Journal of Medical Science*, 73 (2 January 1882), 112–29.

——, 'On micro-organisms and alkaloids which render food poisonous', *Dublin Journal of Medical Science*, 78 (1 December 1884), 473–90.

——, 'Note on the operation in Dublin of the Acts relating to adulteration', *Analyst*, 10 (October 1885), 175–9.

——, *Reminiscences of Sir Charles A. Cameron* (Dublin: Hodges and Figgis, 1913).

Carpenter, M., *Juvenile Delinquents: Their Condition and Treatment* (London: W. And F. G. Cash, 1853).

Carroll, T., 'Education in agriculture', *New Ireland Review*, 4 (February 1896), 336–40.

——, *Introduction to Practical Farming (new edition)* (Dublin: Alex. Thom and Co., 1898).

Carter, R. B., *A Practical Treatise on Diseases of the Eye* (London: Macmillan and Co., 1875).

Colman, H., *European Agriculture and Rural Economy* (Boston: Phillips, Sampson and Company, 4th edn, 1851).

Combe, A., *The Physiology of Digestion* (Edinburgh: MacLachlan and Stewart, 1836).

Commissioners of National Education in Ireland, *Agricultural Classbook, or How Best to Cultivate a Small Farm or Garden: Together with Hints on Domestic Economy* (Dublin: Thom, 1853).

Corrigan, D. J., *On Famine and Fever* (Dublin: J. Fannin, 1846).

Davy, E. W., 'On the scientific principles involved in the feeding and fattening of stock', *Natural History Review*, 6 (1859), 261–8.

Doyle, M., *The Agricultural Labourer viewed in his Moral, Intellectual and Physical Conditions* (London: Groombridge and Sons, 1855).

Drapes, T., 'On the alleged increase of insanity in Ireland', *Journal of Mental Science*, 40 (October 1894), 519–48.

Farr, W. *Vital Statistics, or, the Statistics of Health, Sickness, Diseases and Death* (London, 1837).

Ferguson, K., *Advanced Lessons in Cookery* (Athlone: Athlone Printing Works, 1903).

Foot, A. W., *Symptoms and Treatment of the Cattle Plague* (Dublin and London: McGlashan and Gill, 1866).

Foster, T. C., *Letters on the Condition of the People of Ireland* (London: Chapman and Hall, 1846).

Gallaher, F. M., *Short Lessons in Domestic Science* (Dublin: Browne and Nolan, 1894).

Gamgee, J., *The Cattle Plague* (London: R. Harwicke, 1866).

Gibson, C. B., *Life Among Convicts* (London: Hurst and Blackett, 1863).

Gibson, E., 'Penal servitude and tickets of leave', *Journal of the Statistical and Social Inquiry Society of Ireland*, 3 (April 1863), 332–43.

Gill, T. P., 'Productive thrift', *Journal of the Department of Agriculture and Technical Instruction*, 16:2 (January 1916), 349–52.

——, 'The Department of Agriculture and the food problem', *Studies: An Irish Quarterly Journal*, 6:21 (March 1917), 1–8.

Gogarty, O. St J., 'The need of medical inspection of school children in Ireland', *Irish Review*, 2:13 (March 1912), 12–9.

Gonne, M., 'Responsibility', *Irish Review*, 1:10 (December 1911), 483–5.

Guy, W. A., 'On sufficient and insufficient dietaries, with especial reference to the dietaries of prisoners', *Journal of the Statistical Society of London*, 26 (September 1863), 239–81.

Haughton, J., 'The social and moral elevation of our people', *Journal of the Dublin Statistical Society*, 3 (July 1857), 63–72.

Hodges, J. F., *What Science can do for the Irish Farmer* (Dublin: W. Curry, 1844).

——, *Report of the Composition and Agricultural Value of Kelp* (Belfast: Francis D. Finlay, 1846).

Houston, D., *The Milk Supply of Dublin* (Dublin: Co-operative Reference Library, 1918).

Johnson, J., *An Essay on Morbid Sensibility of the Stomach and Bowels* (London: 1827).

——, *A Tour in Ireland* (London: S. Highley, 1844).

Kane, R., *The Industrial Resources of Ireland* (Dublin: Hodges and Smith, 1844).

——, *On the Importance of Agricultural and Industrial Education* (Dublin, 1845).

Kelly, D., *The War and Ireland's Food Supply, an Appeal to the Irish Farmer* (Dublin: Department of Agriculture and Technical Instruction, 1914).

Lady Aberdeen, *The Sorrows of Ireland* (1916).

Lankester, E., 'On prison and workhouse dietaries', *British Medical Journal*, ii:357 (2 November 1867), 380–2.

Leared, A., *The Causes and Treatment of Imperfect Digestion* (London: John Churchill, 1860).

Lewis, G. C., *Remarks on the Third Report of the Irish Poor Inquiry Commissioners* (London: W. Clowes, 1837).

Liebig, J. von, *Animal Chemistry, or Organic Chemistry in its Application to Physiology and Pathology* (London: Taylor and Walton, 1842).

——, *Research on the Chemistry of Food*, trans. W. Gregory (Lowell: Daniel Bixby and Company, 1848).

Lovibond, F. M. F., 'Women and hygiene in modern life', *New Ireland Review*, 21 (April 1904), 74–82.

Lysaght, E. E., Westropp Bennett, T. W. and Ball, R., 'The farmers and the food problem', *Studies: An Irish Quarterly Review*, 6:21 (March 1917), 21–34.

——, 'Irish agriculture', *Studies: An Irish Quarterly Review*, 7:26 (June 1918), 314–19.

MacSweeney, A. M., *Poverty in Cork* (Cork: Purcell and Company, 1917).

Malone, A. E., 'Peace and potatoes', *New Ireland* (23 December 1916), 110–11.

Mapother, E. D., 'The sanitary state of Dublin', *Journal of the Statistical and Social Inquiry Society of Ireland*, 27 (May 1864), 62–7.

Marsh, H., *On the Preparation of Food for the Labourer* (Dublin: James McGlashan, 1847).

McCormack, M. J., 'A case of land scurvy produced by eating diseased potatoes', *Dublin Hospital Gazette*, 29 (1846), 263–8.

Murray, P. J., *Reformatories in Ireland, and for Dublin in Particular* (Dublin: W. B. Kelly, 1858).

Niemeyer, F. von, *A Text-book of Practical Medicine, with Particular Reference to Physiology and Pathological Anatomy*, trans. G. H. Humphreys and C. E. Hackley (New York: D. Appleton and Co., 1869).

Nulty, T., *The Relations Existing between Convent Schools and the Systems of Intermediate and Primary National Education* (Dublin: Browne and Nolan, 1884).

O'Brien, J. D., 'Cases of a peculiar form of gastro-enteritis resulting from the use of diseased potatoes', *Dublin Hospital Gazette*, 24 (1846), 184–5.

O'Shaughnessy, M., 'The educational and other aspects of the statistics of crime in Dublin', *Journal of the Statistical and Social Inquiry Society of Ireland*, 3 (May 1861), 61–70.

O'Sullivan, A., 'Agriculture in the future', *Journal of Agricultural and Technical Education*, 4:39 (August 1918), 73–4.

Osborne, S. G., *Gleanings in the West of Ireland* (London: T. and W. Boone, 1850).
Paris, J. A., *A Treatise on Diet* (London: Thomas and George Underwood, 1826).
Phibbs, H., *A System of Penal Discipline* (London: Longman, Brown, Green and Longmans, 1850).
Philips, B., *Scrofula: Its Nature, its Causes, its Prevalence and the Principles of Treatment* (Philadelphia: Lea and Blanchard, 1846).
Phillips, G., *The Potato Disease: Its Origin, Nature and Prevention* (London: S. Highley, 1845).
Plunkett, H., *Memorandum on Agricultural Education for Ireland* (Dublin: DATI, 1901).
Redington, J., *The Economic Cookery Book* (Dublin: M. H. Gill and Son, 1906).
Russell G. and A. E., 'The self-supporting community', *Studies: An Irish Quarterly Review*, 7:26 (June 1918), 301–6.
Simpson, J., *On the More Effective Application of the System of Relief by Means of Soup Kitchens* (London: Whittaker and Co., 1847).
Smith-Gordon, L. and O'Brien, C., *Ireland's Food in War Time* (Dublin: Plunkett House, 1914).
——, *Starvation in Dublin* (Dublin: The Wood Printing Works, 1917).
Soyer, A., *Soyer's Charitable Cookery* (Dublin: Hodges and Smith, 1848).
Sproule, J., *Model Farms as Leading to an Improved System of Cultivation: The Appropriate Remedy for the Present Distressed Condition of Ireland* (Dublin: James McGlashan, 1848).
Stanuell, C. A., 'The effect of the war on Irish agriculture', *Journal of the Statistical and Social Inquiry Society of Ireland*, 95 (1914), 223–30.
Taylor, J., *Amalgamation of Unions and Pauper and National Education in Ireland* (Dublin: John Falconer, 1857).
Thomas, E., *Technical Instruction* (Dublin: Browne and Nolan, 1900).
Thompson, W. H., *Food Values, with a note on the Conservation of Irish Food Supplies* (Dublin, 1915).
——, *War and the Food of the Dublin Labourer* (Dublin: Women's National Health Association of Ireland, 1915).
Trafford, F. G., *Maxwell Drewitt* (New York: Harper and Brothers, 1866).
Tyndall, J., 'On dust and disease', *Proceedings of the Royal Institution of Great Britain*, 6 (1870), 1–14.
Walsh, S. B., 'Food and the hungry school children', *Irish Review*, 2:21 (November 1912), 494–501.
Webster, W. B., *Ireland Considered as a Field for Investment or Residence* (Dublin: Hodges and Smith, 1852).
Wilde, W., 'The food of the Irish', *Dublin University Magazine*, 43 (March 1854), 127–46.'
——, Epidemic disease in Ireland', *Dublin Review*, 42 (March 1857), 76–95.
Women's National Health Association, *Lecture on the Health of the Child* (Dublin: Waller & Co., 1909).

Secondary sources

Adelman, J., *Communities of Science in Nineteenth-Century Ireland* (London: Pickering and Chatto, 2009).
——, '*The Industrial Resources of Ireland* by Robert Kane', in J. H. Murphy (ed.), *The Irish Book in English, 1800–1891 Volume IV* (Oxford: Oxford University Press, 2011).

Anderson, W., *Colonial Pathologies: American Tropical Medicine, Race and Hygiene in the Philippines* (Durham: Duke University Press, 2006).

Apple, R., *Mothers and Medicine: A Social History of Infant Feeding, 1890–1950* (Madison, WI: University of Wisconsin Press, 1987).

Armstrong, D., *The Political Anatomy of the Body: Medical Knowledge in Britain in the Twentieth Century* (Cambridge: Cambridge University Press, 1983).

Arnold, D., *Colonizing the Body: State Medicine and Epidemic Disease in Nineteenth-Century India* (Berkeley: University of California Press, 1993).

Banerjee, S., *Muscular Nationalism: Gender, Violence and Empire in India and Ireland, 1914–2004* (New York: New York University Press, 2012).

Barker, T. C., Oddy, D. J. and Yudkin, J., *The Dietary Surveys of Dr Edward Smith 1862–3* (London, 1970).

Bell, J. and Watson, M., *A History of Irish Farming, 1750–1950* (Dublin: Four Courts Press, 2009).

Bielenberg, A., *Ireland and the Industrial Revolution: The Impact of the Industrial Revolution on Irish Industry, 1801–1922* (London: Routledge, 2009).

Bobrow-Strain, A., 'White bread bio-politics: purity, health, and the triumph of industrial baking', *Cultural Geographies*, 15:1 (January 2008), 19–40.

Bourke, J., *Husbandry to Housewifery: Women, Economic Change, and Housework in Ireland, 1890–1914* (Oxford and New York: Oxford University Press, 1993).

Breathnach, C., *The Congested Districts Board, 1891–1923: Poverty and Development in the West of Ireland* (Dublin: Four Courts Press, 2005).

Brock, W. H., *Justus von Liebig: The Chemical Gatekeeper* (Cambridge: Cambridge University Press, 1997).

Burke, H., *The People and the Poor Law in Nineteenth Century Ireland* (Dublin: Women's Education Bureau, 1987).

Burnett, J., *Plenty and Want: A Social History of Diet in England from 1815 to the Present Day* (London: Methuen, 1966 [1979]).

——, 'The rise and decline of school meals in Britain, 1860–1990', in J. Burnett and D. J. Oddy (eds), *The Origins and Development of Food Policies in Europe* (London and New York: Leicester University Press, 1994).

Calder, J., *The Victorian Home* (London: Batsford, 1977).

Carpenter, K. J., 'Nutritional studies in Victorian prisons', *Journal of Nutrition*, 136:1 (January 2006), 1–8.

Carroll, L., *Champion of the Poor: Sir Charles Cameron, Medical Officer of Health, 1862–1921* (Dublin: A. & A. Farmar, 2010).

Carroll-Burke, P., *Colonial Discipline: The Making of the Irish Convict System* (Dublin: Four Courts Press, 2000).

Clark, A., 'Wild workhouse girls and the Liberal Imperial state in mid-nineteenth century Ireland', *Journal of Social History*, 39:2 (Winter 2005), 389–409.

Clark, S., *Social Origins of the Irish Land War* (Princeton, NJ: Princeton University Press, 1979).

Clarkson, L. A., 'The modernisation of Irish diet', in J. Davis, *Rural Change in Ireland* (Belfast: Institute of Irish Studies, Queen's University Belfast, 1999).

——, and E. M. Crawford, *Feast and Famine: A History of Food and Nutrition in Ireland, 1500–1920* (Oxford: Oxford University Press, 2001).

Clear, C., *Nuns in Nineteenth-Century Ireland* (Dublin: Gill and Macmillan, 1987).

Coley, N. G., 'Medical chemists and the origins of clinical chemistry in Britain (circa 1750–1850)', *Clinical Chemistry*, 50:5 (May 2004), 961–72.

Collingham, E. M., *Imperial Bodies: The Physical Experience of the Raj, c.1800–1947* (Cambridge: Polity Press, 2001).

Comerford, R. V., 'Ideas and institutions, 1830–45', in W. E. Vaughan (ed.), *A New History of Ireland V: Ireland under the Union I, 1801–70* (Oxford: Clarendon Press, 1989).

Connell, K. H., *Irish Peasant Society: Four Historical Essays* (Dublin: Irish Academic Press, 1996 [1968]).

Coveney, J., *Food, Morals and Meaning: The Pleasures and Anxiety of Eating* (London: Routledge, 2nd edn, 2006).

Cowen, R., *Relish* (London: Phoenix, 2006).

Crossman, V., *The Poor Law in Ireland 1838–1948* (West Tempest: Dundalgan Press, 2006).

——, 'Cribbed, contained, and confined? The care of children under the Irish Poor Law, 1850–1920', *Éire-Ireland*, 1 & 2 (Spring/Summer 2009), 37–61.

Crotty, P., *Good Nutrition? Fact and Fashion in Dietary Advice* (St Leonards: Allen and Unwin, 1995).

Crotty, R. D., *Irish Agricultural Production: Its Volume and Structure* (Cork: Cork University Press, 1966).

Cullen, C., 'The Museum of Irish Industry (1845–1867): research environment, popular museum and community of learning in mid-Victorian Ireland' (Unpublished PhD thesis, University College Dublin, 2008).

Cullen, L. M., *The Emergence of Modern Ireland 1600–1900* (London: Batsford Academic and Education, 1981).

Cunningham, H., *Children and Childhood in Western Society since 1500* (Harlow: Pearson Longman, 1995).

Daly, M. E., *Social and Economic History of Ireland since 1800* (Dublin: Educational Company of Ireland, 1981).

——, *The First Department: A History of the Department of Agriculture* (Dublin: Institute of Public Administration, 2002).

Davin, A., 'Imperialism and motherhood', *History Workshop*, 5 (Spring 1978), 9–65.

Donnelly Jr., J. S., 'Cork Market: its role in the nineteenth-century Irish butter trade', *Studia Hibernica*, 11 (1971), 130–63.

——, 'Famine and government response 1845–6', in W. E. Vaughan (ed.), *A New History of Ireland V: Ireland under the Union I, 1801–70* (Oxford: Clarendon Press, 1989).

Dunphy, R., *The Making of Fianna Fáil Power in Ireland, 1923–48* (Oxford: Oxford University Press, 2005).

Dwork, D., *War is Good for Babies and other Young Children: A History of the Infant and Child Welfare Movement in England, 1898–1918* (London: Tavistock, 1987).

Elias, N., *The Civilising Process*, trans. E. Jephcott (Oxford: Blackwell, 1978–82).

Ernst, W., *Mad Tales from the Raj: The European Insane in British India, 1800–1858* (London and New York: Routledge, 1991).

Evans, A., 'The Countess of Aberdeen's health promotion caravans', *Journal of the Irish Colleges of Physicians and Surgeons*, 24:3 (July 1995), 211–18.

Fahey, T., 'Nuns in the Catholic church in Ireland in the nineteenth century', in M. Cullen (ed.), *Girls Don't Do Honours: Irish Women in Education in the Nineteenth and Twentieth Centuries* (Dublin: Women's Education Bureau, 1987).

Featherstone, L., 'Infant ideologies: doctors, mothers and the feeding of children in